C0-AOF-637

Common Sense Geriatrics

PROPERTY OF WASHINGTON
SCHOOL OF PSYCHIATRY
LIBRARY

COMMON SENSE GERIATRICS

Edited by

D.W. Molloy, M.B., B.Ch., B.A.O., M.R.C.P.(I), F.R.C.P.(C)

Consultant Geriatrician
Assistant Professor of Medicine
McMaster University
Hamilton, Ontario

Boston
Blackwell Scientific Publications
Oxford   London   Edinburgh   Melbourne   Paris   Berlin   Vienna

Blackwell Scientific Publications

Editorial offices:
Three Cambridge Center, Cambridge, Massachusetts 02142, USA
Osney Mead, Oxford OX2 0EL, England
25 John Street, London, WC1N 2BL, England
23 Ainslie Place, Edinburgh, EH3 6AJ, Scotland
54 University Street, Carlton, Victoria 3053, Australia

Other editorial offices:
Arnette SA, 2 rue Casimir-Delavigne, 75006 Paris, France
Blackwell Wissenschaft, Meinekestrasse 4, D-1000 Berlin 15, Germany
Blackwell MZV, Feldgasse 13, A-1238 Wien, Austria

Distributors:
USA and Canada
    Mosby-Year Book, Inc.
    11830 Westline Industrial Drive
    St. Louis, Missouri 63146
    (Orders: Tel. 800-633-6699)
Australia
    Blackwell Scientific Publications (Australia) Pty Ltd
    54 University Street
    Carlton, Victoria 3053
    (Orders: Telephone: 03-347-0300)
Outside North America and Australia
    Blackwell Scientific Publications, Ltd.
    Osney Mead
    Oxford OX2 0EL
    England
    (Orders: Telephone: 011-44-865-240201)

Designed and typeset by Sheila Walsh
Printed and bound by the Maple-Vail Book Manufacturing Group

© 1991 Blackwell Scientific Publications, Inc.
Printed in the United States of America
91 92 93 94 5 4 3 2 1

Chapters 7, 8, 14, 17–19, 24, 26, 34, 37, 38, and 40 of the present work
appeared previously in *The Canadian Journal of Geriatrics,* and are
adapted with permission.

All rights reserved. No part of this book may be reproduced in any form
or by any electronic or mechanical means, including information storage
and retrieval systems, without permission in writing from the publisher,
except by a reviewer who may quote brief passages in a review.

Library of Congress Cataloging-in-Publication Data
Common sense geriatrics / edited by D.W. Molloy.
            p.   cm.
    Includes bibliographical references and index.
    ISBN 0-86542-107-2 : $29.95
    1. Geriatrics—Case studies.   I. Molloy, D.W.
    [DNLM: 1. Geriatrics—case studies. WT 100 C7335]
RC952.7.C66 1991
618.97'09—dc20
DNLM/DLC
for Library of Congress   90-14502
                                                               CIP

This book is dedicated to Deborah, Jimmy, and Alexander

CONTENTS

CONTRIBUTORS

Jonathan D. Adachi, M.D., F.R.C.P.(C)
St. Joseph's Hospital, Hamilton, Ontario

Efrem Alemeyehu, M.D.
Research Fellow, Division of Geriatric Medicine, McMaster University, Hamilton, Ontario

Ann M. Benger, M.D.
Associate Professor of Medicine, McMaster University; Consultant Hematologist, Hamilton Civic Hospitals, Hamilton, Ontario

Ralph Bloch, M.D., F.R.C.P.(C), Ph.D.
McMaster Faculty of Health Science, Department of Medicine, McMaster University, Hamilton, Ontario

Michael John Borrie, M.B.Ch.B., F.R.C.P.(C)
Assistant Professor, Division of Geriatric Medicine, Department of Medicine, University of Western Ontario, London, Ontario

E. Anne Braun, B.Sc., M.D., M.Sc., D.A.B.I.M., F.R.C.P.(C)
Fellow, Geriatric Medicine, McMaster University, Hamilton, Ontario

Marilyn Cakebread, R.N.
Geriatric Outpatient Department, Chedoke Division, Chedoke-McMaster Hospitals, Hamilton, Ontario

Janice Elizabeth Clark, R.N., B.Sc.N.
Head Nurse, Geriatric Assessment Unit, Chedoke-McMaster Hospitals, Hamilton, Ontario

Roger M. Clarnette, M.B., B.S., F.R.A.C.P.
Consultant Physician, Department of Geriatric Medicine, Osborne Park Hospital, Stirling, Western Australia

Gerald Cohen, M.D.
Professor, Department of Family Medicine, Faculty of Health Sciences, McMaster University, Hamilton, Ontario

May Cohen, M.D.
Professor, Department of Family Medicine, Faculty of Health Sciences, McMaster University, Hamilton, Ontario

Ann B. Cranney, B.Sc., M.B.B.Ch, F.R.C.P.(C)
Fellow in Geriatric Medicine, McMaster University, Hamilton, Ontario

W. Earle DeCoteau, M.D., F.R.C.P.(C)
Professor of Medicine, University of Saskatchewan; Head, Section of
Clinical Gerontology, Former Head, Section of Rheumatology and
Immunology, University Hospital, Saskatoon, Saskatchewan

Roy Alan Fox, M.D., F.R.C.P., F.A.C.P., F.R.C.P.(C)
Professor and Head, Division of Geriatric Medicine, Dalhousie University;
Director, Centre for Health Care of the Elderly, Camp Hill Medical Centre,
Halifax, Nova Scotia

Michael Gross, M.B., B.S., L.M.C.C., F.R.C.S.(C)
Orthopaedic Surgeon, Ambulatory Care Centre, Victoria General Hospital,
Halifax, Nova Scotia

Kevin W. Hall, B.Sc.Pharm, Pharm.D.
Assistant Director, Pharmacy Operations, Health Sciences Centre,
Winnipeg, Manitoba

Lawrence E. Hart, M.B.BCh., M.Sc., F.R.C.P.(C), F.A.C.P.
Assistant Professor, Departments of Medicine and Clinical Epidemiology,
McMaster University, Hamilton, Ontario

Jack Hirsh, M.D.
Director, Hamilton Civic Hospitals Research Centre; Professor of
Medicine, McMaster University, Hamilton, Ontario

David Bryan Hogan, M.D., F.A.C.P., F.R.C.P.(C)
Head, Division of Geriatric Medicine, Department of Medicine,
University of Calgary, Calgary, Alberta

Russell D. Hull, M.B.B.S., M.Sc., F.R.C.P.(C), F.A.C.P., F.C.C.P.
Professor of Medicine and Head, Division of General Internal Medicine,
University of Calgary, Calgary, Alberta

Richard H. Hunt, F.R.C.P., F.R.C.P.(Ed), F.R.C.P.(C), F.A.C.G.
Professor and Head, Division of Gastroenterology, McMaster University
Medical Centre, Hamilton, Ontario

R. Jaeschke, M.D.
Department of Medicine, St. Joseph's Hospital, Hamilton, Ontario

John Lawrence Kelly, MB.Bch., B.A.O.
Medical Student, University College Cork, Cork, Ireland

John S. Kennedy, M.D.
Assistant Professor of Psychiatry, Neurology, and Psychology,
Case-Western Reserve University, Cleveland, Ohio

Louise Lagacé, B.Sc. (Pharm), C.H.C.A.
Pharmacy Department, Hamilton Psychiatric Hospital, Hamilton, Ontario

Andy S.C. Lam, M.D., F.R.C.P.(C)
Consultant, Internal Medicine and Respiratory Diseases, West Lincoln
Memorial Hospital, Grimsby, Ontario

John Kenneth Le Clair, M.D., F.R.C.P.(C)
   Combined Outreach Geriatric Service, Chedoke-McMaster Hospitals,
   Hamilton, Ontario

Judith A. Lever, R.N., B.Sc.N., M.Sc.(A)
   Clinical Nurse Specialist, Geriatrics, Henderson General Hospital,
   Hamilton, Ontario

Gisele M.M. Muir, M.B., B.S., F.R.C.P.(C), D.C.H.
   Assistant Clinical Professor, Department of Psychiatry, McMaster
   University, Hamilton, Ontario

Akbar Panju, M.B., Ch.B., F.R.C.P.(C)
   Clinical Assistant Professor of Medicine, McMaster University; Chief,
   Division of Internal Medicine, Chedoke-McMaster Hospitals, Hamilton,
   Ontario

Christopher Patterson, M.D., F.R.C.P.(C), F.A.C.P.
   Associate Professor and Head, Division of Geriatric Medicine, McMaster
   University, Hamilton, Ontario

Christopher Power, M.D.
   Department of Clinical Neurological Sciences, University of Western
   Ontario, London, Ontario

J.A.H. Puxty, M.B., Ch.B., M.R.C.P.(UK)
   Chief of Geriatrics, Queen's University; Head, Geriatrics and Continuing
   Care Medicine, St. Mary's of the Lake Hospital, Kingston, Ontario

Lee Ramage, R.N., C.I.C.
   Infection Control Officer, Registered Nurse, Chedoke-McMaster Hospitals,
   Hamilton, Ontario

Linda Rees, R.N.A
   Research Nurse/Assistant, Department of Medicine, McMaster University;
   Geriatric Research Group, Hamilton Civic Hospitals, Henderson Division,
   Hamilton, Ontario

M. Rodway-Norman, B.Sc., M.D.
   Fellow, Geriatric Psychiatry, Clarke Institute, Toronto, Ontario

John R. Roy, M.B., Ch.B., F.R.C.P., M.R.C.P., F.R.C.P.(C)
   Professor, Department of Psychiatry and Associate Member, Department
   of English, McMaster University; Medical Director, Division of Geriatric
   Psychiatry, Chedoke-McMaster Hospitals, Hamilton, Ontario

Michel D. Sauvé, M.D., F.R.C.P.(C)
   Clinical Scholar, McMaster University, Hamilton, Ontario

Dina E. Savelli, M.D., F.R.C.P.(C)
   Consulting Neurologist, Hamilton Civic Hospitals; Deputy Chief of
   Neurology, Henderson General Hospital; Assistant Clinical Professor,
   McMaster University, Hamilton, Ontario

Trevor Seaton, M.B., F.R.C.P.(C)
Chief of Medicine and Chief of Gastroenterology, Hamilton Civic Hospitals, Hamilton, Ontario

Sheryl Shoham, M.A., M.D.
Department of Medicine, McMaster University, Hamilton, Ontario

Gurmit Singh, Ph.D.
Associate Professor, Department of Pathology, McMaster University; Career Scientist, Hamilton Regional Cancer Centre, Hamilton, Ontario

Kevin P.D. Smith, B.A.(Psych), B.A.(Gerontology), C.H.E.
Administrator, Health Services, Faculty of Health Sciences, McMaster University, Hamilton, Ontario

Catherine M. Sochasky, B.Sc.Pharm.
Drug Information Pharmacist, Health Sciences Centre, Winnipeg, Manitoba

David Gleeson Stubbing, M.B., B.S., M.R.C.P., F.R.C.P.(C)
Associate Professor, Department of Medicine, Chedoke-McMaster Hospitals, Hamilton, Ontario

Eldon Tunks, M.D., F.R.C.P.(C)
Professor of Psychiatry, McMaster University; Director, Chedoke-McMaster Pain Program, Chedoke-McMaster Hospitals, Hamilton, Ontario

Irene D. Turpie, M.B., Ch.B., F.R.C.P.(C)
Associate Professor of Medicine, McMaster University; Director, Geriatric Services, St. Joseph's Hospital, Hamilton, Ontario

Louise Y. Vitou, B.Sc., M.D.C.M.
Senior Resident, Internal Medicine, McMaster University, Hamilton, Ontario

A. Elizabeth Watson, M.B., B.Ch., F.R.C.P.(C)
Assistant Professor, University of Manitoba; Head, Department of Geriatric Medicine, Seven Oaks General Hospital, Winnipeg, Manitoba

John D. Wells, M.D., F.R.C.S.(C)
Associate Professor of Surgery, McMaster University, Hamilton, Ontario

FOREWORD

I was asked to contribute to this book during my fellowship year in Geriatrics at McMaster. The philosophy is simple — a problem-based practical approach to geriatric patient care. It is designed for use by the general internist, family physician, resident, and nurse. Its greatest application will be in the day-to-day management of common geriatric problems that occur at home, in the consulting room, and in hospital wards. In addition, the bibliographies provide an up-to-date service of further information.

The section on dementia is innovative and thoughtful and contributes greatly to this important area. It provides a very structured and planned approach to management. The importance of managing the caregiver as well as the patient is also stressed. In view of the fact that so much therapy in geriatrics is based on anecdotal information, much of the therapeutic advice has a less than didactic tone. I believe this book will be invaluable for any physician with an interest in the care of the elderly. In addition, many of the chapters provide useful advice for allied health workers.

Roger Clarnette, F.R.A.P.

PREFACE

This book was written as a practical aid for health care professionals who take care of the elderly. I have tried to present a simple, straightforward approach to the management of many of the clinical problems in the elderly. The case presentations are used to illustrate the common presentations of these problems. Readers can test their knowledge by answering the questions at the end of each presentation. The questions also act as a guide so readers can choose to read all or some of the answers. I have set the book up this way to allow readers to focus quickly on their area of interest.

I hope that physicians, nurses, and allied health care professionals who care for the elderly will find this practical approach useful.

ACKNOWLEDGMENTS

I wish to thank my parents and family for their love and encouragement. I would also like to thank my teachers: Mrs. Power, Mary Ann Molloy, Ritchie, and Twink, may God have mercy on them; my teachers at De La Salle, Waterford: Mr. Mullins, Mr. McGrath, Brother Cyprian, Brother Patrick, Brother Athanasius, and Brother Columbus. I would like to acknowledge my teachers in medicine: Professor Jack Sheehan, Professor Doyle, Dr. Jim Walshe, Dr. Brigid Foley, Dr. James Molloy, Dr. Michael Hyland, Professor D.J. O'Sullivan, Dr. Gordon Guyatt, Dr. Dermot Murnaghan, Dr. Dan McCarthy, Dr. Jack Hirsh, Dr. Nick Anthonisen, Dr. Richard Prewitt, Dr. Ron Cape, Dr. Colin Powell, Dr. Stuart MacLeod, and Dr. John Cairns.

Special thanks to Kevin Smith and Geoffrey Price for editing assistance.

Thanks to Karen Mead for her secretarial support and to my nursing colleagues Linda Rees and Judy Lever for their help and support.

Thanks to all the authors and to all members of Division of Geriatrics, McMaster, for their time and assistance in developing and completing this project.

Finally, thanks to Upjohn Canada for a grant to help defray the production costs of this book.

D.W. Molloy

NOTICE

The indications and dosages of all drugs in this book have been recommended in the medical literature and conform to the practices of the general medical community. The medications described do not necessarily have specific approval by the Food and Drug Administration for use in the diseases and dosages for which they are recommended. The package insert for each drug should be consulted for use and dosage as approved by the FDA. Because standards for usage change, it is advisable to keep abreast of revised recommendations, particularly those concerning new drugs.

Part I

COMMON PROBLEMS

1 | ASSESSING DEMENTIA

CASE PRESENTATION

Mrs. Smith, a 72-year-old retired nurse, comes to your office with her daughter. She has lived alone in her house since her husband died five years ago. In the past two or three years, Mrs. Smith has become more forgetful and is now unable to manage her finances. Her daughter reports that her mother's fridge is poorly stocked and she is not coping with the housework.

Mrs. Smith often phones her daughter three or four times to confirm appointments, and she repeats questions and conversations over and over again. Her daughter complains that her mother has become vague, withdrawn, and suspicious.

The daughter is concerned that her mother may have Alzheimer's disease. Mrs. Smith denies any problems with her memory. She scores 19 out of 30 on a Standardized Mini-Mental State Exam. Consider the following statements.

D.W. Molloy
E.A. Braun
R. Clarnette
J. Lever
I.D. Turpie
L. Rees

Consider the following statements (true or false)

1. Patients with senile dementia of the Alzheimer's type usually complain of problems with their memory before the caregivers notice the problem.

2. A complete history and physical are the most important components in an assessment of an elderly individual with cognitive impairment.

3. Comprehensive assessment of elderly patients presenting with cognitive impairment must include objective assessment of cognition, activities of daily living (ADL), mood, behavior, safety, and caregiver function.

4. Every patient who presents with cognitive impairment should have computerized tomography of the head to rule out reversible causes of dementia.

1. FALSE

Definition

Dementia is a common clinical syndrome characterized by a decline in cognitive function from a previously attained intellectual level that is sustained for months or years. There is

1. a deterioration in cognitive function,
2. a decreased ability to perform activities of daily living (ADL), and
3. a change in behavior.

Prevalence

Dementia affects about 10% of those aged over 65 and almost 50% of those aged over 85 years [1]. The primary feature of dementia is a deterioration in intellectual function, for example, comprehension, learning, recent memory, problem solving, reasoning, and judgement.

The diagnosis of dementia has serious implications for the affected individual. These individuals lose their rights and liberties, are deemed incompetent, and are frequently institutionalized. Roughly 11% to 15% of those who present with symptoms of dementia may have a reversible component to their illness and may experience partial or complete recovery if properly diagnosed and treated [2,3].

Etiology

The precise etiology of Alzheimer's disease is uncertain. Although more than 20 factors have been proposed, with the exception of age, no other factors have been consistently reported or proven. Female gender, family history, head trauma, and maternal and paternal age have been suggested but not always shown to be associated with an increased risk of Alzheimer's [4–13].

Presentation

1.   Gradual onset

Many patients with deafness, aphasia or other language difficulties, or depression are misdiagnosed as suffering from dementia. The most common presentation of dementia is a gradual decline in cognition from a previously attained intellectual level of functioning. At first the problem is subtle as family members notice a gradual deterioration in short-term memory and learning. Affected individuals forget names, repeat themselves, and ask the same question over and over. Many patients are aware that their memory is deteriorating. Some patients become depressed, frustrated, or angry if one draws their attention to their memory problems. Patients rarely complain of the memory problem and usually try to cover up the deficit.

In most cases the spouse or family become concerned because the affected individual is showing a gradual, progressive decline in short-term memory. The affected individual slows down, takes longer to perform familiar tasks, and has difficulty with the instrumental activities of daily living—for example, shopping, finances, driving, phone messages—and repeats statements or questions over and over. The spouse or family may note subtle changes in behavior or habits. The individual becomes more irritable, withdrawn, suspicious, angry, or moody.

2.   Acute onset: Catastrophic event

In some cases the family suddenly realizes that there is a problem when the individual behaves in a very inappropriate or uncharacteristic fashion. This may occur when the individual goes to visit a daughter or son for a special event (*e.g.*, a birthday). At the child's house the parent becomes confused and keeps asking to go home. The patient may keep forgetting where the bathroom is, may become anxious, confused, agitated, angry, or disoriented, and may insist on going home. In these cases the patient becomes confused in the new environment and cannot cope with the crowd of people. Because of the learning and short-term memory loss the patient keeps forgetting what he or she is doing there. Finally, the individual walks out or has to be taken home, and the family suddenly realizes that the individual has a serious problem and they must seek help. In these cases, on reflection, they may realize that there had been many clues in the past few months or years that they had ignored or overlooked. This acute catastrophic presentation is not unusual.

2. TRUE

The best diagnostic tests are careful history and physical examination. This is time consuming but necessary. Laboratory tests should be ordered on the basis of the history and physical examination. Over-testing exposes the patient to unnecessary stress, pain, cost, and inconvenience; under-testing may result in missed identification of reversible conditions.

Patients presenting with cognitive impairment or changes in behavior should receive basic diagnostic procedures, as listed in Table 1-1.

Modifications can be made according to individual circumstances. Investigations such as liver function tests, drug levels, chest x-ray, ECG, and EEG may be performed as indicated.

A history of onset, duration, and progression is the single most important factor in the evaluation of a patient with cognitive impairment. Gradual progression of symptoms over years suggests senile dementia of the Alzheimer's type. Ask for a family history of dementia, a previous psychiatric history, and note any precipitating factors such as recent anesthesia, trauma, change in medications, loss of a spouse, or change in mood. A previous history of transient ischemic attacks, stroke, angina, myocardial infarction, and hypertension confirm the presence of arteriosclerosis and make multi-infarct dementia more likely.

Table 1-1 Investigations of Patients with Cognitive Impairment.

Test	*Diseases*
Hemoglobin Complete blood count B_{12}	Pernicious anemia
Erythrocyte sedimentation rate	Giant cell arteritis
Electrolytes Calcium Urea creatine Blood glucose	Metabolic disorders
Thyroid-stimulating hormone (TSH)	Hypothyroidism
Venereal disease research laboratory (VDRL test) (optional)	Syphilis
Computed tomography (CT) scan	Normal-pressure hydrocephalus Space-occupying lesion Subdural hematoma
Drugs (levels)	Toxicity Delirium
Geriatric Depression Score	Depression
Psychiatric assessment	Depression

It is essential to perform a general physical examination, paying particular attention to the central and peripheral nervous system. We routinely examine for tremor, rigidity, reflexes, plantar responses, frontal lobe signs, apraxia, and localizing or lateralizing signs. No examination is complete without assessment of the patient's gait.

3. TRUE

It is essential to assess the level at which this patient is functioning to assess her ability to live safely at home. Mrs. Smith lives alone and has cognitive impairment. Is she shopping, cooking, forgetting to eat, losing weight, or stocking her fridge? Has she been burning pots and pans? How often does she take her medications? Give her the medicine containers and ask her what each medication is for and how often she takes each one. Can she read and understand the directions on the bottle? Can she function safely in her own home?

What activities will need to be supervised, for example, shopping, meals, medications, travelling, cooking, finances, *etc.*? When she travels alone, does she get lost? Mrs. Smith's history may be completely unreliable. Get a collaborative history from her daughter.

In planning Mrs. Smith's care, it is necessary to use all the available resources, including her daughter, community nurses, friends, homemakers, and various services in the community such as Meals on Wheels, Alzheimer's Society. If she refuses help, or enough supervision cannot be organized, she may need to go to a more protected and supervised environment for her own safety. Even if she is functioning safely now, it is necessary to document a baseline to plan for her future.

The assessment of dementia involves six areas where the level of function and disability must be measured:

1. cognition;
2. activities of daily living (ADL);
3. behavior;
4. psychiatric: mood, delusions, hallucinations;
5. caregiver function; and
6. safety.

1. Cognition

The vast majority of patients first present with short-term memory loss and difficulty finding words. Family and friends notice that they repeat themselves and forget recent conversations. They have difficulty finding the right word and forget names of familiar people. We use a Standardized Folstein Mini-Mental State Exam (SMMSE) to screen for cognitive impairment. This standardized version has improved the reliability of this instrument [14]. (See Appendix A.)

Many patients with Alzheimer's are unaware of their memory problems. As the disease progresses, they lose their insight and awareness of their deficits. If some patients are made aware of their deficits, they will have a "catastrophic reaction." These patients will become angry and frustrated, and they will deny that they have any problems. They may accuse the caregiver of "making up lies about them."

It is extremely important never to take a history from the caregiver in the patient's presence. Always interview the caregiver in a different room out of the patient's hearing. Taking a history in front of the patient poses two serious problems.

1. The caregiver may not want to tell all of the patient's problems for fear of embarrassing the patient or making him or her angry. As a result the caregiver will give an incomplete or misleading history, especially regarding alcohol consumption, psychiatric history, *etc.*
2. If the caregiver gives a complete history for a patient who has no insight, the patient may believe that the caregiver is exaggerating or telling lies. This may increase the patient's paranoia, anger, and mistrust of the caregiver and lead to serious behavior problems later.

2.   Activities of Daily Living and Instrumental ADL

Activities of daily living (ADL) may be considered in two categories:

1. instrumental ADL (IADL); and
2. basic ADL (BADL).

Instrumental activities of daily living (IADL)

IADL consists of complex tasks that require planning and problem solving. These tasks include

- handling finances;
- driving, transportation, bus, taxi, *etc.*;
- taking medications;
- cooking;
- using the telephone;
- shopping;
- hobbies—woodwork, cards, mechanics, reading,

gardening; and
- using machines such as washing machine, lawnmowers, dishwashers, TVs, *etc.*

Basic activities of daily living (BADL)

BADL consists of basic tasks that are more automatic. These tasks include
- walking, transfers;
- washing;
- dressing, grooming;
- feeding; and
- toilet.

We compared the relationship between cognitive function and independence in basic activities of daily living (BADL) and instrumental activities of daily living (IADL) in 27 patients with Alzheimer's disease

Figure 1-1 *Effects of Cognitive Impairment on IADL and ADL.*

IADL is affected early. By the time the dementia has progressed to the moderate stages, the person has lost her or his ability to perform IADL, while ADL is maintained. Even in severe dementia the ability to perform some ADL functions, such as feeding and walking, is maintained.

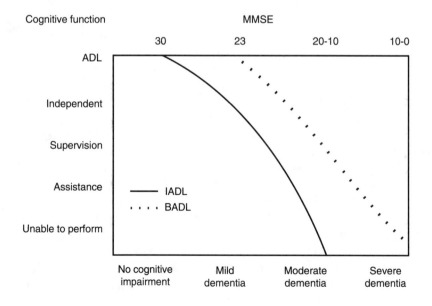

(AD) and 27 patients with stroke. Each had IADL and BADL scored using the Donaldson ADL, Lawton IADL, and modified Lawton IADL (mIADL) instruments. Cognitive function was measured using the MMSE. There was a significantly greater correlation between the mIADL and MMSE scores (r = 0.87) in the Alzheimer's group than in the stroke group (r = 0.58) [15].

It is possible to predict function in BADL and IADL in SDAT from this relatively simple measure of cognitive function. This information will aid in planning care, management, and long-term care requirements.

The more complex instrumental activities of daily living (IADL), require more thinking and planning. IADL is impaired first as cognitive function deteriorates in early (mild) dementia. BADL is affected later, usually in the middle (moderate) and late (severe) stages of dementia. In moderate dementia the patient is usually unable to perform any IADL, but can still perform ADL independently or with assistance. The relationship of IADL and BADL to cognitive function is shown graphically in Figure 1-1. A description of the dementia stages is available in Table 1-2. Reisberg has provided a more accurate and detailed account of seven stages in dementia in the Global Deterioration Scale [16]. This more complex division into seven stages is very comprehensive, but a simple division into three categories—mild, moderate, and severe—is adequate for most clinicians.

3. Behavior

Dysfunctional behavior varies from patient to patient. This problem is nearly always reported by the caregiver, since the patient rarely has insight into the problem. Patients are usually on their best behavior in the doctor's office. The caregiver's previous relationship with the patient, personality, understanding of the disease, and tolerance will dictate what will be interpreted as "dysfunctional behavior."

In the broadest sense, behavior encompasses all the changes in cognition, ADL, social function, and psychiatric disorders in dementia. We define dysfunctional behavior as "an inappropriate action or response for a given social milieu, excluding ADL, that is a problem for the caregiver." This definition is heavily weighted to a change in social function. It is imperfect, but it is an attempt to define dysfunctional behavior simply and to separate it from changes in ADL and cognition. For instance, we would not consider incontinence in moderate or severe dementia as dysfunctional behavior, because it is appropriate for that patient's level of function. However, if the patient was getting angry and

Table 1-2 Stages in Dementia.

SMMSE*	Cognition	Activities of Daily Living (ADL)	Behavior
Stage I Early (mild) SMMSE 20–24	Short-term memory loss, word-finding difficulty Forgetful in conversations Slows down, forgets names of familiar people, for example, friends	*Difficulty with Instrumental ADL* Finances Travelling independently Shopping, hobbies, reading	Repeating over and over Slowing down Anxious or withdrawn Changes in personality May become depressed if insight is maintained
Stage II Middle (moderate) SMMSE 10–20	Disorientation Word-finding difficulties very obvious Conversations become difficult Loss of memory for major life events, forgets names of children	*Difficulty with Basic ADL* Dressing Grooming Washing Gets lost in own home Urinary incontinence	Behavior sometimes has no obvious purpose Blunting in affect and/or more unpredictable Delusions of people stealing things Phobia (fear of being alone) common Hallucinations, for example, a stranger in the house
Stage III Late (severe) SMMSE 0–10	Speech in broken phrases or single words Can't communicate Doesn't recognize spouse	Feeding Fecal incontinence Walking	

*Standardized Mini-Mental State Exam

Figure 1-2 Factors That Contribute to Dysfunctional Behovior.

| Premorbid personality | Psychiatric problems (delusions, depression) | Internal environment (pain impaction, retention) |

```
Premorbid            Psychiatric problems         Internal
personality          (delusions, depression)      environment
                                                   (pain impaction,
                                                   retention)

Dementia with        ↘          ↓          ↙
frontal lobe
involvement      →
                     Dysfunctional     ←    Communication
                 →   behavior               problems
Cognitive
impairment       ↗          ↑          ↖

Drugs
(neuroleptics,       Caregiver                External
beta blockers,       (ill tempered, burnout,  environment
sedatives,           physical disability,     (restraints,
stimulants           no supports)             locked on ward)
```

striking out, that would be considered dysfunctional behavior.

We have developed the Dysfunctional Behavior Rating Instrument, based on Niederehe's Behavioural Problem Checklist [17], for use in the community-dwelling elderly with cognitive impairment. (See Appendix B.)

Dysfunctional behavior is difficult to treat until the cause of this behavior is identified. It does not result solely from cognitive impairment and can be affected by a number of factors (see Figure 1-2). Patients with frontal lobe signs on clinical examination exhibit more dysfunctional behavior than other patients with equal cognitive impairment [18].

It may be possible to predict the behavior problems that will develop in some individual patients. If an angry or violent personality type becomes demented, he or she will respond to an inability to deal with the environment by striking out or being physically aggressive. An assertive, compulsive individual who has always been domineering in the home may have great difficulty taking direction from others. A patient who has insight may become anxious, frustrated, and depressed. A passive husband or wife may have the least difficulty when he or she becomes demented because the relationship with his or her spouse changes the least.

The commonest complaint of demented patients is that they are continually being told what to do. The caregiver should be taught to reward compliant behavior and ignore dysfunctional behavior where possible.

Confirm and document the behavior problems with caregivers. Dysfunctional behavior may cause caregivers to burn out faster than coping with ADL problems. Caregivers can often cope with washing, dressing, preparing food, and generally assisting the patient with their ADL if the patient is pleasant and cooperative. But if the patient is uncooperative, verbally or physically abusive, wanders or keeps the caregiver up at night, the caregiver burns out very quickly. Instruments are available to measure the amount of burden or stress on the caregiver. A high burden score provides a measure of what is often clinically apparent.

4. Psychiatric: Mood, Delusions, Hallucinations

Rule out an underlying psychiatric cause for any dysfunctional behavior. Psychiatric conditions may be the cause of the patient's cognitive impairment, or they may accompany it. The most frequently missed psychiatric cause of cognitive impairment is depression. We use a Geriatric Depression Scale (GDS) [19] to screen patients for depression. Treatment should not be decided on the basis of the score from the GDS alone, but the GDS is a useful adjunct to clinical assessment to confirm or rule out an underlying depression. As the dementia progresses the score on the GDS becomes less reliable.

If depression is present, it is useful to score the GDS before treatment is started. Serial administrations may confirm and measure a response to therapy. Scores above 15/30 are usually indicative of an underlying depression. It may not be possible to use the GDS on all patients, but it is a helpful adjunct to confirm a clinical impression when the diagnosis of depression is considered.

Search for evidence of delusions or hallucinations. Have there been any previous episodes of psychiatric illness? Were these episodes treated? Was the patient institutionalized and what treatments (drugs, *etc.*) did he or she receive?

Paranoid delusions are common in moderate and severe dementia. Demented people keep losing and mislaying things and may come to believe that neighbors, family, friends, or strangers are stealing their possessions. They may become suspicious and angry and accuse family or caregivers of stealing. If the delusions are infrequent and minor they do not require treatment. Confusion and inability to recognize family members, people on TV, voices on the radio, or their own reflection in a mirror may often be mistaken for delusions or hallucinations. Explain this to the caregiver and try to avoid neuroleptics unless the problem becomes unmanageable.

5. Caregiver Function

The burden of caring for a patient with dementia may fall on the spouse, family, or friends. The Alzheimer's Society offers education, support,

Figure 1-3 Effect of Alzheimer's Disease on the Caregiver's Burden.

This figure shows the increase in burden on the Alzheimer caregiver. The caregiver must assume the spouse's role and the burden of caring.

Traditional roles before onset of disease

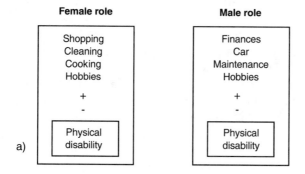

Caregiver role when disease established

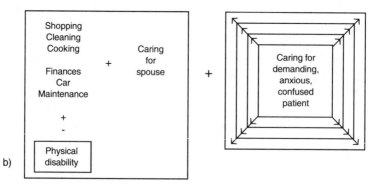

and helpful advice to caregivers. Caregivers must be taught to accept help and take time away from the patient. Structure a care plan to address all the problems. Give the caregiver time off to relax. It is helpful to establish this pattern of care early, so that patient and caregiver get used to other caregivers in the house. This provides a predictable schedule for caregivers that helps them to organize and plan activities.

Providing care to a patient with dementia is extremely exacting and exhausting even for the most resilient individual. Some of the factors that contribute to the burden of caring are listed in Figure 1-3. It is important to recognize stresses in the caregiver, family, and friends and to support and manage the complex psychosocial problems adequately.

Caregivers may require support, counseling and follow-up. Treat any physical problems that limit the caregiver's ability to cope with the patient, for example, arthritis, angina, cardiac failure. Many caregivers are unable to make the decision finally to institutionalize the patient. They often require support, guidance, and follow-up to make this difficult decision and to deal with guilt after they have done so.

Are there any other reversible causes of cognitive impairment that need to be addressed, for example, hyper- or hypothyroidism, B_{12} deficiency? A low dose of chloral hydrate (500 mg), benzodiazepine, or neuroleptic—loxapine 5 mg, haloperidol 0.5 mg, or pimozide 2 mg—at night, may be useful in the short term until this problem has resolved.

Factors that contribute to the caregiver's burden
Many factors contribute to the burden that caregivers in the community carry in caring for an elder with cognitive impairment.

1. *Physical demands:* The caregiver must assume responsibility for the patient's tasks. For example, a husband must start to shop, cook, and perform housework, as well as keeping up with his own tasks, such as gardening.

2. *Uncertain course—more difficult to anticipate:* AD frequently has an uncertain course, which makes it more stressful to cope with than a disease with a predictable outcome (*e.g.*, rate of progression, behavior changes *etc.*).

3. *Increased demands as caregiver wears out:* The patient has gradual sustained deterioration over time—demands for care increase as the disease progresses, and as the caregiver is wearing out.

4. *Accumulation of small losses with gradual loss of control:* Numerous small losses can occur, with progression causing small reactions to each loss, associated with loss of control.

5. *Increased demands in elderly person with decreased coping skills:* Increased financial, social, and physical pressures usually occur at a time of life when the caregiver's coping skills are compromised by age, physical disability, and/or reduced earning capacity.

6. *Disruption in family function/changing roles:* Long-term family disruption due to changing roles in the family is common. Children's and spouse's relationship with the patient dissolve as they are forced to assume a caregiver role.

7. *Decision-making:* Dilemmas about decision-making can occur—institutionalization, accepting care (strangers in the house), experimental treatments, *etc.*

Table 1-3   Safety Checklist Summary.

The results of a survey of 40 caregivers of elderly patients with cognitive impairment who were asked which of the following factors they considered a safety hazard for the patient in the community.

Rank	Factor	% Yes
1	Medication	57.5
2	Transportation	55.0
3	Bathing	52.5
4	Cooking	50.0
5	Mobility	45.0
6	Communication	42.5
7	Nutrition	40.0
8	Mood	32.5
9	Vision	30.0
10	Environment	25.0
11	Transfers	22.5
13	Wandering	20.0
14	Social contact	17.5
15	Transportation	15.0
16	Substance use	15.0
17	Smoking	10.0

8. *Anticipatory grief:* The caregiver may have to deal with prolonged anticipatory grief, anticipating death and loss with mourning, coping, a changing relationship, planning, and psychosocial organization. He or she may need to cope with the loss of a loved one, as he or she recognizes the changes and adjustments in the past, present, and future. The caregiver may disengage from the patient as a spouse, as the patient is deteriorating, but move closer to her or him as a caregiver, as the patient's needs increase.

9. *Loss of social supports affects recovery after death or institutionalization and death:* The caregiver may lose time or energy to follow hobbies, interests, or friendships that refresh. He or she may have to plan for the future without the patient's input. The more involved the caregiver is in the patient's care, the larger the loss when he or she loses the patient through death or institutionalization. Caregivers frequently will have neglected friends or dropped hobbies and are now forced to pick up the pieces and deal with the loss without the benefit of these social supports.

10. *Behavior problems:* Dealing with an angry, aggressive, inappropriate patient is a common problem. Caregivers often find themselves trying to provide support with no recognition from the patient—only arguments, resistance, and/or anger. This problem is often the straw that breaks the camel's back. Dysfunctional behaviors in the patient must be diagnosed and treated promptly.

6. Safety

In a review of 40 patients attending the Memory Clinic at the Henderson General Division, Hamilton Civic Hospitals, we surveyed caregivers of patients living in the community to describe the presence of the factors that they considered safety risks for the patients with cognitive impairment. The results are listed in Table 1-3. This survey revealed that in the majority of cases there were multiple factors that caregivers considered a safety hazard.

4. FALSE

Although dementia is a devastating disease for the individual and family and leads to very expensive institutional care for society, it is not necessary to investigate every patient fully with the expensive, comprehensive battery of investigations listed on Table 1-2. Larson recommended a selective use of diagnostic tests based on the results of a careful history and physical, neurological, psychiatric, and mental status examination [3]. This approach may be as effective and more cost-effective than routinely administering a full battery of tests to all patients with cognitive impairment. Some guidelines for the investigation of dementia are provided as follows.

Patients Who Should Receive Comprehensive Investigation

The following patients should receive comprehensive investigation:
1. those with recent onset with rapid progression,
2. those with atypical presentation,
3. those using multiple drugs, and
4. those exhibiting gait abnormality.

Patients on Whom Investigations May Be Limited

Investigations may be limited on patients with moderate to severe dementia with a history of gradual progressive impairment over three to five years.

REFERENCES

1. Evans DA, Funkenstein HH, Albert MS, Scherr PA, Cook NR, Chown MJ, Hebert LE, Hennekens CH, Taylor JO: Prevalence of Alzheimer's disease in a community population of older persons; higher than previously reported. *JAMA* 262 (18), November 10, 1989.
2. Clarfield AM: The reversible dementia: Do they reverse? *Annals of Internal Medicine* 109:476–486, 1988.
3. Larson EB, Reifler BV, Featherstone HJ, English DR: Dementia in elderly outpatients: A prospective study. *Annals of Internal Medicine* 100:417–423, 1984.
4. Henderson AS: The risk factors for Alzheimer's disease: A review and a hypothesis. *Acta Psychiatr Scand* 78:257–275, 1988.
5. Kay DWK, Beamish P, Roth M: Old age mental disorders in Newcastle up Tyne. Part 1: A study of prevalence. *Brit J Psychiatry* 110:146–158, 1964.

6. Campbell AJ, McCosh LM, Reinken J, Allan BC: Dementia in old age and the need for services. *Age Ageing* 12:11—16, 1983.
7. Schoenberg BS, Anderson DW, Harerer AF: Severe dementia prevalence and clinical features in a biracial U.S. population. *Arch Neurol* 42:740–743, 1985.
8. Hagnell O, Lanke J, Rorsman B, Ohman R, Ojesjo L: Current trends in the incidence of senile and multi-infarct dementia. *Arch Psychiatr nervenkr* 233:423–438, 1983.
9. Heston LL, Mastri AR, Anderson VE, White J: Dementia of the Alzheimer's type: Clinical genetics, natural history and associated conditions. *Arch Gen Psychiatry* 38:1085–1090, 1981.
10. Amaducci LA, Fratiglioni L, Rocca WA, *et al.*: Risk factors for clinically diagnosed Alzheimer's disease: A case-control study of an Italian population. *Neurology* 36:922–931, 1986.
11. Heyman A, Wilkinson WE, Strafford JA, Helms MJ, Sigmon AH, Weinberg T: Alzheimer's disease: A study of epidemiological aspects. *Ann Neurol* 15:335–341, 1984.
12. Shalat SL, Seltzer B, Pidcock C, Baker EL: Risk factors for Alzheimer's disease. *Neurology* 37:1630–1633, 1987.
13. Chandra V, Philipose V, Bell PA, Lazaroff A, Schoenberg BS: Case-control study of late onset "probable Alzheimer's disease." *Neurology* 37:1295–1300, 1987.
14. Molloy DW, Alemeyehu E, Roberts R: A standardized Mini Mental State Examination (SMMSE): Reliability compared to the traditional MMSE. *Am J Psychiatry* 148:102–105, 1991.
15. Molloy DW, McIlroy W, Guyatt G, Lever J: Relationship between cognition, ADL function, and dysfunctional behavior in community-dwelling older adults with cognitive impairment. Submitted for publication.
16. Reisberg B, Ferris SH, DeLeon MJ, Crook T: The Global Deterioration Scale for assessment of primary degenerative dementia. *Am J Psychiatry* 139:1136–1139, 1982.
17. Niederehe G: TRIMS Behavioural Problem Checklist (BPC). *Psychopharmocology Bulletin* 24:771–778, 1988.
18. Molloy DW, Clarnette R, Guyatt G, McIlroy W: Clinical significance of primitive reflexes in Alzheimer's syndrome. Submitted for publication.
19. Yesavage JA, Brink TL, Rose TL: The geriatric depression rating scale: Comparision with other self-report and psychiatric rating scales. *In* Coot T, Ferris S, Bartus R, eds.: *Assessment in Geriatric Psychopharmacology.* New Canaan, Connecticut: Mark Powley Associates Inc., 1983.

2 | MANAGING DEMENTIA

CASE PRESENTATION

Mrs. Smith, a 72-year-old retired nurse, comes to your office with her daughter. They have been living together in Mrs. Smith's house since Mrs. Smith's husband died five years ago. The daughter is concerned because her mother has become more irritable, forgetful, and uncooperative in the past few months. Mrs. Smith has been getting up at night to "go home to her mother's house." (Mrs. Smith's mother has been dead for 20 years.) Sometimes Mrs. Smith does not recognize her daughter and tells her to get out of the house. At night she gets agitated when her daughter tells her that her mother has been dead for 20 years.

Mrs. Smith takes digoxin, calcium, thyroxine, and an over-the-counter sedative containing antihistamines and phenylephrine. The daughter complains that her mother has been wandering around the house at night keeping her awake. The daughter complains that she herself has no energy, her arthritis in her knees is getting worse, and she is losing weight.

D.W. Molloy

Consider the following statements (true or false)

1. Before any care plan is developed for a patient with cognitive impairment, it is essential first to rule out a reversible cause.

2. Refer the daughter to a rheumatologist for assessment and management of her arthritis.

3. Even at this early stage it is important to discuss long-term-care planning for institutionalization at a later date.

4. When the mother wakes the daughter up, the daughter should tell Mrs. Smith to go back to bed because her mother has been dead for 20 years.

5. Cholinergic drugs cause significant improvement in ADL and behavior in patients with Alzheimer's disease (AD).

1. TRUE

When a patient presents with cognitive impairment the first step is to remove or treat any factors that may be contributing to the cognitive impairment, for example, drugs, depression, B_{12} deficiency, deafness.

When any and all possible conditions that may be contributing to the cognitive impairment have been removed or treated, then it is necessary to establish the cause of the cognitive impairment, for example, Alzheimer's, Parkinson's, multi-infarct dementia.

Common reversible causes of cognitive impairment in the elderly:

1. Drugs
2. Depression
3. Metabolism
4. Others, for example, neoplasms, normal pressure hydrocephalus, infections, subdural hematomata

Dementia is a common clinical syndrome produced by many different conditions that affect brain function. It is most likely that senile dementia of the Alzheimer type has many causes and is not a homogeneous disease. AD probably has many predisposing factors and causes. Plaques and tangles in Alzheimer's disease, as in cirrhosis, are most likely the common pathologic endpoint for a variety of insults to the central nervous system. It seems likely that the brain can respond to a variety of insults in only a limited fashion, and Alzheimer's includes a heterogeneous group of clinical syndromes that are presently grouped together. This may account for the differences in neuropathologic, neurochemical, and clinical syndromes presently grouped together as "Alzheimer's disease."

About 10 to 15% of the elderly who present with cognitive impairment have partial reversal of cognitive impairment, and almost 3% have a completely reversible cause [1,2]. This subgroup with reversible cognitive impairment may be better classified as suffering from delirium because the cognitive impairment is transient and reversible [3,4]. The term "dementia" should be reserved for "irreversible cognitive impairment." This terminology avoids problems with terms such as cognitive impairment, delirium, dementia, *etc.* Cognitive impairment occurs in three different syndromes—acute delirium, subacute delirium, and dementia.

1. *Acute delirium:* acute reversible; cognitive impairment, onset rapid; present for less than three months.
2. *Subacute delirium:* subacute reversible; cognitive impairment. Subacute or acute onset present for more than three months.
3. *Dementia*: irreversible, sustained progressive impairment. Cognitive function that has no apparent reversible cause. Clearly there may be many contributors to these syndromes occurring at the same time.

Clarfield reviewed 32 clinical studies of dementia involving 2889 patients. Eleven studies provided follow-up data in 1051 patients. In these studies, 11% had partial reversal and 3% had complete reversal with appropriate diagnosis and treatment [1]. The commonest reversible causes of cognitive impairment are drugs, depression, and metabolic conditions. Other conditions that were associated with reversibility included infections, neoplasm, normal-pressure hydrocephalus, and subdural hematoma. Larsen *et al.* reported that around 20% of patients who presented with cognitive impairment had objective improvement with appropriate diagnosis and treatment [2].

Drug intoxication may result from ingestion of prescription or over-the-counter patent medications. Patients with short-term memory loss are at increased risk of intoxication. They may forget that they had taken a particular drug and take it more often than prescribed. This is more likely in patients taking multiple prescriptions. A large number of medications affect cognitive function, for example, neuroleptics, benzodiazepines, analgesics, steroids, anticholinergic agents, and even drugs for gastrointestinal and cardiovascular disorders. When an elderly person presents with cognitive impairment or a change in behavior, every drug should be considered as a possible cause [5,6,7].

In Mrs. Smith's case, she is taking at least four medications that her daughter is aware of (digoxin, calcium, thyroxine, and an over-the-counter antihistamine). Three of those drugs affect cognitive function (digoxin, thyroxine, antihistamine).

Advise the daughter to inspect her mother's drug cupboard for analgesics, antacids, laxatives, ointments, vitamins, creams, and other over-the-counter "cure alls" and "elixirs of life." The importance of a complete drug history cannot be overstated. Throw out all unnecessary medications.

Discontinue every medication that is not absolutely essential. This can be done slowly over weeks. Every drug should be considered a possible cause of cognitive impairment until proven otherwise. Check digoxin levels and order an ECG. If there is no evidence of atrial fibrillation and there is no history of atrial fibrillation, then discontinue digoxin.

If she has atrial fibrillation and a CT scan of the head is normal, then aspirin or even anticoagulants might be considered. The effects of long-term aspirin or anticoagulatants on cognitive function in patients with atrial fibrillation has not been established. However, the risks of using anticoagulants in an elderly woman with memory loss may out-weigh any possible benefits.

It is also important to determine if the patient has underlying problems with hearing or vision. Would she benefit from hearing or visual assessments?

Metabolic Disorders

Thyroid, adrenal, or pituitary dysfunction or associated malignancy should be considered as possible reversible causes of cognitive impair-ment. Consider pulmonary disease with hypoxia or hypercarbia, renal or hepatic encephalopathy, diabetes, or cancer. Dehydration is the com-monest metabolic abnormality that causes confusion in the elderly. Since Mrs. Smith takes thyroxine, check T3, T4, and TSH levels.

Nutritional Disorders/Alcoholic Dementia

Thiamine deficiency produces Wernickes–Korsakoff encephalopathy, with Korsakoff's dementia. Does Mrs. Smith take alcohol? The patient's history of alcohol consumption is usually very unreliable. It is important to get a collaborative history from the daughter and stop alcohol if Mrs. Smith takes it.

If the patient objects, substitute non-alcoholic beer or wines. Try to stop her supply. Give 50 mg of thiamine daily for at least one month. Her daughter may not be aware of how much alcohol Mrs. Smith takes. Advise the daughter to search the house for hidden caches and monitor the consumption as closely as possible.

Intracranial Conditions

Chronic subdural hematoma may present with progressive loss of cog-nitive function. It may be associated with subtle clinical signs. Benign tumors also produce dementia. If Mrs. Smith's gait is abnormal or unsteady, then consider normal-pressure hydrocephalus, especially if the gait is flat-footed [8]. A CT scan of the head may help to rule out intracranial causes of dementia.

Depression

Elderly with depression may not have any obvious change in mood. In some cases the presentation of depression may mimic dementia or pseudodementia. This is discussed further in Chapter 13, Depression. If there is any doubt, prescribe a sedative antidepressant at night instead of the antihistamine. Start a low dose of antidepressant, for example, nortryptiline 10 mg at bedtime. Increase the dose in 10-mg increments weekly up to about 50 mg. Monitor the patient for side effects and check lying and standing blood pressures. This may improve sleep with less daytime sedation. The following lists the steps that must be taken in developing a care plan in a cognitively impaired elder.

Steps in developing a care plan for patients and family of cognitively impaired elderly:
1. Assess and document
      cognitive deficit,
      ADL function,
      dysfunctional behavior,
      psychiatric problems,
      safety concerns, and
      caregiver function.
2. Rule out reversible cause.
3. Define the caregiver's function, strengths, weaknesses, burnout. Describe denial, anger, depression, or acceptance in the caregiver. Must try to get the caregiver to accept the disease.
4. Educate caregiver(s) about the disease, for example, diagnosis, prognosis, need to accept help, and behavior management. Establish goals of treatment, not to cure but to maintain dignity, independence, and best quality of life.
5. Prioritize problems on the basis of severity, safety, and ability of caregivers to cope. Use a problem-solving approach to individualize care.
6. Get relief for caregivers.
7. Start planning long-term care.

8. Deal with legal issues, for instance, power of attorney.
9. Get directive from patient and caregiver about treatment of reversible or irreversible illness and cardiac arrest.

2. FALSE

Caring for a patient with cognitive impairment can be extremely demanding for even the most resilient caregiver. Patients with cognitive impairment are often very difficult to manage. A caregiver has a difficult role to play because she or he must take over the patient's chores around the house, care for the patient and deal with the loss of a loved one who is suffering repeated losses.

Just as in any chronic illness or death, many caregivers at first deny the illness and go from doctor to doctor looking for "an answer, a miracle, or a definite diagnosis." Many of these caregivers have been told, but they are not ready to listen.

So it is important to deal first with the caregiver's denial until the caregiver has accepted the disease. It is often useless to try to educate the caregiver about management strategies unless he or she has accepted the disease. Many caregivers experience loss, denial, anger, depression, guilt and anxiety, and it is necessary to make them aware of their feelings so they can deal with them. It often helps to explain to them that these feelings are normal, and to take concrete examples of experiences to illustrate this point.

For instance, if a patient keeps asking the same question, the caregiver becomes frustrated answering the question over and over. Finally the caregiver becomes angry and shouts at the patient. Following this the caregiver experiences anxiety and guilt for what he or she has done. It is often helpful to explain to the caregiver that all of this is perfectly natural, but that he or she will be taught behavior strategies to deal with these kinds of problems so that this series of events will be avoided.

Avoid using different terms for the same disease, for example, multi-infarct dementia, strokes, Binswanger's encephalopathy, arteriosclerosis. These terms tend to confuse the caregiver, and as a result he or she may think that the doctor is giving him or her a different diagnosis every time. Explain the diagnosis and prognosis in simple practical terms. For instance, rather than saying the brain will shrink and nerve cells will die, it is more appropriate to say that the patient's speech will get worse and he or she will have greater difficulty dressing, washing, and feeding. Anatomic, physiologic, or neurochemical outcomes are irrelevant to most caregivers, and it makes more sense to describe the disease in terms of speech, behavior, and activities of daily living.

Many caregivers develop significant depressive symptoms, lose weight, or develop stress-related illnesses. It is important to be aware of the caregiver's physical and mental state if one is to manage the disease properly. A depressed caregiver will significantly affect the patient's quality of life. When one treats Alzheimer's disease, one has to manage not only the patient but the whole social unit, which may include spouse, children, other family members, and friends. The whole family unit must be educated to cope with the disease.

Accordingly, it would not be appropriate to refer the daughter to a rheumatologist for x-rays and other investigations for osteoarthritis at this time. It would be more appropriate to explore the caregiver's level of anxiety and/or burnout. This complaint of arthritis may be a call for help. The daughter has already complained that she can't sleep because her mother is wandering around the house at night. The priority here is the daughter's loss of sleep, and not arthritis, which may get better when she gets a night's sleep. Explore any factors in the history that may be contributing to the patient's insomnia (see Chapter 7, Sleep).

We use the Zarit Burden Scale as a screening instrument at our clinic to assess the level of stress and burnout in caregivers [9]. In our experience the instrument is a valid measure of caregiver stress. The Dysfunctional Behavior Rating Instrument also gives a measure of stress and burden in the caregiver (Appendix B).

3. TRUE

The vast majority of caregivers are unable to care for a severely demented adult alone in their own homes. In the late moderate and in severe stages of dementia, the physical and psychological demands are too much for an elderly spouse or middle-aged son or daughter. The task is too demanding, and the average person who has not received nursing training is unable to cope alone.

Therefore it is likely that nearly all caregivers will have to give up the patient to an institution in the final stages of the disease. Some caregivers cannot cope with this burden and have to give up the patient earlier. The obsessive compulsive caregiver, or one who refuses to accept the disease, gives up earlier. We usually try to deal with denial as early as possible before developing a care plan for the caregivers.

I usually ask the caregiver if he or she plans to let the patient go to an institution. The majority emphatically reply, "No." Then I ask these questions:

1. If the time comes when your mother does not recognize you any more and does not know that she is in her own house, will you continue to care for her?
2. If your mother loses control of her urine and feces and is unable to wash, dress, feed herself, or even walk, will you continue to care for her?
3. If your mother cannot understand even simple sentences and loses her ability to speak, and if you have to lift her in and out of bed, will you continue to care for her?

When the caregiver realizes that the patient's condition is going to deteriorate to a point where the patient will require heavy care and will be unable to communicate or recognize the caregiver, then the caregiver usually accepts institutionalization. This informs the caregiver that this disease is finite and that he or she will most likely survive the patient. The caregiver realizes that he or she will have a life after the patient has been institutionalized.

At this time we inform the caregiver that his or her most important responsibility is to stay healthy. If Mrs. Smith's daughter's health breaks down, then she will be admitted to a hospital and the patient will be institutionalized prematurely. Then we tell the caregiver that she must accept help and allow the patient to go out to day care, or have home-makers or other health professionals come into the home to give care.

In this way we give the caregiver a general time frame, a rough concept of when the patient will require institutionalization, and a general idea of what resources are available in the community. We tell the caregiver that he or she will have to give up the patient eventually and will only have a certain period of time to care for the patient. We challenge the caregiver to take the best possible care of the patient to make the patient's last months or years at home as dignified and as happy as possible. We also tell the caregiver that he or she will have complete control of these decisions, and he or she will decide when the patient will be institutionalized. We emphasize the fact that this must be the caregiver's decision.

To face this challenge we advise the caregiver that he or she must learn how to manage the variety of problems that will be faced. We then challenge the caregiver to take on this task and keep the patient at home as long as possible. Only by remaining healthy and coping will the caregiver do this job properly. A burned out caregiver cannot help anyone. This approach is the most practical, straightforward, and successful strategy in managing the demented elderly in the community.

We make it clear to all caregivers that we are merely giving advice, but all the important decisions will be theirs. We will help them to cope, to get help in any way at all. We emphasize that our goal is to

1. preserve the patient's dignity,
2. improve the patient's and caregiver's quality of life as much as possible,
3. keep the patient at home as long as possible until the caregiver tells us that he or she has had enough.

4. FALSE

Once the caregiver has accepted the diagnosis and has a general idea about the prognosis and possibility of institutionalization, only then is it possible to deal with the problems at hand. It is necessary to list in order of importance the problems the caregiver is having in coping with the patient. These can be written in specific and general terms and need to be individualized for each patient and caregiver.

Dysfunctional behavior has significant negative consequences for the patient and caregiver. It is necessary to be aware of these consequences if one is to manage this disease adequately.

We advise the caregivers to keep diaries listing the problems they have with the patient and describing the steps they have taken to deal with it. We also ask them to prioritize their problems so we can deal with a few problems at a time. This makes the caregivers adapt an objective approach to the management of the problem. The diaries are invaluable because caregivers can monitor their progress and we can see how effective our interventions have been. After they have successfully managed the first few problems, it is usually unnecessary to continue using the diary. In managing any behavior problem in the demented elderly, a few simple rules must be followed. These simple "golden rules" are listed as follows and can be adapted for just about any situation.

Golden rules in managing the elderly individual with cognitive impairment:

1. Do not argue or contradict. Patients with cognitive impairment cannot learn because of short-term memory loss, so reasoning

does not work.

2. Reality orientation and negative reinforcement do not work. There is no point in telling the patient that this is 1990 and not 1942. There is also no point punishing a demented person who does something wrong. The person will not remember why he or she is being punished.
3. Validation therapy helps; it makes more sense to deal with patients on an emotional level rather than trying to reason.
4. Distract rather than arguing—get her off the subject.
5. If all else fails, remove yourself from the situation (losing your temper just makes it worse).
6. Learn physical responses to stress, for example, tightness in chest, clenched teeth, making a fist. Caregivers must recognize their physical manifestations of stress and learn to relax the body by walking, opening hands, relaxing jaw, deep breathing, visualization to unwind and control stress.

Tell the daughter not to tell her mother it is 3:00 a.m., 1990, and Mrs. Smith's mother has been dead for 20 years. Instead, the daughter must

1. go to where her mother is, rather than trying to bring her mother to where she is. Validate, do not attempt reality orientation;
2. get out of bed;
3. not try to reason with her mother (for example, "But it's 3:00 a.m.");
4. calm her mother down and soothe her, for example, put her arm around her, rub her back, hold her hand;
5. talk quietly to her;
6. slowly get her back to bed—it may be helpful to give warm milk, talk to her for a little while, *etc.*;
7. tell her that she will be able to visit her mother later, but basically try to distract her so the mother will get off that subject and on to a more relaxing, calming topic. Arguing or trying to reason with a patient with short-term memory loss is a waste of time. The caregiver becomes frustrated, angry, and resentful. The patient may also become angry and uncooperative. Later the caregiver feels guilty and can't sleep anyway. Some of the consequences of dysfunctional behavior are listed in Table 2-1.

Table 2-1 Effects of Dysfunctional Behavior on Patient and Caregiver.

Patient behavior	Consequence to patient	Caregiver	Consequence to caregiver
Confusion and delusions at night, for example, people in house	Up at night, sleeping in day, anxiety	Up at night, loss of sleep	Exhausted, angry, resentful, depressed
Fear of being alone	Fear, anxiety, panic attacks, demanding	Patient requires attention 24 hours per day	No privacy, exhausted, feels trapped
Wants to go home, wanders	Wanders gets lost, lack of safety with cars, etc.	Must watch patient all the time	Exhaustion, anxiety, fear

5. FALSE

Neuropathologic studies have consistently reported a decrease in cholinergic nuclei in patients with senile dementia of the Alzheimer's type [10–15]. Neurochemical findings have confirmed a decrease in choline acetyltransferase, the enzyme that synthesizes acetylcholine, which acts as a marker for the presynaptic cholinergic system in patients with Alzheimer's disease. However, other studies have shown a decrease in other neurotransmitters in patients with AD [16–19]. Neuropharmacologic studies have demonstrated a deterioration in memory and cognitive function in individuals given anticholinergic drugs, preparations widely used in the elderly [6].

Although a few reports have described a significant improvement in ADL and/or cognitive function with the anticholinesterases physostigmine and tetrahydroaminoacridine, the majority of properly controlled, randomized, double-blind trials have failed to show a significant clinical improvement in ADL and/or cognitive function with cholinergic drugs [20,21].

Cholinergic drugs cause significant toxicity, which limits their effectiveness. Recently "nootropic" agents have been tested in patients with

Alzheimer's disease with limited success [22]. The place of these agents in the routine management of AD has not yet been established.

To date the indications for benzodiazepines, antidepressants, and/or neuroleptics have been poorly studied. There is a shortage of properly controlled clinical trials to establish the indications, doses, toxicity, and side effects of these agents in the routine management of dementia [23].

REFERENCES

1. Clarfield AM: The reversible dementia: Do they reverse? *Annals of Internal Medicine* 109:476–486, 1988.
2. Larson EB, Reifler BV, Featherstone HJ, English DR: Dementia in elderly outpatients: A prospective study. *Annals of Internal Medicine* 100:417–423, 1984.
3. Lipowski ZJ: Delirium (acute confusional states). *JAMA* 258:1789–1792, 1987.
4. Lipowski ZJ: Transient cognitive disorders (delirium, acute confusional states) in the elderly. *Am J Psychiatry* 140:1426–1436, 1983.
5. Molloy DW, Seliske JM, Cape RDT: Survey of the prescribing pattern and use of anticholinergic medications in the institutionalized elderly. *J Clinical Experimental Gerontology* 9(3):231–242, 1987.
6. Molloy DW, Brooymans MA: Anticholinergic medications and cognitive function in the elderly. *J Clinical Experimental Gerontology* 10(3 and 4):89–98, 1988–1989.
7. Molloy DW: Memory loss, confusion and disorientation in an elderly woman taking Meclizine. *J Am Geriatric Soc* 35:454, 1987.
8. Power CN, Wilson D, Patterson C, Molloy DW: Diagnostic clues to normal pressure hydrocephalus. *Diagnosis* 4(11):83–97, 1987.
9. Zarit SH, Reever KE, Poach-Peterson J: Relatives of the impaired elderly: Correlates of feelings of burden. *Gerontologist* 20:649–655, 1980.
10. Davies P, Maloney AJR: Selective loss of central cholinergic neurons in Alzheimer's disease. *Lancet* 2:1403, 1988.

11. Rogers JD, Brogran D, Mirrs SS: The nucleus basalis of Meynert in neurological disease: A qualitative morphological study. *Ann Neurol* 17:163–170, 1985.
12. Tagliavani F, Pilleri G: Neuronal counts in basal nucleus of Meynert in Alzheimer's disease and in simple senile dementia. *Lancet* 1:469–470, 1983.
13. Bowen DM, Allen SJ, Benton JS, Goodhardt MJ, Haan EA, Palmer AM, Sims NR, Smith CC, Spillane JA, Esihi MM, Neary D, Snowden JS, Wilcock GK, Davison AN: Biochemical assessment of serotonergic and cholinergic dysfunction and cerebral atrophy in Alzheimer's disease. *J Neurochem* 41:261–272, 1983.
14. Davies P: Neurotransmitter—related enzymes in senile dementia of the Alzheimer's type. *Brain Res* 171:319–327, 1979.
15. Perry EK: The cholinergic hypothesis—Ten years on. *Br Med Bull* 42:63–69, 1986.
16. Davies P, Katzman R, Terry RD: Reduced somotostatin-like immunoreactivity in cerebral cortex from cases of Alzheimer's disease and Alzheimer senile dementia. *Nature* 288:279–280, 1980.
17. Adolfsson R, Jootfries CG, Roose BE, Winblad B: Changes in brain catecholamines in patients with dementia of Alzheimer's Alzheimer type. *Br J Psychaitry* 135:216–223, 1979.
18. Yates C, Allison Y, Simpson J, Maloney AFS, Gordon A: Dopamine in Alzheimer's disease and senile dementia. *Lancet* 2:851–852, 1979.
19. Rossor MN, Garret JN, Johnson AL, *et al.*: A post mortem study of the cholinergic and GABA systems in senile dementia. *Brain* 105:313–330, 1982.
20. Molloy DW, Cape RDT: Acute effects of oral pyridostigmine on memory and cognitive function in SDAT. *Neurobiology of Aging* 10:199–204, 1989.
21. Molloy DW, Guyatt G, Wilson D, Duke R: Effects of THA on cognition, activities of daily living, and behavior in Alzheimer's disease: Results of a double-blind randomized trial. *Can Med Assoc J* 144(1):29–34, 1991.
22. Molloy DW, Guyatt G, Brown G, Johnston M, Rees L: Effects of Oxiracetam on cognitive function, activities of daily living, and behavior in dementia: Results of a controlled randomized double-blind trial. Submitted for publication.
23. Cummings JL, Miller BL: Disease-specific therapies in Alzheimer's disease: Treatment and long-term management. Marcel Dekker Inc., New York, 1990.

3 | MANAGING BEHAVIOR PROBLEMS

CASE PRESENTATION

Mrs. Smith, an 82-year-old woman, comes to your office with her daughter. Her daughter is concerned because her mother has become more forgetful in the past three years. Her daughter complains that Mrs. Smith has become more argumentative and constantly repeats the same questions over and over again.

Mrs. Smith is unaware of any problems with her memory. When asked why she came to your office, she replies that her daughter wants to get a check-up, and she came to keep her company.

Mrs. Smith lives with her daughter. The daughter works all day, and Mrs. Smith is on her own. The daughter is concerned for her mother's safety. Mrs. Smith has been burning pots and pans on the stove and has been mixing up her medications. Mrs. Smith denies any episodes of wandering, perseveration, agitated behavior, or burning utensils on the stove. She repeatedly says, "Well, what do you expect at my age?"

The daughter says that recently while shopping, her mother wandered off for about two hours. The daughter also complains that her mother gets up at night and wanders around the house. This keeps the daughter awake. She has to get up repeatedly to make sure her mother has not wandered off. The daughter asks if there is anything that can be done to stop her mother from asking the same questions over and over again [1,2]. Mrs. Smith's daughter mentioned that her mother often complains that there is a stranger in the house.

D.W. Molloy
L. Rees

After you have taken the history from her daughter, Mrs. Smith becomes very agitated, complains that her daughter is telling a pack of lies, and storms out. She refuses to be examined or to have anything to do with you because she says, "All you want to do is put me in a home."

You consider prescribing flurazepam 30 mg at bedtime.

Consider the following statements (true or false)

1. This type of reaction is rarely seen in patients with dementia because they usually cannot follow conversations when people are talking about them.
2. The most appropriate management of Mrs. Smith's tendency to burn pots and pans is to advise her to stop cooking while her daughter is away.
3. When Mrs. Smith asks the same questions again and again, her daughter should tell her that she has asked that question before. When Mrs. Smith hears this, she will stop asking the same question.
4. Mrs. Smith's complaint that there is a stranger in the house may not be a real hallucination and may not require any antipsychotic drug.
5. The most appropriate course of action to address Mrs. Smith's wandering about the house at night is to give her a sedative such as flurazepam 30 mg PO QHS.

1. FALSE

Mrs. Smith had a "catastrophic reaction" in your office because you talked about her problems while she was present. Mrs. Smith had no insight into her condition and was not aware of any problems with her memory. She probably did not remember any of the episodes her daughter talked about—getting lost, burning pots and pans, taking medication inappropriately. So she had to sit there and hear her daughter tell all those "lies" about her to the doctor.

Understandably, Mrs. Smith became very upset. If we take a history from a caregiver in front of a patient who has no insight into her or his condition, this type of catastrophic response will be seen again and again. Behavior changes are common in dementia [3–7]. It is important to establish the type, frequency, and severity from the caregiver. Do this privately when the patient is not present.

When you first meet a patient with memory loss, dementia, or confusion, interview the patient and family at the same time. This allows you to observe how they interact. *Always interview the patient first.* The patient will often not complain of any memory loss but may tell you in great detail about some other problem he or she may have, such as arthritis, *etc.*

Gently prod the patient and ask if he or she has noticed if "your memory has let you down recently." If the patient has no insight into the problem, then it is not worth taking a history from the patient.

At first interview the patient with the family. It is useful to watch how the family reacts to the patient when the patient is giving a history. If a family member continually corrects the patient—"It's not Tuesday, it's Wednesday," or "It's not the fourth floor, it's the second floor," this may eventually provoke aggressive, angry, or abusive behavior in the patient. Observing this interaction may permit the health care professional to advise family members how to deal with the patient and modify their behavior if necessary.

Advise the family to refrain from continually correcting the patient. There is little to be gained from continual correction since the corrections are quickly forgotten. If caregivers make demented patients angry, they can remain that way for hours or days and become impossible to reason with. Do not make the patient aware of her or his problems. This can provoke anxiety, anger, frustration, depression, and aggressive behavior.

After the patient interview is complete, the patient should leave the room and be taken to a different area so the family can be interviewed separately.

Many arguments arise when caregivers try to reason with patients with short-term memory loss. It is often useless to try to reason with a person who has short-term memory loss. The caregivers will just get frustrated and angry, and this will make the patient angry and frustrated too. It is better to avoid arguments, and to distract the patient when she or he makes unreasonable demands.

What do you do when a patient wants to go shopping at 3:00 a.m.? It often doesn't help to tell the patient that it's 3:00 a.m. and the stores are closed. A better approach to take is to say to the patient, "Just relax for a while. I'll make you a nice cup of hot milk and a sandwich (or turn on some music, play a game of cards, or whatever the patient would like), and we will go for a walk later." Avoid confrontation and attempt to reassure in these situations.

By distracting the patient we hope that the patient will forget what he or she wants. In this way, one is using the memory loss to one's advantage. Some simple suggestions and changes in the way a patient and family interact will often help to modify behavior problems.

Patients' most frequent complaint in dementia is that they are always being "told what to do." Demented people *are* always being told what to do. It is necessary so they can perform the simple activities of daily living. They must be told to wash, dress, feed, eat, *etc*. Caregivers must be taught how to get patients to do these things by asking in a nonthreatening fashion, but never by "telling."

Caregivers must be educated about the disease. This is done best by the Alzheimer's Society. Advise caregivers to contact their nearest Alzheimer's Society.

2. FALSE

It is probably a complete waste of time to tell Mrs. Smith to stop cooking. You may want to try it, but it is unlikely that it will work. She is not aware that she is burning pots and pans to begin with, and would probably forget the instructions after a few minutes anyway. If her daughter tells her, this will most likely cause arguments and resentment. Some of the following suggestions may help:

1. Get a master switch on the stove so the daughter can switch it off when she leaves in the morning—the mother will not be able to switch it on.
2. Purchase an electric kettle that automatically switches off when it boils.
3. Cover or disconnect all the elements on the stove except one, so that Mrs. Smith will have only one element to worry about. This may help to reduce the risk of fire.
4. Leave prepared food for her so she does not have to cook during the day.
5. Leave food that can be heated in the oven.
6. Phone after meals to remind her to switch off the stove.
7. Get a neighbor or friend to drop in at meal times to supervise.
8. Disconnect the stove! Get Meals on Wheels.

3. FALSE

Being asked the same question repeatedly can be very annoying for the caregiver. Demented elderly get stuck on a topic and often cannot seem to move on. It is important to talk to the family to discuss this problem. Although one often cannot stop the problem, one can offer the family and caregiver some simple strategies for coping with it.

1. When the patient asks the same questions repeatedly, offer a simple "yes" or "no" and hope she or he will stop.
2. If the patient continues to ask the question or stay on the same topic, leave the room, go to another part of the house, and hope he or she will have changed the topic by the time you come back.
3. Get the patient's mind off it—distract him or her; for example, say, "Look what's on TV," "Have you seen your old wedding photos lately?" or "Would you like to go for a walk later?"

By getting the patient to do something else, it may help to get his or her mind off the subject. Do not try to reason, saying things like, "You have asked that question already and I told you . . ." This is likely to lead to arguments. Distract, postpone, change the subject.

Finally, if none of these strategies works, then, before you get angry with the person, get out of her or his space.

We routinely advise our caregivers, "Never expose the problem." Never remind or tell the patient that he or she has problems with memory. We always advise the caregiver to "play down" the problem. There is little to be gained from giving the patient insight into his or her forgetfulness. This may lead to depression and anger, and it may worsen behavior problems.

It is also important not to argue with the patient. The patient will forget what the argument was about but may stay angry for hours afterwards. It may not be possible to reason with a patient. Trying to do this may just cause the caregiver and patient to become frustrated. Ignore the behavior. The caregiver who becomes angry and resentful will change his or her behavior too. There is little point in telling the patient that he or she has asked the same question over and over again. It is better to distract or get the patient off the subject. This is a good rule of thumb to use in dealing with any repetitive behavior.

Exercise [8,9] and stimulation [10,11] in a regular daily schedule may help to maintain and maximize function.

4. TRUE

Patients with cognitive impairment may often mistake their reflection in the mirror or photographs of others for a stranger. They are unable to process information and interpret their environment logically and reasonably. Patients often wonder how people "go into those small boxes," that is, photographs.

As a result, they have recognition problems; they do not understand how a TV works, and they will think that there are "strangers in the house." Many patients get upset when there are panel discussions on TV—they get angry or confused by all the strangers in their living room. A radio playing in the house may account for "voices." With regard to inpatients, families complain that the patients are "seeing things." Patients have told them that there are police or little children on the ward. This may often be explained by maintenance people, security men, or grandchildren visiting other patients. Always give the patient the benefit of the doubt. Strangers outside the door may be a letter carrier, a neighbor whom the patient does not recognize, or perhaps even a picture on the wall. When there are "strangers in the house," does it occur in any room in particular where there is a mirror or big picture on the wall? Cover pictures, cover mirrors, and shut off the TV and/or radio for a few days and see if the problem solves itself. Even if the problem persists, it can often help to reassure the family. These "delusions" should not be treated.

Be cautious using antipsychotics as they may produce harmful side effects, and the anticholinergic properties may make matters worse. Use antipsychotics as a last resort.

To cope in the comunity, the demented patient needs the caregiver. The goal of the physician should be to educate the caregiver about the disease, solve problems, and provide support. The burden of care on the caregiver depends on the level of function of the patient—his or her personality and behavior changes. The ability of caregivers to cope depends on their coping skills, personality, medical problems, and their social support from families, friends, and health professionals [20–24].

5. FALSE

Wandering at night or insomnia is a common problem in the demented elderly [24–26]. If a caregiver starts to lose sleep (particularly if the caregiver is elderly), if a caregiver has medical problems or has to work during the day, she or he will burn out very quickly. Caregivers frequently become medically ill from coping with the stress of caregiving. The burned out caregiver may even take the patient to the nearest Emergency Room and refuse to take the patient home. It is essential to deal with the problem quickly and effectively.

First try to establish why Mrs. Smith is up at night. Is she looking for the bathroom? Mrs. Smith may need to urinate frequently and may be confused and disoriented, which may cause her to get lost at night in the house. Would a light in the hallway or bathroom, or a commode beside her bed solve the problem?

Does she have arthritis pain or is she sleeping all day while her daughter is at work? If she has day/night reversal and sleeps all day, this cycle may be difficult to reverse. Regular exercise during the day may help, and a regular routine—going to bed at the same time and getting up at the same time every day—may help to re-establish a normal pattern.

Put a hook and eye lock at the top or bottom of exit doors. This will enable the daughter to confine her mother. It is very unlikely her mother will be able to get past either of these locks. With these measures in place, if her mother is up at night, the daughter doesn't have to worry about her walking out. The daughter can sleep knowing that her mother cannot wander away.

Some simple questions about sleep hygiene may also help. Stopping the use of stimulants such as cola drinks, chocolate, coffee, and tea, may help. These not only keep Mrs. Smith awake at night but they also act as diuretics. Chloral hydrate 500–1000 mg at bedtime can help. If tolerance develops, alternate with a short-acting benzodiazepine such as triazolam 0.125–0.25 mg. Flurazepam 30 mg is a large dose of sedative for such an elderly woman.

If Mrs. Smith is at risk of wandering during the day, make sure she has her name and address on her at all times. A Medic Alert bracelet or locket on a chain may suffice. Keep her address in her handbag at all times. Inform neighbors that if they ever see Mrs. Smith wandering around, they should introduce themselves, talk pleasantly to her, and walk with her. In this way they can try to direct her home, if she is lost. It may help to give Mrs. Smith's photograph to the local police in case she does get lost.

Advise the daughter to contact the Alzheimer's Society—they may have a registry for wandering patients, and they provide invaluable information, support and counseling. *The 36-Hour Day* is an invaluable aid for caregivers and health professionals [27].

REFERENCES

1. Sandson J, Albert ML: Perseveration in behavioural neurology. *Neurology* 37:1736–1741, 1987.
2. Fuld PA, Katzman R, Davies P, *et al*.: Intrusions as a sign of Alzheimer's dementia chemical and pathological verification. *Ann Neurol* 11:155–159, 1982.
3. O'Connor M: Disturbed behaviour in dementia—Psychiatric or medical problem? *Med Jour Avst* 147:481–485, 1987.
4. Rubin EH, Morris JC, Storandt M, Berg L: Behavioural changes in patients with mild senile dementia of the Alzheimer type. *Psychiatry Research* 21:55–62, 1987.
5. Zimmer JG, Watson N, Treat A: Behavioural problems among patients in skilled nursing facilities. *AJPH* 74(10):1118–1121, 1984.

6. Rubin EH, Morris JC, Berg L: The progression of personality changes in senile dementia of the Alzheimer type. *JAGS* 35:721–725, 1987.
7. Maletta GJ: Management of behaviour problems in elderly patients with Alzheimer's disease and other dementias. *Clinics in Geriatric Medicine* 4(4):719–747, 1988.
8. Molloy DW, Beerschoten DA, Borrie MJ, Crilly RG, Cape RDT: Acute effects of exercise on neuropsychological function in elderly subjects. *JAGS* 36:29–33, 1988.
9. Molloy DW: The effects of a three-month exercise programme on neuro-psychological function in elderly institutionalized women: A randomized controlled trial. *Age and Ageing* 17(5):303–310, 1988.
10. Gibson AJ, Moyes IC, McKendrick DC: Cognitive assessment of the long stay patient. *Br J Psych* 137:551–557, 1980.
11. Leng H: Behavioural treatment of the elderly. *Age and Ageing* 11:235–243, 1982.
12. Breitner J, Foldi N, Rabins P, Sunderland T, Butler RN: Practical considerations in managing Alzheimer's disease: II *Geriatrics* 42(10):55–65, 1987.
13. Maletta GJ: Medications to modify at-home behaviour of Alzheimer's patients. *Geriatrics* 40(12):31–42, 1985.
14. Windgrad CH, Jarvik L: Physician management of the demented patient. *JAGS* 34:295–308, 1986.
15. Helms PM: Efficacy of antipsychotics in the treatment of the behavioural complications of dementia. *JAGS* 3(3):204–209, 1985.
16. Risse GC, Barnes R: Pharmacologic treatment of agitation associated with dementia. *JAGS* 34:368–376, 1986.

17. Peabody CA, Walner MD, Whiteford HA, Hollister LE: Neuroleptics in the elderly. *JAGS* 35:233–238, 1987.
18. Granagher RB: Agitation in the elderly. *Postgraduate Medicine* 76(6):83–96, 1982.
19. Stewart RB, May FE, Hale WE, Marks RG: Psychotrophic drug use in the ambulatory elderly population. *Gerontology* 28:325–328, 1982.
20. Zarit SH, Reever KE, Bach-Peterson J: Relatives of the impaired elderly: Correlates of feelings of burden. *Gerontologist* 20:655–679, 1980.
21. Zarit SH, Cole KD, Guider RL: Memory training strategies and subjective complaints of memory in the aged. *Gerontologist* 21:158–164, 1981.
22. Zarit SH, Zarit JM, Reever KE: Memory training for severe memory loss: Effects on senile dementia patients and their families. *Gerontologist* 22:373–377, 1982.
23. Zarit SH, Zarit JM: Families under stress: Interventions for caregivers of senile dementia patients. *Psychotherapy: Theory, Research and Practise* 19(4):461–471, 1982.
24. Cornbleth T: Effect of a protected hospital ward area on wandering and non-wandering geriatric patients. *J Gerontology* 32(5):573–577, 1977.
25. Dawson P, Reid DW: Behavioural dimensions of patients at risk of wandering. *Gerontologist* 27:104–107, 1987.
26. Snyder LH: Rupprecht P, Pyrek J, Brekhus S, Moss T: Wandering. *Gerontologist* 18(3):272–280, 1978.
27. Mace NL, Rabins PV: *The 36-Hour Day*. London: Johns Hopkins University Press, 1981.

4 | AGITATION

CASE PRESENTATION

You receive a call late Saturday night from a local residential home concerning a confused resident who is shouting and screaming uncontrollably. The patient is described as a pleasant 84-year-old female who is mildly forgetful but fully independent. She became confused earlier today. Her daughter had visited her this afternoon and noted to the staff that her mother seemed more confused than usual. The patient was drowsy earlier in the evening and slept for a few hours. Upon waking she refused to stay in bed. She is presently walking up and down the corridor, shouting, "You better get a doctor before it's too late because I'm going to have a baby." She is pulling off her clothes and will not let the nurses put her back to bed. There have been no previous episodes of disturbed behavior.

The patient is on no medications. A neurological consultation, performed six months ago, included CT scan, EEG, and blood work. Early mild senile dementia of the Alzheimer type (AD) was diagnosed.

Her vital signs this morning were: temperature, 37.4°C; BP, 120/70; heart rate, 72, regular. The nurse has been unable to determine vital signs this evening due to the agitated state of the patient. Over the telephone you hear the patient shouting in the background, "Ma, ma, ma—I want my mother," and yelling at the nursing staff. The nurse requests you to prescribe a sedative since this patient's behavior is disturbing other residents.

___

Consider the following statements (true or false)

1. The most likely cause of this patient's agitation is dementia, that is, senile dementia of the Alzheimer's type.

2. The underlying cause of agitation is usually identified in the majority of elderly demented patients who present with an acute onset.

3. History and physical examination is unlikely to reveal any treatable cause for this woman's agitation.

4. This woman should be put in bed with restraints and bedsides to prevent her from falling and hurting herself.

5. The most appropriate treatment would be to give haloperidol 0.25–1.0 mg IM, or thioridazine 12.5–50 mg IM Q4H, with review in the morning.

1. FALSE

Agitation may be defined as "observed inappropriate verbal or motor activity which cannot be explained by need or external need alone" [1]. Agitated behavior is usually repetitive and frequently consists of repeated questions, complaints, words, or movements (Table 4-1). Agitation may be a manifestation of delirium. Delirium, "a transient disorder of cognition and attention, accompanied by disturbances of the sleep–awake cycle and psychomotor behavior" [2,3] is estimated to occur in 30% to 50% of patients over the age of 70 at some point during hospital admission [4,5].

Up to 10% of hospitalized elderly medical and surgical patients are delirious at any given time [2,6]. Features that make a diagnosis of delirium more likely are listed in Table 4-2.

Content of the complaint should never be ignored. The complaint can frequently provide an important clue to the underlying cause of agitation. In this case, the patient expressed that she is going to have a baby. This may represent an attempt to explain or verbalize abdominal discomfort that may be a result of obstruction, urinary retention, fecal impaction, perforation, or biliary or urinary colic. Some patients with dyspnea and confusion complain that they are being smothered. The pacing of this patient also suggests that she is experiencing physical discomfort.

Table 4-1 Verbal and Physical Characteristics of Agitated Behavior.

	Repetition	*Abuse*	*Behavior*
Verbal	Calling out Questions Complaints Single Words Phrases	Cursing Threats Screams	Strange noise Grunts Coughs
Physical	Walking Pacing Wandering Dressing Undressing Pounding Rattling the bed	Biting Fighting Striking out Throwing objects	Bizarre movements Twitches

Table 4-2 Clinical Features of Delirium.

Features in the presentation of an illness that make delirium more likely:

Rapid onset of symptoms and/or signs
Symptoms and signs that fluctuate
Reduced awareness of environment
Memory loss and disorientation
Presence of organic factor(s) that may be related from history,
    physical exam, or investigations
Two or more of the following:
    perceptual disturbance (delusions, hallucinations)
    change in psychomotor activity
    change in sleep–wake cycle
    incoherent speech

Adapted from *Diagnostic and Statistical Manual of Mental Disorders.* 3rd ed., Washington, DC: American Psychiatric Association, 1980.

This woman suffers from mild forgetfulness from senile dementia of the Alzheimer's type. Acute deterioration in her condition cannot be explained by AD alone. Alzheimer's disease usually causes a gradual, relentless deterioration in cognitive function over years. An acute insult to her nervous system is the most likely cause of her confusion and agitation, for example, hypoxia, infection, dehydration, stroke, myocardial infarction, metabolic abnormality, or drug-induced delirium (Table 4-3).

2. TRUE

Agitation is not a diagnosis but a symptom of an underlying abnormality. If the underlying cause of agitation is identified quickly and treated, the agitation may be reversed.

In this case the vital signs taken earlier this morning are not helpful, since the onset of confusion and agitation occurred hours later. Normal vital signs in an elderly patient do not rule out an underlying infection. Some elderly patients with pneumonia or septicemia don't even have an elevated white cell count.

The elderly may have various causes for acute confusion that must be considered and investigated (see Table 4-3). Incorrect diagnoses and management of diseases manifesting agitation may prove fatal or cause irreversible damage.

Table 4-3   Causes of Delirium in the Elderly.

1. *Drugs*
   Any drug can cause delirium in
      the elderly but especially drugs
      with anticholinergic properties.
   Digitalis, sedatives, levodopa,
      steroids, antihypertensives, anti-
      convulsants, cimetidine, drug
      withdrawal

2. *Cardiovascular system (CVS)*
   Myocardial infarction,
      congestive heart failure
   Arrythmias

3. *Metabolic*
   Dehydration
   Electrolyte abnormality
   Hypothyroidism/
      hyperthyroidism
   Diabetes mellitus
   Renal /liver abnormalities
   Nutritional deficiencies

4. *Respiratory*
   Pneumonia
   Acute exacerbation of chronic
      obstructive pulmonary disease

5. *Central nervous system (CNS)*
   Subdural hematoma, stroke,
   transient ischemic attacks (TIA),
   epilepsy, neoplasm, infection

6. *Mechanical*
   Fecal impaction
   Urinary retention

7. *Environmental*
   Any change in environment

8. *Infection*
   Urinary tract
   Biliary tract

9. *Hematologic*
   Anemia, especially following
      an acute/subacute bleed
   B_{12} deficiency
   Myeloma

10. *Other*
    Giant cell arteritis
    Concussion without subdural
    Alcohol withdrawal or
       intoxication
    Over-the-counter medications
    Pain
    Fracture

3. FALSE

Taking the History

It is important to determine if the patient has had her temperature taken regularly in the past few days in order to determine a baseline. If the patient normally has a temperature of 35.5–36.0°C and it is 37.5°C today, this represents a significant increase in body temperature.

Note if any new medications have been started recently, or if there have been changes in the doses of maintenance medications. Medications, which frequently cause delirium in the elderly, must be carefully prescribed and monitored. Drug-induced delirium and confusion may be completely reversed by altering or discontinuing medications.

Ask about changes in the frequency of urination and defecation. Urinary retention or fecal impaction may cause confusion and agitation in the elderly. Is her urine cloudy or foul smelling? Has she had new episodes of incontinence? Has she fallen recently? Is the patient in bed and refusing to get out? It is easy to overlook a fractured hip, and the possibility of subdural hematoma must always be considered. Consider a fracture, no matter how trivial a history of falls or injury.

Ask if she has been drinking more than usual or if she is gaining weight. Are her ankles more swollen than usual? It is very important to ascertain if she has had similar episodes of confusion and agitation in the past, and if so, how they were investigated, diagnosed, and/or treated.

Clinical Examination

A general examination should be performed on all agitated or confused patients. Take your time talking to the patient to develop confidence and trust before you begin your exam. Establish physical contact at the start by stroking her hair, holding her hand, or adjusting her clothing. Explain that you are the doctor and that you have come to help. Be patient and go slowly and gently. Agitated patients forget who you are and may think you mean them harm. It may help to wear a white coat in order to alleviate her anxiety.

General inspection may reveal anemia, cyanosis, pigmentation, bruising from falls, edema, tachypnea, neglect, or weakness on one side from a recent stroke, dehydration, or evidence of hypothyroidism. Try to get vital signs if possible. Examine the cardiovascular system for heart rate, rhythm, elevated jugulovenous pulse (JVP), or evidence of failure. Percuss the chest carefully since the patient may not cooperate and breathe when you want. Dullness in a base is easier to find than decreased breath sounds in an uncooperative patient. Dullness in both bases with an elevated JVP is very suggestive of cardiac failure.

In this case the patient believes she is going to have a baby. This is very significant and should prompt you to examine her abdomen carefully. An agitated patient will not localize pain in the abdomen but may display rigidity and guarding over the affected viscus. Listen for bowel sounds. If they are increased, get a straight abdominal film to help in the diagnosis of obstruction. If they are absent, get a straight film and a surgeon. Always do a rectal exam.

Rectal examination may reveal fecal impaction, evidence of rectal bleeding, or prostatic hypertrophy in males. Fecal impaction may cause confusion and agitation in the elderly. Urinary retention is also commonly overlooked as a cause of confusion with agitation in elderly patients. Men with prostatic hypertrophy are particularly at risk. If you have any doubts, especially in obese patients, catheterize them to check the residual volume. Catheters should be removed immediately and not left in situ, since agitated patients do not tolerate catheters, and it can even make them worse.

In-and-out catheterization serves two purposes:

1. to rule out urinary retention, and
2. to get a catheter specimen of urine for routine microscopy and culture.

On examination of the nervous system, look closely for localizing or lateralizing signs. Check for neck stiffness, tone, and reflexes and do the plantar responses. If you can, observe the fundi for papilledema; however, funduscopic examination is usually impossible in agitated patients.

Investigations

If after your examination you still cannot diagnose the cause of the agitated patient's confusion, some simple tests may help. Hemoglobin and complete blood count will detect anemia or leucocytosis if they are present. Blood sugar, electrolytes, urea, and creatinine will detect acute renal failure, hyponatremia, acidosis, or glucose abnormalities. If there is some concern that the patient has intra-abdominal pathology, order liver enzymes and a serum amylase. Be sure to check thyroid function since hypothyroidism or thyrotoxicosis are easily overlooked in the elderly due to atypical presentations.

An ECG is mandatory. Myocardial infarction can be "silent" and may present with confusion in the elderly. Do a chest x-ray to rule out pneumonia or cardiac failure, and do a flat plate, erect abdomen, and/or ultrasound if you suspect intra-abdominal pathology.

Check the patient for recent fractures. Consider an x-ray of lumbosacral spines and/or hip as patients with vertebral fractures may complain of pain in the abdomen or lower limbs, which can be misleading.

All patients who present with acute delirium should have blood cultures done since sepsis in the elderly may not cause fever or leucocytosis. Dehydration commonly causes confusion, so if you are in doubt, give intravenous fluids. This may be easier said than done in combative patients. In all cases, staff should be encouraged to ensure adequate fluid intake by mouth, and, where feasible, urinary output should be measured.

4. FALSE

Restraints are absolutely contraindicated in this patient at this time. It would be completely inappropriate to confine her to bed with bedsides. If restrained she may struggle to escape and choke herself. If she escapes from the restraints she may climb out over the bedsides and fall from a greater height, suffering even greater trauma than if she just fell from the bed.

If a patient becomes extremely agitated in bed and attempts to climb out over the sides, remove the bed and place the patient on a mattress on the floor. Bedsides often make agitation worse, because patients may feel imprisoned, which increases their paranoia, frustration, and confusion.

In this case, you might wish to call the patient's daughter and ask her to come in and sit with her mother. Family members can supply support, reassurance, and comfort to distressed elderly patients in these situations. A familiar voice and face may work wonders in calming the patient.

Restraints frequently make confusion, paranoia, and agitation worse. Patients can get tangled in them, choke themselves, or cut off the circulation to their limbs. Restraints have a limited place in the management of agitated patients. If one feels it is necessary to give intravenous fluid, nasogastric suction, or catheterization in a thrashing, agitated patient, then chemical or physical restraints are often necessary to facilitate treatment or monitoring. However, use of restraints in a patient such as this is inappropriate, cynical, and cruel without having first seen her or examined her for a reversible cause of her agitation. Putting her in restraints may allow the underlying process to go unchecked and could even prove fatal.

5. FALSE

This woman was seen by her family doctor, who referred her promptly to the Emergency Room. She had acute cholecystitis and dehydration. She was treated with intravenous fluids and rehydrated, and appropriate antibiotics were started. She was given "boxing gloves," that is, her hands were taped in a clenched position grasping a roll of bandage. She was put on a mattress on the floor of a well-lit, quiet, private room and had an aide sit with her for 24 hours until her delirium/agitation resolved. She was given haloperidol 0.5 mg IM Q4H PRN and settled on this therapy.

There is a limited place for physical and chemical restraints in the treatment of agitation [7,8,9]. They may be used after careful assessment of the patient and/or initiation of treatment. It is inappropriate to use chemical restraints without first seeing the patient.

REFERENCES

1. Lipowski ZJ: Transient cognitive disorders (delirium, acute confusional states) in the elderly. *Am J Psychiatry* 140:1426–1436, 1983.
2. Lipowski ZJ: *Delirium: Acute Brain Failure in Man.* Springfield, Ill.: Charles C. Thomas Publishers, 1980.
3. *Diagnostic and Statistical Manual of Mental Disorders.* 3rd ed., Washington, D.C.: American Psychiatric Association, 1980.
4. Gillick MR, Serrell NA, Gillick LS: Adverse consequences of hospitalization in the elderly. *Soc Sci Med* 16:1033–1038, 1982.
5. Warshaw GA, Moore JT, Friedman SW, *et al.*: Functional disability in the hospitalized elderly. *JAMA* 248:847–850, 1982.
6. Lipowski ZJ: Delirium (acute confusional states). *JAMA* 258(13):1789–1792, 1987.
7. Helms PM: Efficacy of antipsychotics in the treatment of behavioural complications of dementia: A review of the literature. *J Amer Geriatric Soc* 33(3):204–209, 1985.
8. Molloy DW, Turpie ID, Powell C: Treating agitation. *Can J Geriatric* 6(6):44–46, 1990.
9. Cummings JL, Miller BL: *IV Long Term Care in Alzheimer's Disease: Treatment and Long Term Management.* New York and Basel: Marcel Dekker Inc., 1990.

5 | PRESSURE SORES

CASE PRESENTATION

Mrs. Jones, an 85-year-old frail woman, was admitted to the hospital one week ago with a fractured neck of the left femur. She had fallen several times at home in the past few months and had bruises on her arms and legs. She had a Moore's prosthesis five days ago and has had an uneventful recovery. Today, she has reactive hyperemia on her right lateral malleolus and right greater trochanter, and blisters on her heels.

J. Lever
D.W. Molloy

Consider the following statements (true or false)

1. With aging, the epidermis and dermis thin; there is loss of subcutaneous fat and reduced blood supply to the skin.

2. The distributions of the areas of hyperemia and blisters suggest that the problem is caused by Mrs. Jones sitting in a chair too long.

3. Mrs. Jones has Grade 1 ulcers on both heels.

4. Comprehensive assessment of this woman's ulcers would include a description of the lesions and a care plan emphasizing the need to change her position regularly.

5. Any treatment in this patient should include vigorous massage over the areas of hyperemia and application of povidone iodine over the blisters to prevent bacterial infection.

1. TRUE

The normal physiologic changes in the skin with aging make the elderly more vulnerable to developing pressure sores (decubitus ulcers—bed sores) and slow the rate of healing once an injury has occurred.

Wrinkling of the skin and graying of the hair are among the most universally recognized signs of aging. With aging, the cell layers of the epidermis and dermis are thinned; the remaining cells are larger, more irregular in shape, and reproduce more slowly. Normal cell replacement is reduced by about 50%, and healing is significantly slower. Epidermal macrophages are also reduced, and this may contribute to cellular immunity and sensitivity to antigens [1].

Associated with the loss of superficial capillaries, there is an increase in vessel wall fragility, which increases the likelihood of purpura. Elastin loses its elastic nature, and collagen bundles become larger and stiffer. There is also a decrease in subcutaneous fat, which is more marked in the extremities.

There is a decrease in size and number of sweat glands. Sebaceous glands decrease in function. Both of these factors contribute to the problem of dry skin, which affects many as they age.

The thinning of the skin, slowed cellular replacement, loss of subcutaneous fat, increased dryness, and reduced blood supply, in combination with an increased tolerance for pain and pressure as well as poor nutritional habits, increase the risk of decubitus ulcers in the elderly.

Risk factors in aging and decubitus ulcers

Some of the factors that increase the risk of decubitus ulcers in the elderly are

1. poor general condition;
2. decreased mobility and activity;
3. poor nutritional intake;
4. cognitive impairment;
5. decreased sensation of pain and pressure;
6. urinary and/or fecal incontinence;
7. dryness, itching and rashes;
8. moisture buildup in skin folds;
9. edema;
10. anemia; and
11. decreased level of consciousness.

2. FALSE

A pressure sore is "an area of cellular necrosis, usually over a bony prominence, that has been subjected to pressure greater than capillary pressure for a period of time sufficient to cause cell death" [2]. The primary factors normally contributing to breakdown are pressure and shearing, followed by decreased capillary flow. Ischemia results, which causes increased capillary permeability. If the ischemia is unrelieved, the local tissue remains anoxic, and this leads to cell death.

Common sites for skin breakdown include the following:

1. *Supine position*: scapulae, elbows, posterior iliac crests, coccyx, and heels.
2. *Side lying position*: ear, shoulder, elbow, greater trochanter, lateral and medial aspects of the knees and ankles.
3. *Prone position*: elbows, anterior iliac crests, knees, and toe tips.
4. *Sitting position*: coccyx and ischial tuberosities (heels if sitting in bed).

The sacrum, greater trochanters, and ischial tuberosities are the commonest sites for decubitus ulceration.

3. TRUE

When the skin of an elderly person breaks down, assessment of the wound is necessary to develop a care plan that includes preventive measures and treatment strategies. Decubitus ulcers (pressure sores) have been assessed in many ways over the past few years. A comprehensive approach presently being used by many skin care nursing experts is Shea's classification of pressure sores [3], listed in Table 5-1.

Mrs. Jones's areas of hyperemia are over the right greater trochanter, heels, and right lateral malleolus. These areas are at risk while Mrs. Jones is in bed in the supine and right lateral position. It would be appropriate to keep her in the chair as long as possible to relieve pressure on these areas. However, it would be important to use a foam padded cushion on the chair and adjust her position every two hours. Mobilize as quickly as possible and monitor the areas that are now at risk from sitting in the chair, that is, ischial tuberosities and coccyx.

While she is lying in bed, discourage her from lying in the right lateral and supine positions. Lay her in a 30° oblique position on the right and left sides.

Table 5-1 Shea's Grading Classification of Pressure Sores.

Threatened	Evidence of erythema, warmth, and congestion of blood, producing a slowness to blanch when pressed by finger (reactive hyperemia).
Grade 1	Involvement of epidermis with some extension into the dermal layer.
Grade 2	Involvement of most of epidermis and dermal layers, extending into the adipose tissue. Shows an inflammatory response.
Grade 3	Deeper progression down to and including muscle. The superficial layers slough off.
Grade 4	Ulcer communicates with bone or joint. All skin, fat, and muscle have necrosed.

4. FALSE

Careful attention must be given to the elderly patient's appetite, skin condition, and energy and activity levels in order to identify the risk factors. The risk must be evaluated regularly and plans set up to reduce the risk areas where possible. For example, if assessment shows you that the patient is emaciated and incontinent of urine and has a rash on the buttocks, the care plan may include such interventions as

1. high-protein, high-carbohydrate diet if not contraindicated;
2. adequate fluid intake;
3. frequent changes for incontinence, including cleansing the skin with a pH balanced cleanser;
4. remoisturizing the skin after each cleansing with a moisturizer;
5. use of barrier products;
6. encouraging position changes to avoid prolonged pressure points on the areas at risk; and
7. possible treatment of any rash if it has not cleared with the interventions listed above.

Assessment of impaired skin should include the following:

1. *Describing and measuring the area*: The description should include the location of the site, the size (measured accurately) and shape (draw a picture or take a photograph), and should list the

presence of discharge, erythema, sinus formation, *etc.*
2. *Grading the area*: Use of Shea's classification is helpful in standardizing terminology.
3. *Listing the causative factors*: Consider the risks to skin breakdown present in the situation and list these, for example, immobility, stroke, poor blood supply, straps, belts, creams, *etc.*
4. *Develop a comprehensive care plan* that includes continuity of treatment and outcome measures.
5. *Reassessment date*: Any care plan should be re-evaluated at reasonable intervals and altered according to the outcome.

5. FALSE

The care plan varies with the type and extent of skin impairment. Several rules of thumb may be used as a guide:

1. Strong disinfectants or antiseptics are best avoided because products such as Proviodine, hydrogen peroxide, and Hygeol, can damage new cells and slow healing. If such solutions are required, thorough cleansing with saline should follow their use.
2. Topical antibiotics are best avoided because they can cause allergic reactions and increase inflammation. Topical antibiotics are generally not effective in the treatment of infected pressure sores. (Systemic antibiotics may be indicated if there is evidence of cellulitis or systemic infection related to the ulcer.)
3. Normal saline is probably the safest cleanser to use on pressure sores.
4. Grade 1 and 2 ulcers may respond well to an occlusive dressing such as DuoDerm or Opsite. Gentle massage around the site may improve the circulation to the area. Never massage directly over the site because this may cause already compromised tissue to break down further.
5. Grade 3 and 4 ulcers require more intensive dressings with debriding agents until the base is healthy and pink. These ulcers may take several weeks to several months to heal.
6. The single most important factor to promote healing is the *complete removal* of pressure on the affected site. Foam pieces, sheepskin protectors or alternating air mattresses may be helpful. Repositioning the immobile patient every two hours is essential to prevent breakdown of other areas at risk.

7. Controlling incontinence either with adult pads or catheterization may be necessary to keep the site dry and free of urates and bacteria, which assist in the process of skin breakdown.
8. Debriding agents such as papaya or elase will be required for the black, hard, necrotic tissue often evident in Grade 3 or 4 ulcers. These agents should be used *only* until the black tissue lifts off. If not effective within one to two weeks, surgical debridement may be required.

The treatment of decubitus ulcers can be quite time-consuming and costly to the health care system. Although there are many products on the market today, many pressure sores require months of expert nursing care to heal. They are often quite debilitating, especially for the elderly. Mortality in the elderly is higher for those with pressure sores [4]. It seems, therefore, extremely important to utilize all of the knowledge we possess to prevent such difficulties from occurring.

REFERENCES

1. Carnevali DL, Patrick M, eds.: *Nursing Management for the Elderly*. Philadelphia: J.B. Lippincott Co., 1986.
2. King RB: Assessment and management of soft tissue pressure. *In* Martin N, Holt NB, Hicks, D, eds.: *Comprehensive Rehabilitation Nursing*. Toronto: McGraw-Hill, 1986.
3. Shea JD: Pressure sores—Classification and management. *Clinical Orthopedics and Related Research* 112:89–100, 1975.
4. Eliopoulos C: *A Guide to the Nursing of the Aging*. Baltimore: Williams & Wilkins, 89–94, 1987.

SUGGESTED READINGS

Monk BE, Graham-Brown RAC, Sarkany I, eds.: *Skin Disorders in the Elderly*. Oxford: Blackwell Scientific Publications, 97–111, 1988.
Gomez, EC, Berman B: The aging skin in clinics. *Geriatric Medicine* 1(1):285–305, 1985.

6 | URINARY INCONTINENCE

CASE PRESENTATION

You are in hospital attending Mrs. M., an 82-year-old moderately obese woman who has been under your care for several years. She suffers from mild osteoarthritis in her hips and shoulders and had become a little forgetful in the past year. She lives alone; she was not taking any medication prior to admission and was completely independent. She was admitted to the hospital with pneumonia seven days ago with confusion and disorientation. She was kept in restraint because the staff were afraid she might fall if she walked independently. Her confusion has now cleared, and she is alert, oriented, and cooperative. Her chest x-ray has cleared, but she is still taking cefamandole 500 mg IV; chloral hydrate 1 gm PO, QHS; haloperidol 0.5–1.0 mg PO, Q4H PRN; heparin 5000 SC BID; lactulose 30 cc PO BID PRN; acetaminophen 650 mg 2 TAB PO Q4H PRN; and dextrose saline infusing at 60 cc per hour.

Mrs. M is in bed, and both of her bedsides are up. The nurse states that Mrs. M. is incontinent of urine and diapers are being used to cope with the problem. Mrs. M. tells you that she was continent at home; her daughter, who is visiting, confirms this.

D.W. Molloy
L. Vitou
M.J. Borrie

Consider the following statements (true or false)

1. Significant urinary incontinence affects 5% to 10% of community-dwelling and 50% of institutionalized elderly.

2. Over 50% of urinary incontinence in the elderly is attributable to age-related changes and is irreversible.

3. The commonest cause of transient or reversible urinary incontinence in the elderly is urinary tract infection.

4. Only selected patients with urinary incontinence should have cystometry.

5. A short trial of oxybutynin (Ditropan) would be useful in this patient.

1. TRUE

Terminology

Clinically significant urinary incontinence is an involuntary loss of urine of sufficient severity to cause a social, hygiene, or health problem. Incontinence may occur

- infrequently (less than once weekly),
- occasionally (less than once daily),
- frequently (one or more episodes per day), or
- continuously.

The severity will depend on the frequency and amount of urine loss during incontinent episodes.

1. Minimal incontinence does not necessitate the use of extra laundry and/or pads, does not restrict the patient's activities, and requires no extra expense.
2. Moderate incontinence, in addition to extra laundry, necessitates the regular use of pads, and the patient's activities are restricted.
3. Severe incontinence, in addition to causing problems associated with moderate incontinence, requires outside help for the patient.

Prevalence

Incontinence is common in the elderly, and its prevalence increases with age [1,2]. The fact that only 20% of incontinent elderly are known to medical services emphasizes the hidden nature and social stigma of incontinence [3]. It behooves doctors to be more aware of the possibility of this problem in their elderly patients.

Incontinence can usually be improved or even resolved without resorting to invasive tests or surgery and without the need for indwelling catheters. Urinary incontinence is found in about 5% to 10% of the community-dwelling elderly, increasing to about 10% to 20% in those with chronic illness or disability. About 20% to 40% of elderly in acute-care institutions have urinary incontinence, rising to 40% to 60% for those in nursing homes, and beyond in chronic care institutions [4,5].

2. FALSE

This is a myth. Many elderly people believe that incontinence is an accompaniment of old age. This is often reinforced by the nihilistic attitudes of peers, families, and physicians.

The storage of urine in the bladder and voluntary expulsion at the appropriate time is controlled by complex reflex arcs involving the sacral plexus, with conscious control occurring through a micturition center at the cerebral cortical level. As the bladder fills, alpha sympathetic tone increases pressure on the urethral sphincter closure and beta sympathetic stimulation relaxes the dome of the bladder. Parasympathetic tone is inhibited, and somatic tone maintains pelvic and voluntary urethral musculature. When micturition occurs, sympathetic and somatic tone are inhibited, while parasympathetic impulses cause the bladder (detrusor) muscle to contract. As the detrusor contracts, the intrinsic bladder pressure rises until it exceeds urethral closure pressure and voiding occurs. The urge to void is felt at volumes between 250 ml and 600 ml [1,6,7,8].

Post-voiding residual urine volume is normally less than 50 ml in the elderly. In some elderly, however, up to 100 cc may be considered normal, depending on the voided volume.

Age may cause a decrease in bladder capacity, a decline in maximum urethral closure pressure, and an increase in the frequency of involuntary bladder contractions. When combined with impaired mobility and mental impairment, these changes make the elderly particularly vulnerable to incontinence. It is important to realize that at least one-third of incontinence encountered in the community-dwelling elderly is transient [4].

3. FALSE

Although urinary infection may be associated with transient incontinence in the elderly, it is not a common cause [10]. The common causes of reversible incontinence are
- drugs (see Iatrogenic Incontinence),
- restricted mobility or access,
- acute illness,

- fecal impaction,
- delirium or confusional state,
- infection,
- atrophic urethritis,
- vaginitis,
- psychiatric disorders (especially depression),
- hyperosmolar states, hypercalcemia, or hyperglycemia.

Many of the drugs prescribed in the elderly can cause incontinence by precipitating urinary retention; by sedation; by causing a prompt diuresis; or, rarely, by causing sphincter weakness. Neurological or mental impairment, immobility, depression, previous gynecologic or urological surgery, drugs, and hospital admission are independent risk factors for incontinence. There is no clear association between age, chronic bacteriuria, or urinary infection [4,6].

Although the pathophysiology of persistent urinary incontinence is complex, for practical purposes it may be divided into the following five categories:

1. *Urge incontinence* (detrusor instability, unstable or uninhibited bladder). This is the commonest cause of urinary incontinence in the elderly [5]. Bladder contractions that escape central control (due to neurologic diseases such as Alzheimer's disease, multiple sclerosis, Parkinson's disease, or cerebrovascular disease) cause involuntary voiding. This may be preceded by a brief warning period of minutes or seconds. Voiding frequency may be normal or increased. The volume is moderate to large, and post-void residuals are low.

Nocturnal frequency and incontinence are common. Sacral sensation and spinal reflexes are normal.

Detrusor instability may be idiopathic, secondary to outlet obstruction or any of the neurologic conditions listed above.

2. *Stress incontinence.* Stress incontinence is a symptom or sign, with loss of urine following stress such as coughing, laughing, sneezing, or jumping. It may be due to urethral sphincter incompetence (genuine stress incontinence) or to stress-induced detrusor instability. It occurs predominantly in young to middle-aged females [7]. In men, it may occur after transurethral prostatectomy (TURP) if the urethral sphincter is compromised. People with this condition will void small volumes frequently by habit to reduce the likelihood of leakage with coughing, laughing, or sneezing. Nocturnal incontinence is infrequent, and post-

void residual volume is low. Cystometry is necessary to differentiate between genuine stress incontinence due to sphincter incompetence and "stress-induced" detrusor instability.

3. *Overflow incontinence* (outlet obstruction and/or poorly contractile detrusor). This results from obstruction of the bladder outlet, underactive detrusor muscle contractions, or impaired afferent sensation. It occurs at high bladder volumes when intravesicular pressure exceeds urethral closure pressure. Common causes of outlet obstruction in men are prostatic hypertrophy or urethral stricture. Diabetic autonomic bladder is a common cause of a poorly contractile detrusor. Small amounts of urine are lost throughout the day and night.

The patient may complain of the symptoms of prostatism (hesitancy, frequency, small voided volumes, post-micturition dribbling, and the sensation of incomplete emptying). Clinically, the bladder is markedly distended and may be palpable on percussion. It may be tender if the condition is acute. Residual volume is large (more than 200–250 ml).

If the incontinence is neurologically mediated, perineal sensation to pinprick, sacral reflexes (cremasteric and bulbocavernosus), and control of the anal sphincter tone are often impaired. Prolonged obstruction can cause hydronephrosis and impaired renal function.

4. *Functional incontinence.* Functional incontinence implies the inability of a usually continent person to reach a toilet in time. This is usually related to unfamiliarity with one's surroundings, musculoskeletal abnormalities, or cognitive impairment. The toilet may be located too far from the bed, or bedrails or an IV severely restricts the patient's mobility. Joint abnormalities or pain and muscle weakness may predispose an otherwise continent person to "accidents."

5. *Iatrogenic incontinence.* A large number of prescribed drugs may precipitate or exacerbate urinary incontinence in the elderly. These include loop diuretics, sedatives, and hypnotics (especially long-acting agents). Agents with anticholinergic properties such as antipsychotics, antidepressants, antihistamines, (including over-the-counter drugs), antiparkinsonian medications, and antidiarrheal drugs precipitate or can worsen incontinence. Another common cause of persisting incontinence in the elderly is the use of diapers. They are often difficult to remove and may actually promote incontinence. Psychologically, they are a disincentive to regaining continence.

4. TRUE

The most important first step in the assessment of urinary incontinence in the elderly is to take a careful history. Try to identify any reversible components that contribute to the incontinence. Establish the duration and severity of the problem. It is important to inquire about irritative symptoms of urinary tract infection as well as obstructive symptoms. Fluid intake, mobility, and mental state need to be documented. A corroborative history from a caregiver is often helpful where dementia, depression, or denial may be present.

A comprehensive drug history including all over-the-counter medication must be obtained from patient and caregiver. The patient's proximity and access to the toilet should be documented and barriers noted. The patient in the Case Presentation had, in addition to her acute illness, an IV and bedrails. Determine whether the patient is incontinent as a result of her acute illness and hospitalization, or whether she has been incontinent in the past and her problem has only been unmasked by the admission.

Voiding/incontinence records are available and very helpful for use in institutions or for outpatients. They document frequency of urinary incontinence as well as response to therapy. Measured voided volumes give some idea of bladder capacity. Appendix C has a bowel/bladder record that may be used in institutions or in the community.

Every patient should have a complete physical exam with emphasis on the urogenital, neurologic, and musculoskeletal systems. A rectal examination should be performed. The findings for each type of persistent incontinence are found in Tables 6-1 and 6-2. In-and-out catheterization should be carried out in all patients primarily to determine post-void residual volume. This can also be used for urine analysis and culture. A residual volume of greater than 100 ml (supine) is considered abnormal and would tend to point to a diagnosis of overflow incontinence [9].

If after a history, physical examination, and residual volume estimation, the incontinence is clearly one of the five types of incontinence, a trial of appropriate therapy is worth undertaking.

Urodynamic studies may more clearly define bladder and urethral dysfunction. The role of these studies in the evaluation of urinary incontinence is controversial. They are somewhat invasive, expensive, uncomfortable, and not always readily available [8,11]. The patient should be referred for urodynamic tests including cystometry if

1. a working diagnosis cannot be reached with an appropriate history, physical examination, residual volume determination, and urine culture; or
2. if there seems to be a mixed picture; or
3. if an empiric trial of treatment based on a working diagnosis fails.

Because of the possibility of obstruction and the long-term consequences of urinary retention, all patients with a residual volume of greater than 100 ml should have outlet obstruction ruled out and relieved, if possible. If obstruction is excluded, the bladder can be decompressed via intermittent or indwelling catheterization over the course of 10 to 14 days. This will often restore detrusor contractile function. If the initial residual volume is large and the distension is painless, then a regular program of intermittent catheterization may be needed for up to several months. Referral may be necessary if a uterine prolapse, cystourethrocele or rectocele, or recurrent or refractory symptomatic urinary tract infections are detected.

5. FALSE

Successful treatment of urinary incontinence involves considering all the contributory factors. It is essential to establish an accurate diagnosis. The use of drugs should be limited in the elderly. Side effects may make the problem worse or even create an additional problem, for example, confusion and postural hypotension may cause a fall and a fractured hip. Nonpharmacological interventions are often very effective, so drugs should be used only as an adjunct and added when simpler measures fail.

TREATMENT

Urge Incontinence

Common-sense measures often cure the problem. Any toilet regimen must be based on analysis of an incontinence chart [7,10]. Is the incontinence worse at particular times, for example, after meals, in the morning, or after diuretics? The patient is asked to void about every two hours or more often, if necessary, to reestablish continence. Once continence has been established and confidence is regained, the intervals

Table 6-1   Historical Features Differentiating Types of Incontinence in the Elderly.

	Urge	Stress	Functional	Overflow
Causes	Uninhibited detrusor activity	Sphincter insufficiency	Musculoskeletal Environmental Psychological	Outlet obstruction Underactive detrusor Impaired sensation
History				
Amount of urine loss	Moderate to large	Small to moderate	Variable, often	Small
Frequency	Normal or increased	Increased, voids preventively	Normal	Increased
Nocturnal	Common; accidents on way to toilet	No	Accidents on way to toilet Restraints IV Bedrails Change in environment or cognition	Common
Triggers	Short warning Stress induced	Coughing Laughing Sneezing Exercise		
Associated	Urgency	Obesity Multiparity Unsuccessful bladder repairs		History of diabetes Symptoms of prostatism
Palpable bladder	No	No	No	Yes, when gross retention present

Table 6-2 Physical Examination to Establish Types of Incontinence

	Urge	Stress	Functional	Overflow
Physical Examination				
Gynecological	Normal	Atrophic vaginitis Weak musculature Uterine prolapse Cystocele Urethrocele	Normal	Normal
Rectal	Normal	Normal	Normal	Prostatic hypertrophy
CNS	None	Intact	Cognitive impairment Depression	Impaired perineal sensation Impaired sacral reflexes (cremasteric and bulbocavernosus) Impaired anal sphincter tone
Special	None	Stress imposed on full bladder will result in incontinence	Joint anomalies Muscle weakness	None
Residual volume	Low	Low	Low	High

between toileting may be gradually increased. Bedside commodes, urinals within easy reach, and improved access to the bathroom are important. Bladder retraining will often improve or resolve incontinence in this group.

Restriction of fluids in the evening and at night may help nocturnal frequency and incontinence. How much coffee or tea is the patient drinking? Caffeine is a diuretic that may be overlooked.

Oxybutynin, a smooth-muscle relaxant with anticholinergic properties, may be tried. A week's trial of 2.5 mg BID PO may be used before the dose is increased to 5 mg BID PO with a maximum of 5 mg TID [7,9,12].

Imipramine is also used to treat urge incontinence in the elderly. It has an alpha agonist action that increases urethral tone, and its anticholinergic effect stabilizes the detrusor muscle. Give at 10 mg PO QHS and increase slowly by 10 mg weekly up to 50 or even 100 mg [7,9,12]. It has a theoretical advantage in depressed women with detrusor instability and genuine stress incontinence. In men with subclinical prostatic hypertrophy and detrusor instability, it may precipitate retention.

For both oxybutynin and imipramine, side effects to watch for include confusion, orthostatic hypotension, dry mouth, and constipation. Lying and standing blood pressures should be measured, and a repeat residual volume should be obtained if the incontinence is not improved.

Flavoxate, a smooth-muscle relaxant with low anticholinergic activity, should be less likely to cause confusion. Starting at 200 mg BID, the dose can be gradually increased to QID.

Stress Incontinence

Treatment of cough (and stopping smoking) will reduce frequency of stress incontinence. Kegel pelvic floor exercises are useful and more successful if the patient can cooperate with a physiotherapist [7,9]. Weight loss in obese patients is important to reduce abdominal pressure. Colposuspension or the Marshall-Marchetti bladder suspension may be used in moderate to severe cases of genuine stress incontinence and may have up to 80% success. Vaginal pessaries are a nonsurgical option for urovaginal prolapse and may reduce genuine stress incontinence.

Atrophic vaginitis responds to estrogen replacement therapy orally or vaginally. Estrogen may be given orally as Premarin. A one-month trial is worthwhile, but if prolonged use is planned, estrogens should be cycled with progestogens. This treatment should be strongly considered in women with osteoporosis. Premarin is given on days 1–21, and Provera is given on days 15–25 of each month.

Overflow Incontinence

Diagnosis is made by measuring the bladder residual urine. This condition may occur post-surgery, for example, for a hip fracture, with prostatic hypertrophy or urethral stricture, or following use of anticholinergic drugs. Obstruction due to prostatic hypertrophy or urethral stricture needs urologic assessment and possible surgery.

Bethanechol may be used in stepwise increments up to 50 mg TID as an adjunct to intermittent catheterization. Any anticholinergic drug should be discontinued after this diagnosis is made.

Functional Incontinence

Attention should be paid to optimizing mobility and cognitive function. Verbal cueing for cognitively impaired people and regular toileting is important. Attention to environmental factors that may contribute to the incontinence is often helpful. Demented patients in a hospital or in the community may become incontinent because they cannot find the bathroom and are unable to communicate a desire to micturate. Bathrooms should be clearly labeled, and even photographs or visual clues may be helpful for the visually or cognitively impaired. Communication boards may help dysphasic patients or those who do not speak English.

For the patient in our scenario, it would be common sense to remove any restraints, take out the intravenous infusion, and remove the bedsides. Make sure the bed is neither too high nor too low to allow the patient access to a toilet or bedside commode. If this woman is in a four-bed room, put her in the spot next to the bathroom or put a commode next to the bed. Regular prompting may be helpful to maintain continence in those who are not aware of their normal bladder cues.

Treatment Can Be Summarized as Follows

For urge incontinence:
1. Bedside commode or urinal, decreased fluid intake in the evenings, increased frequency of voiding
2. Bladder drill retraining
3. Biofeedback
4. Oxybutynin, imipramine, flavoxate

For stress incontinence:
1. Weight loss, treatment of cough
2. Kegel pelvic floor exercises, biofeedback
3. Estrogen
4. Vaginal pessary for prolapse
5. Bladder suspension surgery

For functional incontinence:
1. Attention to mental state, mobility, adjustment of environment

For overflow incontinence:
1. Correction of outflow obstruction
2. Stop anticholinergic drugs
3. Intermittent catheterization
4. Bethanecol as an adjunct to intermittent catheterization

REFERENCES

1. James MH: Disorders of micturition in the elderly. *Conference on the Aging Brain, Age and Ageing* 7:285–287, 1978.
2. Resnick NM, Yalla SW: Management of urinary incontinence in the elderly. *N Engl J Med* 313(13):800–805, 1985.
3. Thomas TM, Plymat KR, Blannin J, Meade TW: Prevalence of urinary incontinence. *British Medical Journal* 1243–1244, November 1980.
4. Yarnell JWG, St Leger AS: The prevalence, severity and factors associated with urinary incontinence in a random sample of the elderly. *Age and Ageing* 8:81–85, 1979.
5. Williams ME, Pannill FC, 3d: Urinary incontinence in the elderly. Physiology, pathophysiology, diagnosis and treatment. *Ann Intern Med* 97:895, 1982.
6. Burton JR: Managing urinary incontinence—A common geriatric problem. *Geriatrics* 39(10):46–60, 1984.
7. Eastwood HDH: Urodynamic studies in the management of urinary incontinence in the elderly. *Age and Ageing* 8:41–48, 1979.
8. Ouslander JG: Urinary incontinence: Geriatric challenge. *Geriatrics* 31–43, Oct.–Nov., 1986.
9. Brocklehurst JC: *Geriatric Medicine and Gerontology.* London and New York: Churchill Livingstone, 1978.
10. Geuidcen RG: Using urodynamic studies to diagnose voiding dysfunction. *Geriatrics* 43–47, Feb.–March, 1986.
11. Borrie MJ: Bladder and urethral dysfunction—when drugs indicated. *New Ethicals* 89–108, July, 1985.

7 | SLEEP

CASE PRESENTATION

A 72-year-old woman with osteoporosis comes to your office for a routine check-up. She is in good health. Apart from calcium (1 g daily), she takes no other medications. She complains that in the last few years she has been sleeping poorly. She takes a long time to fall asleep, awakens frequently during the night and before 6 a.m. every morning, and cannot go back to sleep. She does not nap or feel tired during the day. She has no symptoms of depression.

Occasionally during the past few months, she has taken one of her husband's sleeping pills and reports sleeping very well afterward. She asks you for a prescription for sleeping pills.

D.W. Molloy
J. Clark
M. Cakebread
J.R. Roy
C.J. Patterson

Consider the following statements (true or false)

1. The elderly report more dissatisfaction with sleep than younger people.

2. With aging, there is an increase in the sleep-onset latency (time taken to fall asleep).

3. Normal elderly people awaken often during the night. Generally, these are related to physical discomfort or bladder requirements.

4. With aging, there is a significant decrease in the proportion of rapid-eye-movement (REM) sleep, and a slight decrease in the deeper levels of sleep (stage-four non-REM sleep).

5. In this patient, a short trial (two to three weeks) of chloral hydrate or a short-acting benzodiazepine would be appropriate. This will help to reestablish a normal sleeping pattern and can be discontinued in two to three weeks.

1. TRUE

A number of studies have compared subjective assessments of sleep across different ages. These studies confirm that the elderly are generally more dissatisfied with their sleep than younger individuals [1]. Complaints of nonspecific sleep disturbances, awakenings during the night, and the use of sedatives/hypnotic medications increase with age.

One British study surveyed 2466 subjects, aged 15 to 75 years. In respondents aged 65 or more, there was a significant increase (up to 15%) in the proportion who claimed to sleep less than five hours a night. Early morning awakenings were reported more often in the elderly than in the younger age groups. Fifteen percent of the elderly subjects reported arousal before 5 a.m. Elderly females report sleeping difficulties more often than elderly males.

2. TRUE

Sleep latency refers to the time from the decision to sleep to sleep onset. Complaints of prolonged sleep latency are approximately twice as prevalent in females of all age groups. Females over age 55 reported prolonged sleep latency more often than younger females [2]. Although some studies have found that elderly subjects have increased sleep latency [3–5], one group of researchers reported that sleep latency changed little between ages 3 and 70 for men, and 3 and 80 years for women [6]. The largest increase in sleep latency occurred in men after age 70, but there is considerable variation between individuals. In females, difficulty falling asleep has been related to both age and use of hypnotic drugs. Another study found increased sleep-latency times in healthy elderly subjects, aged 73 to 92 years (39.8 minutes), compared to young females (11.5 minutes) [7].

3. TRUE

Wake after sleep onset (WASO) refers to the time spent awake between sleep onset and final awakening. Many studies have found that the elderly have increased WASO [8]. Between the ages of 20 and 70 years, the number of WASO was higher in men than in women. In males, the number of awakenings increases after puberty, and again after age 40. Females show a general increase after age 39, with a more rapid increase during old age. Very brief arousals may parallel daytime function closely.

Nocturnal arousals without complete awakening may be associated with shifts into stage-one sleep, or the total number of changes from one sleep stage to another.

One investigator noted that nocturia was a significant factor contributing to awakenings in the elderly [4]. Other researchers have attributed 38% of nocturnal arousals in the elderly to physical discomfort or bladder requirements [9]. Other causes of nocturnal arousals in the elderly were pain, restless legs, and dyspnea.

4. FALSE

Sleep is divided into two stages: REM and non-REM (NREM) sleep. NREM sleep may be further divided into four stages. Stage one is the lightest, and stages three and four are the deepest levels of sleep. With aging, there is little change in the ratios of REM and NREM sleep. The most significant changes with aging are the absolute and relative reduction in time spent in stage-four sleep. In general, stage-three sleep tends to be normal, or even increased in elderly females, and normal or reduced in elderly males. In the sixth decade, one may find little or no stage-four sleep in some elderly people. In the very elderly, sleep stages three and four are reduced markedly. In general, absolute amounts of REM sleep fall slightly, but relative amounts of REM (to total sleep time) are well maintained until extreme old age, when they show some decline [8].

5. FALSE

Elderly patients report insomnia as well as the use of sleeping medications more often than any other age group. Hypnotics are useful in patients suffering pain, grief, or temporary anxiety. Drug treatment may not be the optimal solution for all elderly subjects who complain of sleep disturbance. Hypnotics may cause dizziness, light-headedness, staggering, ataxia, and falls in the elderly. Hypnotics lose their effectiveness within two weeks of use [10], and withdrawal from hypnotic drugs can lead to rebound insomnia with increased sleep disturbance [11].

Hypnotics may also cause daytime drowsiness in elderly subjects [12]. When an elderly person complains of insomnia, a careful history will help rule out organic causes of sleep disturbance, such as depression, drugs, arthritis, frequency, dyspnea, pain, or anxiety. Advise the patient to keep a diary for two or three weeks to allow more definitive analysis of the quality and distribution of sleep.

Some simple tips on sleep hygiene may be helpful (Table 7-1). Explain to the patient that sleep disturbance is a normal consequence of aging. This may help alleviate anxiety associated with the sleep disturbance [13].

In this case, the patient should be encouraged to adopt a regular sleep schedule and avoid daytime naps. Education and reassurance may be helpful, and may diminish anxiety and eliminate the need for hypnotics.

A prospective study in 1964 of 1,057,398 subjects over age 30 reported that insomnia was associated with significantly increased mortality rates in males, but not in females. Males and females who ingested sleeping pills often, died 1.5 times more frequently than matched subjects who never used sleeping pills. This also appeared true for the elderly [14]. Therefore, avoid prescribing hypnotics to elderly patients.

REFERENCES

1. Dement WC, Laughton ME, Carskadon MA: White paper on sleep and aging. *J Geriatr Soc* 30:25, 1982.
2. McGhie A, Russell S: The subjective assessment of normal sleep patterns. *J Ment Sci* 108:642, 1962.
3. Agnew H, Webb N: Sleep latencies in human subjects—age, prior wakefulness, and reliability. *Psychosom Sci* 24:253, 1971.
4. Feinberg I, Koresko R, Heuer N: EEG sleep patterns as a function of normal and pathologic aging in man. *J Psychiatr Res* 5:107, 1967.
5. Prine P, Obrist W, Wang H: Sleep patterns in healthy elderly subjects: Individual differences as related to other neurologic variables. *Sleep Res* 4:132, 1975.
6. Williams R, Karacan I, Hursch C: *Electroencephalography of Human Sleep: Clinical Applications.* New York: John Wiley & Sons, 1970, p. 1.
7. Hayashi Y, Otomo E, Endo S, *et al.*: The all night polygraphies for healthy aged persons. *Sleep Res* 8:122, 1979.
8. Miles LE, Dement WC: Sleep and aging. *Sleep* 3:119, 1980.
9. Webb W, Swinburne H: An observational study of sleep in the aged. *Percept Mot Skills* 32:895, 1971.
10. Kales A, Allen C, Scharf MB, *et al.*: Hypnotic drugs: Drugs and their effects. All night EEG studies of insomniac subjects. *Arch Gen Psychiatry* 23:226, 1970.
11. Kales A, Scharf MB, Kales JD, *et al.*: Rebound insomnia: A potential hazard following withdrawal of certain benzodiazepines. *JAMA* 241(1):692, 1979.
12. Frost J, DeLucchi M: Insomnia in the elderly: Treatment with flurazepam hydrochloride. *J Am Geriatr Soc* 27:541, 1979.

Table 7-1 Patient Tips.

Do's

Do establish a routine

Do relax for an hour before going to bed every evening. Watch television, read, knit, sew, or do a relaxing hobby to soothe yourself

Do go to bed at the same time every night

Do exercise daily. Walking, swimming, or cycling are recommended

Do keep a soothing environment—a comfortable mattress, clean linen, and loose-fitting night clothes

Do go to your doctor for advice about problems that wake you during the night, such as frequency in voiding, pain, arthritis, or shortness of breath

Don't's

Don't write letters or watch television while in bed. Keep the bedroom for sleeping

Don't eat or drink excessively before going to bed, as you may have to awaken to go to the bathroom. Digesting food also may interfere with sleep

Don't drink coffee, tea, colas, or ingest any other caffeine-containing foods after midday

Don't nap during the day. This steals from your night's sleep. If you feel drowsy during the day, do something stimulating (walking)

Don't worry because you can't sleep

Don't stay in bed worrying or feeling anxious because you cannot go back to sleep. If you are awake for about 30 minutes and cannot go back to sleep, go to another room, have a drink of hot milk, read, try to relax, and then go back to bed. Do not stay in bed or drink tea or coffee.

13. Caranosos GJ: Use of hypnotics for sleep disturbances in the elderly. *Geriatric Medicine Today* 3:43, 1984.
14. Hammond E: Some preliminary findings on physical complaints from a prospective study of 1,064,004 men and women. *Am J Public Health* 54:11, 1964.

8 CHRONIC OBSTRUCTIVE PULMONARY DISEASE

CASE PRESENTATION

A 74-year-old man with a history of chronic bronchitis complains of dyspnea, a two-day history of worsening cough that produces large amounts of purulent sputum, and low-grade fever. He does not complain of chills, hemoptysis, or flu. He had been a heavy smoker until five years ago when he was diagnosed as having chronic obstructive lung disease. He has mild exacerbations of bronchitis two or three times a year, usually during winter. He takes salbutamol and a diuretic for "ankle swelling."

The patient has tachypnea (respiratory rate 30 per min) and cyanosis. His heart rate is 84 beats per minute and regular. He uses accessory muscles of respiration. Chest examination reveals diminished breath sounds and low-pitched wheezes. Right ventricular heave is evident and heart sounds are loudest in the xiphoid region. A trace of ankle edema is present. Chest x-ray shows no evidence of pneumonia.

A. Lam
D.G. Stubbing
D.W. Molloy

Consider the following statements (true or false)

1. Antibiotics are not useful treatments for exacerbation of chronic obstructive pulmonary disease (COPD).

2. Corticosteroids are useful in treating acute exacerbations of COPD.

3. Digoxin should be prescribed to improve this patient's cardiac failure.

4. Long-term oxygen therapy improves survival in patients with severe COPD.

5. Intravenous aminophylline should be administered should the patient be admitted to the hospital.

1. FALSE

COPD occurs in 10% to 15% of men over the age of 65. Patients often have an average of one to four exacerbations per year. Antibiotic therapy is frequently employed but until recently its benefit had not been proven [1].

Anthonisen *et al.* reported 362 exacerbations in 173 patients over 3.5 years [2]. Exacerbations were defined as increased breathlessness and increased sputum production and purulence. Patients were given oral antibiotics (trimethoprim/sulfamethoxazole, doxycycline, or amoxicillin) or placebo. They reported significant benefits associated with antibiotic use. Patients who received antibiotics were more likely to recover within 21 days and their peak flow rates improved more rapidly than in those who did not receive antibiotics.

This study suggests that COPD exacerbations that result in increased dyspnea, sputum, and sputum purulence should be treated with a 7 to 10 day course of oral antibiotics. Obtaining sputum cultures prior to treatment is not necessary.

2. TRUE

The benefit of corticosteroids was demonstrated by Albert *et al.* [3]. They studied 44 patients with COPD exacerbations; 22 received intravenous methylprednisolone (0.5 mg/kg every six hours for 72 hours), and 22 received placebo. Both groups received the usual regimen of oxygen, inhaled bronchodilators, antibiotics and theophylline. Corticosteroid therapy was associated with a more rapid improvement in airway obstruction as measured by daily forced expiratory volume in one second (FEV_1).

Whether corticosteroid treatment reduced mortality or hospital stay was not clear. The study also did not identify any particular subset of patients that benefitted from corticosteroid therapy. Therefore, it would be reasonable to treat this patient with a brief course of corticosteroids.

3. FALSE

Right heart failure, as evidenced by peripheral edema and elevated jugular venous pressure, often complicates severe COPD. Right-sided failure is thought to be related to underlying pulmonary hypertension. This condition frequently is treated with digoxin, although use of this agent is controversial [4]. In a recent trial, 15 patients with clinical features of right ventricular dysfunction were given digoxin orally for eight weeks [5]. Ejection fractions were measured by radionuclide angiography. The study showed that right ventricular ejection fractions increased only in patients who also had abnormal (but clinically silent) left ventricular ejection fractions.

Pulmonary disease increases susceptibility to digoxin toxicity [4]. Reserve digitalis for the treatment of concurrent left heart failure and supraventricular arrhythmias. Do not use digitalis if cor pulmonale alone is present. Supplemental oxygen and diuretics (if necessary) probably constitute the best treatment for pulmonary hypertension and associated cor pulmonale, and hypoxemia. Therefore, this man should not receive digoxin.

4. TRUE

Recent clinical trials indicate that the use of long-term oxygen therapy in selected patients with COPD improves the duration of survival [6,7]. A British study compared hypoxemic and hypercapneic patients with COPD who were given oxygen for 15 hours daily with a group that was not treated with oxygen. After a five year follow-up, mortality rates were 45% and 67%, respectively. This difference was statistically significant.

An American trial compared hypoxemic men who received nocturnal oxygen (12 hours per day) with hypoxemic men who received continuous oxygen (at least 19 hours per day). After a follow-up of 19 months, 40% of COPD patients treated with nocturnal oxygen died; only 23% of patients treated with continuous oxygen died. These differences were statistically significant.

Consider long-term oxygen therapy in patients with hypoxemia and an arterial oxygen tension less than 56 mm Hg or in patients with cor pulmonale or erythrocytosis and an arterial oxygen tension of 56 mm Hg to 69 mm Hg [8]. Decisions regarding long-term oxygen therapy should be made when the patient is stable (usually at least six weeks after an exacerbation).

5. FALSE

Patients with COPD in severe exacerbations of their disease often are treated with oxygen, parenteral antibiotics and steroids, inhaled bronchodilators, and intravenous aminophylline. Aminophylline provides a longer period of bronchodilation than β-adrenergic agonists alone. This practice, however, has not been studied critically.

A recent study suggests that intravenous aminophylline treatment is unnecessary when treating patients hospitalized for COPD exacerbations [9]. Researchers studied 30 patients; 15 received intravenous aminophylline, and 15 received placebo. Both groups were given the usual adjunctive treatment as outlined above. Measurements included pulmonary function tests, arterial blood gas determinations, and subjective evaluation of breathlessness. All three parameters improved to an equal extent in both groups; however, patients given aminophylline reported a higher incidence of side effects.

Most patients with acute exacerbations of COPD may be treated effectively with oxygen, antibiotics, steroids, and large doses of inhaled bronchodilators. Parenteral aminophylline probably is of little benefit, and the risk of toxicity associated with its use may be substantial, particularly in patients with impaired cardiac or hepatic function. Elderly patients may be at increased risk of side effects; therefore, intravenous aminophylline is not necessary in this patient.

REFERENCES

1. Nicotra MB, Rivera M, Awe RJ: Antibiotic therapy in acute exacerbation of chronic bronchitis: A controlled study using tetracycline. *Ann Intern Med* 97:18, 1982.
2. Anthonisen NR, Manfreda MD, Warren CPW, *et al.*: Antibiotic therapy in exacerbation of chronic obstructive lung disease. *Ann Intern Med* 106:196, 1987.
3. Albert RK, Martin TR, Lewis SW: Controlled clinical trial of methylprednisone in patients with chronic bronchitis and acute respiratory insufficiency. *Ann Intern Med* 92:753, 1980.
4. Lertzman MM, Cherniack RM: Rehabilitation of patients with chronic obstructive lung disease. *Am Rev Respir Dis* 114:1145, 1976.
5. Mathur PN, Powles ACP, Pugsley SO, *et al.*: Effect of digoxin on right ventricular function in severe chronic airflow obstruction. *Ann Intern Med* 95:283, 1981.
6. British Medical Research Council Working Party: Long-term domiciliary oxygen therapy in chronic hypoxemic cor pulmonale complicating chronic bronchitis and emphysema. *Lancet*, 1981, p. 681.
7. Nocturnal Oxygen Therapy Trial Group: Continuous or nocturnal oxygen therapy in hypoxemic chronic obstructive lung disease: A clinical trial. *Ann Intern Med* 93:391, 1980.
8. Timms RM, Kvale PA, Anthonisen NR, *et al.*: Selection of patients for long-term oxygen therapy. *JAMA* 245:2514, 1981.
9. Rice KL, Leatherman JW, Duane PG, *et al.*: Aminophylline for acute exacerbation of chronic obstructive lung disease. *Ann Intern Med* 107:305, 1987.

9 | CONSTIPATION

CASE PRESENTATION

Mrs. C., a pleasant 73-year-old widow, presents with fatigue, weakness, arthritis, and constipation. She is a tea and toast eater. She takes two Tylenol #3 (acetaminophen (paracetamol) and codeine 30 mg) three or four times daily for arthritis, and hydrochlorothiazide 25 mg daily for ankle edema from venous stasis. She takes about 8 to 10 calcium carbonate antacid tablets daily as required for indigestion. She self-medicates with the laxatives Ex-lax (phenolphthalein) and Dulcolax (bisacodyl) for constipation. Lately she has had irregular bowel motions which are hard and painful.

On examination, she had some joint tenderness. Bowel sounds are normal, she is slightly distended, and rectal exam reveals hard stool in the rectum. Routine blood screen shows low potassium 3.2 mmol/L (normal 3.5–4.5 mmol/L) and borderline calcium 2.7 mmol/L (normal 2.14–2.62 mmol/L). You are concerned about abdominal neoplasm with bony metastasis causing hypercalcemia.

T.L. Seaton
D.W. Molloy
J. Kelly
K. Smith
L. Lagacé

Consider the following statements (true or false)

1. Order an abdominal ultrasound, fecal occult bloods, barium enema, and bone scan to rule out malignancy.

2. Continue Tylenol #3 for pain control.

3. Fecal impaction can present with spurious (watery) diarrhea and fecal incontinence.

4. Refer this patient to a dietitian for dietary counseling.

5. Increase the doses of phenolphthalein and bisacodyl, and give enemas twice weekly. Review in one week's time.

1. FALSE

Before expensive, time-consuming, and needless investigations are undertaken, some simple measures may help. Changes in her fluid intake, diet, medications and over-the-counter medications may resolve the constipation and relieve her problems.

Constipation is the commonest disorder of the gastrointestinal tract in old age [1]. It is defined as the passage of hard, dry fecal matter. About 25% of the elderly suffer from constipation, but more than half take laxatives regularly [2]. A large proportion of the institutionalized elderly receive laxatives [3]. Cost of cathartics in chronic care institutions usually accounts for about 15% of their drug budget.

The inactive elderly are particularly liable to develop constipation. Overloading of the rectum, incomplete evacuation, diminished awareness of rectal distention, and neglecting the call to defecate can precipitate or worsen constipation [4].

Other factors that contribute to the risk of constipation include inadequate dietary fiber and diminished fluid intake. Mrs. C. is a tea and toast eater. Poor dietary intake can often be a feature of depression. Inquire about other symptoms of depression. This woman's only fluid intake is tea, which contains caffeine (a diuretic), which may contribute to dehydration.

Certain drugs should be used with caution in the elderly because of their tendency to cause or worsen constipation. Analgesics, particularly codeine and morphine, iron salts, calcium, aluminum, and anticholinergic drugs should be avoided. Many over-the-counter patent medicines used for allergies, coughs, colds, or insomnia contain anticholinergic drugs. Always ask what over-the-counter medications the patient takes.

Hypothyroidism, immobility, carcinoma, anal fissures, hemorrhoids, and cognitive impairment are also associated with constipation. These factors should be considered in the history, investigation, and management of an elderly person with constipation.

Hypercalcemia may result from the consumption of thiazide diuretics, lithium, and large doses of vitamin D. This patient may also be abusing antacids. It is essential to advise her that excessive use of antacids may be contributing to her constipation. Hypercalcemia may develop as a result of ingestion of calcium-containing antacids. Constipation may worsen from precipitation of calcium salts in the bowel. If she must take an antacid, then advise her to take one with a magnesium base.

Discontinue the calcium carbonate and thiazide and repeat her serum calcium in about four weeks. Will she wear elastic stockings for her ankle edema or keep her legs elevated? This simple and practical maneuver may allow you to discontinue the thiazide.

Patients should not be maintained on stimulant laxatives for prolonged periods because they cause dehydration from excessive electrolyte and fluid loss. Hypokalemia may cause muscle weakness, arrhythmia, and precipitate digoxin toxicity in patients on maintenance digitalis.

2. FALSE

Tylenol #3 (acetaminophen or paracetamol and codeine) has analgesic and antipyretic effects but no anti-inflammatory actions. This patient had joint tenderness, and a comprehensive work-up of her arthritis might be more productive at this time than investigations for hypercalcemia. A salicylate, nonsteroidal anti-inflammatory drug or low dose of steroid drug may be more useful than a pure analgesic in the elderly with evidence of joint inflammation. Because of the danger of gastric ulceration with nonsteroidal anti-inflammatory drugs, a cytoprotective agent is often prescribed at the same time. In this patient Sulcrate may worsen constipation; Misoprostol should be considered instead.

3. TRUE

In the presence of fecal loading or impaction, a flat plate radiograph of the abdomen should be performed to assess the level of loading in the large bowel. Fecal loading may often be visualized in the ascending, transverse, and descending colon. The impaction usually occurs in the lower part of the rectum, and the fecal matter may protrude through the anal ring.

If the impaction is limited to the rectum and sigmoid colon, then enemas and manual disimpaction may be sufficient to clear the problem. However, if the impaction is present in the transverse and descending colon, then oral agents will be required for complete evacuation. Enemas are usually required in the initial treatment of fecal impaction. However, if this patient has extensive impaction and enemas fail to resolve the problem, then one may even consider admitting this patient to the hospital. Whole gut irrigation with saline [5] was reported to be successful, but in the elderly, the danger of salt and water overload makes it inappropriate. Balanced polyethylene glycol/electrolyte solutions (Golytely) have been developed to achieve the same effect without the problems of saline irrigation [6].

An alternative regimen for this woman with fecal loading would be to use lactulose 15 ml BID, increasing until effective, with Microlax or Fleet enemas daily. Many elderly have difficulty retaining enemas, so large bulk enemas are impractical. The use of bulk enemas, like soap suds, are irritating and potentially dangerous.

Fecal impaction is a common sequel of constipation in the elderly. The feces becomes rounded and molded, resembling large gall stones. Fecal impaction can present in different ways and has serious consequences if it is missed.

1. *Fecal incontinence/diarrhea.* The impacted feces act like a ball valve. Stool above the impaction is passed by "spurious diarrhea," or watery diarrhea. The rectum is distended, and sensation is diminished. Incontinence persists as leakage around the impacted stool through a stretched and dilated anal canal.

2. *Urinary incontinence.* A distended rectum can press against the bladder neck and affect bladder emptying. Fecal impaction can precipitate urinary incontinence or retention in the elderly.

3. *Confusion/delirium.* Patients with cognitive impairment are at increased risk to develop fecal impaction. In turn, fecal impaction can exacerbate cognitive impairment and delirium. Preliminary findings suggest that patients with fecal impaction often develop delirium. When relieved, there may be improvement in their delirium [7].

4. *Intestinal obstruction.* Patients with fecal impaction frequently have abdominal distention and increased bowel sounds. They may even develop vomiting and dehydration and may show fluid levels on abdominal x-ray. Unless rectal examination is performed they may even be considered for surgery.

Chronic fecal impaction can cause ulceration of the bowel wall with bleeding. When fecal impaction is present it is essential first to establish how extensive it is. Abdominal radiography should be requested, specifically stating the problem and the reason for the investigation. Rectal examination is mandatory in any patient with constipation. Its necessity cannot be overstated.

4. TRUE

A dietary consultation is often the single most useful intervention in the elderly who are constipated. Practical advice, education, and common sense often solve the problem without the need for laxatives. Some simple dietary manipulations—practical advice about what brands of cereal, bread, and other foodstuffs—are more likely to be effective than vague general advice to "increase the amount of fiber in the diet and eat fresh fruit."

Dietitians can provide patients with detailed lists of "good" and "bad" foods. Dietary follow-up, diaries, and support alone are often successful in dealing with chronic constipation in the elderly. The dietitian can provide the patient with a list of natural laxatives such as dates and fresh fruit.

The physician should rule out underlying problems, avoid medications that worsen the problem, and provide on-going support and advice. Advise patients to

1. increase fluid intake, mainly water if possible (at least 1500 cc),
2. eat a high fiber diet,
3. exercise as much as possible,
4. develop a regular bowel habit, and
5. avoid medications or foods that exacerbate constipation.

Advise patients to keep a diary of their bowel motions, diet and fluid intake. This helps the dietitian and physician and gives the patient insight into the factors that improve and worsen the problem.

The management of constipation often requires the patient to change lifelong habits. It is essential to educate the patient and make her or him see constipation as her or his own problem and not the doctor's. We use a high fiber cocktail that has proven useful in the management of constipation in the elderly [8,9]. It is part of a protocol that includes increased dietary fiber, increased fluids, increased exercise, and regular toileting. The secret ingredients are

- 2 cups applesauce
- 2 cups All Bran (Kellogg's All Bran cereal)
- 1 cup 100% prune juice

Blend mixture, keep refrigerated, and give 1 to 3 ounces (30–90 ml, 2–6 tablespoons) daily. Start at 30 cc per day; increase to 60 or even 90 cc as required. Give as a pre-lunch cocktail. It is much cheaper than, and as effective as, regular laxatives. In a hospital chronic care unit each patient received an average of 9.8 doses of a pharmaceutical weekly for constipation. Use of this supplement reduced the need for laxatives.

5. FALSE

It is essential to disimpact this patient's rectum and order a flat plate of the abdomen. Then, if she is impacted throughout the colon, she may even require admission to be disimpacted. Chronic use of laxatives really should be avoided because of the problems associated with their use. Laxatives may be the single most abused drug in our society, and more elderly are addicted to laxatives than to any other drug. Their use should be discouraged because they often have serious side effects. A brief description of the various types of laxatives is given below.

In particular, bulk-forming laxatives can cause intestinal obstruction when the expanded mass blocks the gut lumen. They should always be administered with adequate fluid.

Bowel perforation and peritonitis may result when laxatives are given in the presence of inflammatory bowel disease. Chronic use of liquid paraffin can cause osteomalacia by interfering with vitamin D absorption. Mineral oils may be aspirated.

LAXATIVES

Many of the preparations are ancient, their mode of action is poorly understood and, as a result, the classification of laxatives continues to be debated.

There has been renewed interest in defining the mechanisms of action of laxatives, but the clinical pharmacology has not been clarified enough to allow the old classifications to be abandoned. The discussion will therefore use the old classification, but we will refer to the current theories on the physiological bases of the specific laxative action [10,11,12,13].

All the laxative agents appear to work by promoting mechanisms similar to those that cause diarrhea [11,12,13]. These involve a net increase in the water content in the stool either by active secretion of electrolytes and water into the gut, decreased absorption of water, or increased intraluminal osmolarity.

This is an important consideration in the elderly because most laxatives increase intraluminal water in the gut in competition with the demands for fluid in the rest of the body. In the elderly, where fluid intake is often inadequate or where there is already volume depletion from diuretics, *etc.*, laxatives may fail for this reason or may aggravate dehydration.

Enemas

Soap suds
Enemas using various concentrations of soft soap probably should be abandoned. They can cause mucosal damage and deliver a large amount of sodium and potassium to the colon. They may even lead to hypovolemic shock or severe electrolyte imbalance.

Tap water enemas
Tap water enemas are safer but should be used with caution in patients who have renal impairment. They may cause hyponatremia and/or water intoxication in the elderly.

Saline enemas
A variety of enema preparations use hypertonic solutions of sodium phosphate—biphosphate. These are usually mild enemas that act by breaking up particles of stool and attracting fluid to the gut. They are usually safe but can cause sodium absorption, which may be hazardous in patients with renal impairment.

Oil retention enemas
Enemas using various volumes of mineral oil have been popular in the management of severe constipation. Their action seems to be entirely mechanical, where the oil coats the stool and acts as a lubricant to promote expulsion.

Mineral oil taken orally may coat the stool and block the colon from absorbing fluid and dehydrating the stool. When taken orally, it may interfere with the absorption of fat-soluble vitamins. Aspiration of mineral oil may also lead to lipoid pneumonia. Oil is messy, often leaks out through the anal sphincter, and it is difficult to manage for those who have any problem with continence. All of these are important considerations in the elderly.

Bulk Laxatives

Bulk laxatives vary from foods that are high in fiber to commercial preparations that contain complicated carbohydrates, cellulose derivatives, or polysaccharides.

Low-fiber diets have been implicated in the etiology of many of the degenerative disorders of Western civilization, such as coronary artery disease, diabetes, gallbladder disease, and even colon cancer [14]. There is significant controversy as to whether these problems result from the Western diet's low fiber or high cholesterol and saturated fat content. There is no doubt that a high-fiber diet prevents constipation.

However, the definition of fiber and its components and the importance of the different components remain somewhat controversial. Wheat fiber in various preparations of bran contains cellulose as well as lignin and various gums, while psyllium hydrophilic mucilloid preparations are mainly cellulose and hemi-cellulose. Fiber products act by increasing the water content in the stool. This causes a bulkier, softer stool, which is associated with a reduction in intra-colonic pressure and a decrease in gastrointestinal transit time.

This simple explanation has been questioned, however. The most hydrophilic products, such as pectin, are not as effective in constipation as bran, which holds comparatively little water. Instead, the action of fiber may be based on metabolism of some components to volatile fatty acids and also the action of fiber in changing bacterial flora [15].

The target is to increase the dietary fiber by 10 to 20 g per day.

The major concern with fiber products is intestinal obstruction. These products should not be used in patients with intestinal stenosis and should always be taken with extra fluid. They may even worsen constipation and cause obstruction if additional fluid is unavailable.

Fiber supplementation is the only strategy recommended for long-term use in the treatment of constipation. Patients should always be educated about their use and advised to increase their fluid intake simultaneously.

Stimulant Laxatives

This group of laxatives was once thought to act by irritating or stimulating intestinal motility. It is much more likely that they act by increasing the secretion of fluid into the gut lumen [11]. There are three commonly used stimulant laxatives, the diphenylmethane laxatives, the anthracene glycosides and castor oil.

Diphenylmethane derivatives

Phenolphthalein is the active constituent in many of the popular over-the-counter laxatives. It is tasteless and odorless and is often used in chocolate and other candy preparations. The drug is absorbed from the intestine and is excreted in the bile as a glucuronide. Although listed as a stimulant laxative, it causes accumulation of fluid and electrolytes in the intestinal lumen. The drug is moderately potent with relatively few side effects, but because of its wide availability, it is very commonly abused.

Oxyphenisatin is related to phenolphthalein, and its use is related to chronic active hepatitis. It is no longer available in North America or Great Britain, but it may still be available elsewhere. This may be a problem especially with elderly people who obtain laxatives from "the old country" that they were familiar with in their youth. It is not recommended [17].

Bisacodyl is effective as a suppository and as an oral preparation. Free bisacodyl is absorbed from the small intestine and colon and is conjugated in the liver and excreted in the bile as a glucuronide. The conjugate is not absorbed in the small bowel, but it is deconjugated in the colon by bacterial action. It was once believed that it acted through direct stimulation of nerve plexuses in the colon, but now it is more likely that it mediates its effect by increasing the accumulation of fluids and electrolytes in the small bowel [18].

Anthracene glycosides (anthraquinones)
The commonly used anthraquinones include senna, cascara sagrada and danthron. Danthron is not very potent, and both senna and cascara are more potent than danthron and phenolphthalein.

These substances are glycosides, and the molecule requires hydrolysis by colonic bacteria for its action. These compounds stimulate peristalsis of the colon after direct application to the mucosa; the effect can be prevented by application of topical local anesthetic [19]. However, these compounds cause sodium and water accumulation in the gut. The relative importance of the effects on sodium transport and the effect on the colon are not known [19,20]. Chronic use of senna may cause pigmentation of the colonic mucosa (melanosis coli). This is reversible with withdrawal of the drug, but it is controversial whether chronic use causes bowel damage.

Castor oil
Castor oil is a very potent laxative that has been extensively investigated. The active ingredients are ricinoleic acid and hydroxy fatty acid, which have potent effects on fluid secretion in the small bowel. Its action is similar to the cholera toxin in stimulating cyclic AMP in the small bowel,

producing active secretion of fluid and electrolytes. This is a very potent laxative that has an unpleasant taste, rapid onset of action, and is associated with violent cramps. It is best avoided in clinical practice [21].

Stool Softeners

Docusate/dioctyl sodium sulfosuccinate

These agents are widely promoted as laxatives because of their detergent effect. They promote mixing of water and fatty substances in the stool, which softens it.

This simple mechanism of action has been questioned. These substances may inhibit the enzymes of sodium and potassium ATPase and stimulate cyclic AMP with increased accumulation of sodium and water in the intestine [22,23].

The detergent action of these drugs may disrupt the gastric and intestinal mucosa and increase the absorption of other drugs administered concurrently. In the elderly who often take several medications, this potential to increase toxicity may be an important consideration [24,25,26].

Osmotic Laxatives

This group of laxatives acts by providing a hyperosmolar solution with small molecules within the gut lumen that draw fluid into the bowel. Compounds such as magnesium sulfate and sodium phosphate-biphosphate are commonly used in this way. This simple explanation for their action may not be the complete story because magnesium sulfate releases cholecystokinin, which may account in part for the laxative action [27,28].

Lactulose

This laxative is a synthetic disaccharide for which there is no disaccharidase enzyme in the small bowel. The compound is therefore presented to the large bowel, where bacterial action breaks it down into small organic acids. This acidification of the stool is one of the reasons why this compound is effective in hepatic encephalopathy; it traps ammonia in the bowel as the ammonium ion [29]. The unabsorbed lactulose in the small bowel has an osmotic effect, which is significantly enhanced in the colon, where the smaller molecules are produced by bacterial action. Like the other osmotic laxatives, lactulose holds extra fluid in the bowel.

Lactulose is an effective and relatively safe laxative. Its dose can be adjusted to provide the desired degree of laxation over a fairly wide range. Its main undesirable effects are its sweet taste and its tendency to produce "gas and bloating" [30,31].

Polyethylene glycol/balanced electrolyte solutions (Golytely, Colyte, Klean Prep, and others)

This agent was developed and used mainly in preparation for colonoscopy and barium enema. It has also been used in preparation of the large bowel for surgery. It was a development from the technique of whole gut lavage, which required passing a nasogastric tube and infusing large volumes of saline that exceed the intestine's ability to absorb. Although successful, the patients retain considerable amounts of salt and water, and cardiac failure has been reported.

The P.E.G./electrolyte solutions are designed to produce no net absorption of fluids or electrolytes by balancing the osmolarity with the unabsorbed P.E.G. and using sulfate ion to block sodium transport [31]. The experience in using these solutions for gastrointestinal investigation is that patients need to drink an average of 4 liters over a short time (four hours). This produces a completely clean colon, and it is safe even in cardiac patients [32,33].

In controlled trial for fecal impaction, 2 l seemed to be effective [34]. Our preliminary experience is that 1 l per day may also be effective. These agents have some promise in even smaller volumes (250 mg) for managing constipation and merit controlled trials.

Summary

Laxatives are very commonly abused in the elderly. Their toxicities range from aggravating fluid and electrolyte imbalance, to some direct toxicity and enhancing the toxicity of other drugs. None is recommended for long-term use. The main contribution the clinician makes is often to help the patient discontinue chronic use of any laxatives and to maintain a regular bowel habit with an enhanced fiber and fluid intake. Enhancing the fluid intake is particularly important in the elderly.

REFERENCES

1. Exton-Smith AN. Constipation in geriatrics. In F. Avery Jones and E.W. Godding (eds.), Management of Constipation. Oxford: Blackwell, 1972.

2. Connell AM, Hilton C, Irvin G, Lennard-Jones, JE, Misiewicz JJ: Variations in bowel habit in two population samples. *Brit Med J* 2:1095-1099, 1965.
3. Molloy DW, Seliske JM, Cape RDT: Survey of the prescribing pattern and use of anticholinergic medications in the institutionalized elderly. *J Clin Exp Gerontol* 9(3):231–242, 1987.
4. Brocklehurst JC: Gastrointestinal system. *In* J.C. Brocklehurst (ed.), *Geriatric Pharmacology and Therapeutics.* Oxford: Blackwell Scientific Publications, 1984.
5. Smith RG, Curry AEJ, Walls ADF: Whole gut irrigation. New treatment for constipation. *Brit Med J* 3:396–397, 1978.
6. Fox RA: Managing constipation. *Geriat Med* 85–89, Apr. 2, 1986.
7. Puxty JAH, Fox RA: Constipation and confusion. (In preparation.)
8. Behm RM: A special recipe to banish constipation. *Geriat Nursing* 6(4):216–217, 1985.
9. Everett I, Brown M, Caulfield PA, Yong P: Evaluation of the use of a "special recipe fiber supplement" in the management of constipation in the elderly. *Geriatric Nursing.* (In press.)
10. Binder HJ, Donowitz M: A new look at laxative action. *Gastroenterology* 69:1001–1005, 1975.
11. Ewe K: Physiological basis of laxative action. *Pharmacology* 20 (Suppl.1):2–20, 1980.
12. Donowitz M: Current concepts of laxative action. Mechanisms by which laxatives increase stool water. *Clinical Gastroenterology* 1:77–84, 1979.
13. Tedesco FJ: Laxative use in constipation. *American Journal of Gastroenterology* 80:303–309, 1985.
14. Burkitt DP, Walker ARP, Painter NS: Effect of dietary fibre on stools and transit times and its role in the causation of disease. *Lancet* 2:1408–1411, 1972.
15. Cummings JH: Constipation, dietary fibre and the control of large bowel function. *Postgrad Med J* 60:811, 1984.
16. Surawicz C, Saunders, *et al.*: Effects of phenolphthalein on structure and function of intestinal mucosa. *Gastroenterology* 72:1137(A), 1977.
17. Cooksley WGE, Cowen AE, Powell LW: The incidence of oxyphenisatin ingestion in chronic active hepatitis: A prospective controlled study of 29 patients. *Aust NZ J Med* 3:124, 1973.
18. Ewe K, Przybylski P, *et al.*: Intestinal secretion induced by the laxative bisacodyl. *Gastroenterology* 72:1056(A), 1977.

19. Hardcastle JD, Wilkins JL: The action of sennosides and related compounds on the human colon and rectum. *Gut* 11:1038–1042, 1970.
20. Thompson WG: Laxatives: Clinical pharmacology and rational use. *Drugs* 19:49–58, 1980.
21. Binder HG, Dobbins JW, Whiting DS: Evidence against the importance of altered mucosal permeability in ricinolic acid induced fluid secretion. *Gastroenterology* 72:1029(A), 1977.
22. Binder HJ, Donowitz M: Effect of dioctyl sodium sulphasuccinate on colonic fluid and electrolyte movement. *Gastroenterology* 69:941–950, 1975.
23. Rachmilewitz D, Karmeli F: Effect of bisacodyl and dioctyl sodium sulphasuccinate on rat intestinal prostaglandin E. 2, content sodium Na-K-ATPase and adenylcyclase activities. *Gastroenterology* 76:1221A, 1979.
24. Bernier JJ, *et al.*: Cell loss under laxatives in human jejenum. *Gastroenterology* 76:1099a, 1979.
25. Cochran KM, Nelson L, Russell RI, *et al.*: Laxative and gastric mucosal damage—The danger of dioctyl sodium sulphasuccinate. *Gut* 18:422(A), 1977.
26. Safety of stool softeners: *Medical Letter.* 195:46, 1977.
27. Harvey RF, Read AE: Saline purgatives act by releasing cholecystokinin. *Lancet* 2:185–187, 1973.
28. Harvey RF, Dowsett, *et al.*: A radioimmunoassay for cholecystokinin-pancreozymin. *Lancet* 2:826–827, 1973.
29. Conn HO, Leevy CM, *et al.*: Comparison of lactulose and neomycin in the treatment of chronic portal systemic encephalopathy. *Gastroenterology* 573–583, 1972.
30. Wesselius-De Casparis A, Braadbaart S, *et al.*: Treatment of chronic constipation with lactulose syrup. *Gut* 9:84–86, 1968.
31. Davis GR, Santa Ana CA, *et al.*: Development of a lavage solution associated with minimal water and electrolyte absorption or secretion. *Gastroenterology* 78:991–995, 1980.
32. Ambrose NS, Keighley MRB: Physiological consequences of orthograde lavage bowel preparation for elective colorectal surgery: A review. *Journal of the Royal Society of Medicine* 76:767, Sept. 1983.
33. *Medical Letter* 27:39–40, 1985.
34. Puxty JAH, Fox RA: Golytely: New approach to fecal impaction in old age. *Age and Ageing* 15:182–184, 1986.

10 FALLS

CASE PRESENTATION

You are the attending physician in an emergency department. At 11:00 p.m. your attention is called to a 79-year-old man who has been brought in with a history of falls. He presented to the department about two weeks ago, also with a fall. On that occasion he had fallen down a flight of stairs. Apart from superficial contusions to the right shin, he suffered no serious injury, appeared well, and was discharged home.

At the time of presentation he is very anxious and disoriented with regard to time and place. He is unable to give an accurate account of the events of the last two weeks. He lives alone and has no next of kin. He has evidence of contusions in the right supra-orbital area, left upper and lower forearm, and left leg. The contusions appear to be of varying ages. Careful examination does not show any apparent bony injuries.

You note some rigidity in the right arm in all directions of movement. On attempting to stand he becomes anxious, grabbing for people and furniture. He is very unstable and unable to use the walker you provide. In view of the probability of recurrent falls, the confusional state, and lack of caregivers, you decide to admit him overnight.

On examination of his personal belongings you find an unlabeled bottle with three different types of tablets. You manage to identify

J. Puxty
D.W. Molloy
E.A. Braun

these tablets as Sinemet 100/25, haloperidol 1 mg tablets, and Lasix 40 mg tablets. His pharmacy confirms that he has been taking them for at least six months.

Consider the following statements (true or false)

1. Falls are such a common problem in the elderly that they are rarely worthwhile investigating.

2. It is likely that these medications are implicated in the present problem even though he has taken them for six months.

3. Impaired vibration sense appreciation bilaterally below the knees suggests that this is the single most important cause of this man's falls.

4. In the hospital, his medications were discontinued. His mental state improved and no further falls were observed after three days. It is now appropriate to discharge him home with no further follow-up.

5. Poor nutrition secondary to his confusional state explains his serum albumin of 29 g/l (normal 37–52 g/l).

1. FALSE

Falls have a particularly bad prognosis in the elderly. They are associated with increased morbidity and some lethal complications. In one study, 65% of independent elderly who had six or more falls died within 2.2 years [1]. In a study of falls in the home, with treatment at a community hospital, 42% of victims were admitted to hospital, 61% of whom had fractures [2]. The average duration of stay was 27.3 days. Of these patients, 9% died.

Of all accidents in long-term care facilities, 75% are falls [3]. In a Canadian hospital studied, 11.4% of accidents in the elderly required treatment and 3.2% resulted in fractures [4]. Margules *et al.* reported a total injury rate of 51 per 1000 residents per year in homes for the aged. Other studies have found falls comprising 95% of injuries [5]. The incidence of severe injury was 34 per 1000 residents per year.

Survey of acute admissions to a Manchester teaching hospital for fractured femurs found that 40% of patients attended local accident and emergency units within the preceding three months because of falls [6]. Of these patients, 75% were discharged to the same environment without any detailed search for remedial medical or environmental factors. Subsequent fractures may have been preventable.

A large number of conditions should be considered as possible causes of falls (Table 10-1). It is important to get an accurate history from the patient. Loss of consciousness suggests syncope, with a specific differential diagnosis. Did the patient grasp for furniture or support while falling? Did the patient simply pass out and fall down? It is crucial to establish this from the history if possible. A careful comprehensive examination is essential on admission.

Test for orthostatic hypotension. Take the patient's blood pressure after he or she has been lying quietly for 15 to 20 minutes. Leave the blood pressure cuff on the arm and have the patient stand up. Measure the blood pressure again immediately on standing and again after 3 to 5 minutes. Note any symptoms of dizziness or weakness. Observe the patient's balance upon standing. Postural hypotension is defined as a 20 mmHg or greater drop in systolic blood pressure on standing. Although frequently asymptomatic, it is an important risk factor for falls and syncope. Following blood pressure measurement, walk the patient and observe gait, balance, strength, and maneuverability.

On admission, blood work including CBC, ESR, electrolytes, urea, creatinine, thyroid function, B_{12}, protein electrophoresis, creatine phos-

Table 10-1 Causes of Falls.

Accidents
 	
Environmental hazards
Changes in gait
Poor stability from disease
(arthritis, Parkinson's) or judge-
ment (dementia, vision)
 	
Orthostatic Hypotension
 	
    Low cardiac output
        Autonomic dysfunction
        (Parkinson's, diabetes)
        Bed rest
        Impaired venous return
 	
    Drugs
        Antihypertensives
        Tricyclics
        Sedatives
        Antipsychotics
        Hypoglycemics
        Alcohol
 	
Cardiovascular
 	
Arrhythmia
Myocardial ischemia/infarction
Valvular heart disease
Carotid sinus syncope
 	
Syncope (sudden loss of conscious-
ness, spontaneous recovery)
 	
    Vasomotor
        Orthostatic hypotension
        Carotid sinus syndrome
        Micturition, defecation,
          cough syncope
        Vasovagal
        Volume depletion, drugs
	Cardiac
	    Valvular
	    Ischemic
	    Arrhythmia
	
	Cerebral
	    Seizures
	    Vascular (stroke, TIA)
	
	Metabolic
	    Hypoglycemia, hypoxemia,
	      hyponatremia
	
	Acute Illness (presentation of)
	
	Infection
	Hyper/hypoglycemia
	Fracture (vertebra, hip)
	Pulmonary embolism, etc.
	
	Neurological
	
	    Central
	        Transient ischemic attack
	        Stroke
	        Seizure
	        Parkinson's
	        Dementia/normal-pressure
	          hydrocephalus
	        Cerebellar disease
	
	    Vestibular
	
	    Peripheral
	        Peripheral neuropathy
	        Cervical/lumbar spondylosis
	        Muscle weakness
	
	Idiopathic

phokinase, blood cultures, and liver function tests should be performed. Abnormalities of liver enzymes, an increased MCV, or low urea suggest alcohol abuse. This is often overlooked in the elderly.

A chest radiograph may reveal pneumonia or neoplasm. An ECG may show evidence of a myocardial infarction and/or arrhythmias. Holter monitoring may reveal significant arrhythmias. A history of drowsiness after a fall should suggest the possibility of a seizure, and an EEG must be considered. Seizures may not be accompanied by incontinence, tongue biting, or visible jerking in the elderly.

In addition to this work-up, radiographs of the skull, vertebrae, pelvis, femur, *etc.*, should be considered to rule out fractures. Further radiological investigation may include a CT scan of the head to rule out subdural hematomas.

2. TRUE

Although this patient has been taking medications for several months, one cannot assume they are not contributing to the present problem. Since the patient is confused and disoriented he may have been taking them inappropriately. The finding of all three medications mixed in one unlabeled bottle raises a high suspicion of problems with drug compliance. The furosemide may be contributing to falls by producing hyponatremia and/or postural hypotension. Sinemet may produce delirium and/or postural hypotension. Haloperidol may have sedating effects or exacerbate Parkinsonian features. Any or all of these may be causing the falls.

3. FALSE

Impaired sense of vibration in the lower limbs is common in the elderly. However, it is unlikely that this is the most important single factor causing this man's falls. Falls are usually multifactorial in the elderly. Surveys of community-dwelling elderly with falls reveal that each had an average of three to four chronic co-existing diseases. Falls in the elderly are more likely due to combinations of disorders than to a single disease. It is important to recognize that falls are often a symptom of an underlying disease [7]. In the absence of visual impairment, proprioceptor mechanisms alone are relatively unimportant contributors to falls [8].

Sheldon suggested that the inability to control sway in advancing years played a part in the tendency to fall [9]. Fallers sway more than nonfallers, especially when the fall was not a result of tripping or slipping [10]. The speed of sway is greater for those who fall one or more times in a year than those who do not fall [11]. The speed of sway is also greater in the institutionalized elderly than in community-dwelling elderly. Fernie *et al.* concluded that "postural sway was an indicator of tendency to fall, but the difference was less than might have been expected" [11]. No correlation in the amount of postural sway to the frequency of falls was found.

Standing from the sitting position has been studied by Yoshida *et al.* [12]. The elderly needed more time to stabilize the antero-posterior sway in the standing-up motion. The grade of sway was greater in females than males, perhaps since the center of force in females was located more posteriorly. To avoid falling down accidentally, hemiparetics should lean their bodies forward and grasp supports while standing. Pathological changes in gait have been repeatedly reported in the elderly. Ataxic, hemiplegic, spastic, equine, and many other gaits are readily recognized clinically in falling seniors.

Even healthy old people show slower walking speeds, shorter step length, and lower frequency of stepping. Little change in stride width, when compared to younger people, exists [13]. Although the velocity of walking has been shown to decrease slightly with advancing age, this was found to be more dependent on associated pathology than on age itself.

The elderly are more prone to trips and falls, particularly in the presence of one or more of the precipitating factors listed in Table 10-1.

4. FALSE

A fall is not a diagnosis. It is merely a symptom or sign of an underlying problem. Medical factors account for 50% of falls. Contributing environmental factors must be considered. The value of environmental modification is often neglected in the investigation and management of falls. Rodstein [14] has suggested manipulations to make the environment safer for the impaired elderly. This potentially important and relatively cheap method of reducing the decline in function, commonly seen following a fall, has not been adequately investigated. Information from medical examination and gait analysis can be properly evaluated only in the context of the individual's immediate environment. An elderly person often stops falling in a safe environment such as a hospital. But on return to the previous environment, he or she will fall again.

It is important to get a physiotherapist to assess this patient's gait and assess his risk of future falls. An occupational therapist should be consulted to do a home assessment for environmental hazards. This should be a routine part of the work-up of a recurrently falling patient. Inadequate lighting, cluttered furniture, loose carpet edges, steps, rugs, and slippery surfaces all increase the risk of falling. Simple preventive measures in the home will often solve the problem.

Consider an alarm system that the patient can carry to let caregivers or neighbors know if he or she has fallen. A simple checklist and guide to treatment is provided in Table 10-2. This table describes the common causes of falls in the community-dwelling elderly that can be assessed and corrected in the home. The assessment can be performed by an occupational therapist, physiotherapist, or visiting nurse. Family doctors can order these assessments through community-based programs.

5. FALSE

The serum albumin is a poor guide to the nutritional state in the elderly, unless there has been long-term protein-calorie malnutrition [15]. This patient was noted to be well only two weeks previously. A protein-losing nephropathy must be excluded by urinalysis. The other likely cause of

Table 10-2   Falls Checklist.

Problem	Assessment by	Strategy
Poor lighting Clutter Slippery floors Loose steps Stairways	Physiotherapist Occupational therapist	Replace, fix
Aids Walkers Sticks Chairs	Occupational therapist Physiotherapist Community nurse	Educate about correct use
Problem Poor vision Postural hypotension Arthritis Heart rate and rhythm Drugs	Physican Community nurse	Evaluate/treat Provide alarm system in home for emergencies

hypoalbuminemia in this man is sepsis. In sepsis the liver may preferentially synthesize globulin at the expense of albumin synthesis. Infection in the elderly may present with delirium and falls. Symptoms of infection may exacerbate Parkinson's disease. It is important to consider infection as a possible cause of this man's hypoalbuminemia and falls. A thorough search for a focus should be undertaken. The elderly may not have some of the more common symptoms and signs, for example, fever, leucocytosis. It is important to be alert to the possibility of infection at all times, and keep a high index of suspicion. Therefore blood cultures must be included in the work-up.

REFERENCES

1. Gryfe CI, Amies A, Ashley MJ: A longitudinal study of falls in an elderly population. 1. Incidence and morbidity. *Age and Ageing* 6:201–211, 1977.
2. Lucht U: A prospective study of accidental falls and resulting injuries in the homes among elderly people. *Acta Socio-Medica Scandinavia* 2:105–120, 1971.
3. Pablo RY: Patient accidents in a long term care facility. *Canada J Public Health* 68:237, 1977.
4. Berry G, Fisher RH, Lang S: Detrimental incidents, including falls, in an elderly institutional population. *J Am Geriatr Soc* 29:322, 1981.
5. Margules I, Librach G, Schadel M: Epidemiological study of accidents among residents of homes for the aged. *J Gerontology* 25:342, 1970.
6. Puxty JAH: Unpublished observation concerning a study of patients admitted with fractured necks of femurs to Hope Hospital, Manchester, England, 1986.
7. Tinetti ME, Williams TF, Mayewski R: Fall risk index for elderly patients based on number of chronic disabilities. *Am J Med* 80:429, 1986.
8. Brocklehurst JC, Robertson D, James-Groom P: Clinical correlates of sway in old age—sensory modalities. *Age and Ageing* 11: 1–10, 1982.
9. Sheldon JH: The effect of age on the control of sway. *Geront Clin* 5:129–138, 1963.
10. Overstall PW, Exton-Smith AN, Imms FJ, Johnson AL: Falls in the elderly related to postural imbalance. *Br Med J* 1:261–264, 1977.
11. Fernie GR, Gryfe CI, Holliday PJ, Llewellyn A: The relationship of postural sway in standing to the incidence of falls in geriatric subjects. *Age and Ageing* 11:11–16, 1982.
12. Yoshida K, Iwakura H, Inoue F: Motion analysis in the movement of standing up from and sitting down on a chair. *Scand J Rehab Med* 15:133–140, 1983.
13. Guimaraes RM, Isaacs B: Characteristics of the gait in old people who fall. *Int Rehab Med* 2:177–180, 1980.
14. Rodstein M: Accidents among the aged. *In* Reichel W (ed.): *Clinical Aspects of Aging*. Baltimore: Williams and Wilkins, 1978, p. 499.
15. Munro HN, Young VR: Protein metabolism and requirements in metabolic and nutritional disorders in the elderly. *In* Exton-Smith AN, Caird FI (eds.). John Wright and Sons Ltd., 1980.

11 | SEXUAL BEHAVIOR

CASE PRESENTATION

A 68-year-old man, widowed for two years, is looking forward to remarrying in two months. His fiance is a 65-year-old widow whom he has known for many years, as both couples had been close friends. He presents to you because on attempting intercourse with his fiance for the first time, he was unable to achieve an erection. His marital and sexual life had been very satisfying, although in the last year prior to his wife's death, they had no intercourse because of her illness.

G. Cohen
M. Cohen

Consider the following statements (true or false)

1. An elderly man in good health achieves erections just as readily as he did earlier in life.

2. As people age, they lose interest in sexual activity.

3. Prior patterns of sexual expression at a younger age are important determinants of sexual activity in the elderly.

4. The elderly are frequently seen as asexual.

5. This patient should be referred to a urologist for a penile implant.

1. FALSE

A number of physiological changes occur in the sexual responses of most aging males. It takes longer to develop an erection, the erection is usually less firm than earlier in life, and more direct tactile stimulation to the penis is required to achieve the erection. Most elderly men are able to maintain a high state of arousal for a longer time prior to orgasm, and there is a less intense feeling of ejaculatory inevitability. With orgasm there is a decrease in the number of contractions, in the pulsatile sensation, in the force of ejaculation, and in the amount of seminal fluid. The resolution phase occurs faster, and the refractory period lengthens. There also appears to be less of a drive for orgasm or ejaculation to occur every time intercourse or other sexual activity is attempted [1].

Similarly in women, a number of physiological and anatomical changes occur. These include thinning of the vaginal mucosa, decrease in length and width of the vagina, decrease in the fat covering the mons, relatively more exposure of the clitoris, and a thinning of the pubic hair. During the arousal phase of sexual response, lubrication begins more slowly and is decreased in amount. There may be decreased pelvic vascular engorgement resulting in a decreased sensation of vulvar and vaginal fullness. When orgasm occurs the orgasmic contractions are generally shorter and sharper, although the capacity for multiple orgasms remains. The resolution phase tends to be more rapid [2,3].

For both sexes, understanding and adjusting to these changes as well as regular sexual activity is critical in maintaining sexual capacity and effective performance.

2. TRUE

A number of studies [4,5,6,7] have demonstrated generally decreasing levels of both sexual activity and interest with aging. However, some comments are important. Among those surviving into their 80s and 90s, continued sexual activity is not a great rarity, especially when this is defined broadly to include masturbation, erotic dreams, and nocturnal orgasms. Although sexual interest declines as well, it does so to a lesser extent than activity, and indeed some patients may experience an increased level of interest. In their study, Adams and Turner [8] reported that masturbatory activity in elderly women increased from 10% to 26%

compared to when they were younger. Hite [9] found that at least some of the women between 40 and 80 years of age reported an increasing desire for and enjoyment of sex with aging. Mullens [7] in a study of residents of nursing homes and public housing in Saskatchewan, found that arousal, interest, dreams, sexual thoughts and fantasies, and the desire for knowledge about sexuality in the elderly was two to three times higher than reported genital sexual activity, thus indicating ongoing sexual interest in the absence of such activity. Brecher [6] found that much, though not all, of the sexual decline among sexually active men and women involved the frequency of various sexual activities, yet enjoyment was still identified by many subjects.

3. TRUE

It has been reported that individual differences in sexual function before middle age were likely to be maintained past middle age [10]. A number of other factors influence and affect sexual expression in the elderly. These include:

1. *Marital status or the availability of a partner.* Societal standards appear to influence the behavior of unmarried men and women differently. Substantially more unmarried men than unmarried women are sexually active, with sexual activity continuing at least into the 70s for half of the unmarried women but for three-quarters of the unmarried men [6]. In another study [7], 43% of married respondents were sexually active as compared to 5% of the widowed, 12% of the never married and 11% of the separated and/or divorced. As well, of those who indicated a reason for lack of sexual activity, 68% of these respondents stated that this was due to the unavailability of a spouse or partner. Cessation of sexual activity by women was usually attributed to problems of their partners, whereas males attributed their cessation of activity to themselves [4].

2. *Belief systems.* These may exert either a permissive or a restrictive attitude toward sexuality.

3. *Knowledge about sexuality.* Awareness of the normal physiological changes described earlier in this chapter will facilitate adaptation to these changes.

4. *Religiosity.* It has been shown that a higher religious adherence is associated with poorer overall sex information.

5. *Economic and living status.* The opportunity to meet people and to engage in sexual activity is highly dependent on economic status and the availability of privacy. Institutionalized patients are particularly disadvantaged since few nursing homes or chronic care facilities provide opportunities for individuals to engage in solitary or shared sexual activity.

6. *Sexual repertoire.* The willingness to express sexual intimacy in ways other than intercourse is an extremely important determinant of the continuation of sexual satisfaction and activity in the elderly.

7. *Physical and emotional well being.* Sexual expression may be affected by both physical and emotional illness, or by psychological stress of severe or protracted illness impacting on either the patient or on the partner. Illnesses may be acute or chronic. They may impact on sexual function because of their interference with the physiology of the sexual response (endocrine, vascular, or neurologic disorders), because of their general debilitating or depressing effect, or because of their effect on body image. Common diseases that may cause sexual difficulties include cardiac disease, diabetes, stroke, arthritis, alcoholism, depression, and hypertension [11]. Not infrequently the treatment for these diseases, such as the drug treatment for hypertension, may be instrumental in contributing to the sexual problems and dysfunctions in the elderly (Table 11-1)[12,13].

4. TRUE

In our society the elderly are not generally perceived to be sexual people. As a result, the sexual concerns of the elderly are frequently overlooked or disregarded by doctors and other health professionals. The cultural taboo about sexuality in the elderly is a result of several factors:

1. The widely disseminated belief that sex is for reproduction and must not be separated from that role. The elderly are unable to fulfil this reproductive function; therefore it follows that they are asexual.

Table 11-1 Drugs That Can Cause Sexual Dysfunction.

	Erectile Dysfunction	Ejaculatory Dysfunction	Decreased Libido
Antihypertensive Agents			
Frequent offenders			
Thiazide diuretics	+		
Central sympatholytics (Methyldopa, Clondine)	+		
Peripheral sympatholytics (Guanethidine)	+	+	
Beta-blockers (including Hydralazine)	+		+
Likely nonoffenders			
ACE inhibitors (Captopril, Enalapril)			
Calcium-channel blockers			
Arteriolar dilator (Apresoline)			
Histamine H₂ Receptor Antagonists			
Cimetidine	+		+
Ranitidine	+		+
Famotidine	0		0
Psychotropic Drugs	+	+	+
Antipsychotics			
Tricyclic antidepressants			
MAO inhibitors			
CNS depressants (in large doses) (sedatives, anti-anxiety drugs, cannabis, alcohol, heroin)			

Adapted from *The Medical Letter on Drugs and Therapies* 29 (744), July 1987; and Wein AJ, Van Arsdalen KN: Drug-induced male sexual dysfunction. *Urologic Clinics of North America* 15(1):23–31, 1988.

2. The belief that sex equals intercourse. As a result, other forms of sexual intimacy which may be equally pleasurable and stimulating, such as caressing, hugging, and mutual masturbation are devalued. Thus those who cannot or do not wish to have sexual intercourse perceive themselves as being unable to have sex and

therefore as sexless individuals.

3. Since our society equates youth with beauty, and sexual desirability with beauty, the elderly are seen as devoid of beauty and therefore as sexless individuals.

Kass [14] describes the concept of the "geriatric sexuality breakdown syndrome," in which she traces the breakdown of sexual expression in the elderly as a negative cycle beginning with increased susceptibility resulting from physiologic changes and loss of roles, friends, and self-esteem. Then, negative societal cues about geriatric sexuality lead to discounting the importance of sex in later years, to labeling of sex as bad or dirty, and to a diminution of sexual skills. Eventually these pose a threat to the older person's identification of his or her own masculinity or femininity. Thus, it is hardly surprising that for many elderly, the commonest cause of sexual dysfunction is not physiologic but performance anxiety and the fear of failure.

5. FALSE

Satisfactory management must utilize a multifactorial approach. This consists of:

1. *Education.* The patient should be provided with information about physical and emotional factors that might be contributing to his or her difficulty. Not only must he or she be aware of the physiological changes which may have affected him or her during the past few years, but also those involving his or her partner. For example, her decreased vaginal lubrication during arousal may make intromission more difficult for him. The association between emotional factors and inhibited sexual responses must be explained to both. These might include an inadequate grieving process, negative feelings about sex prior to marriage, or socialization factors that have led him to expect that as a male he must always be ready to perform sexually whenever the opportunity presents, even though he may not wish to include intercourse in his present relationship.

2. *Assessment of total health,* looking for illnesses that may affect sexual function, such as diabetes, atherosclerotic disease, or significant emotional disease. As well, an inventory of drug use is essential, looking for those agents which are known to interfere with sexual responses.

Excess alcohol usage must be included in this category.

3. *Counseling/advice.* In the case of this patient it may involve advice re seeking sufficient genital stimulation by his partner as a necessary requisite for attaining erection. The message must be given that it is permissible to try a broader repertoire of sexual expression, which may include noncoital pleasuring and intimacy. This may necessitate the need for increased communication and negotiation with his partner. Brecher [6] found that a majority of his respondents were able to make use of effective measures, which included a variety of new approaches, such as changes in stimulation, position, and timing and nature of sexual activity to adapt to the changes associated with aging.

4. *Medical and surgical treatment* [15]. With improved investigative techniques, penile blood flow can now be measured; and where found to be deficient, such techniques as intracavernosal injections of papaverine or selective transluminal angioplasties may produce a desired effect. Finally, some patients may wish to explore the possibility of having a penile implant. However, any of these should be considered only after full exploration of all of the above factors with both members of the couple, as these therapies are not invariably successful and are not without hazard.

Health-care providers to the elderly must recognize that the sexual needs of older men and women are the same as those of younger people, namely the need for warmth, closeness, intimacy, and body contact. Thus to be instrumental in helping the elderly deal with their sexuality, some tasks for health professionals include:
- acknowledging sexual expression as a basic need through-out the life span;
- educating self and public about the need to discuss sexual expression in the elderly with openness and honesty;
- educating the elderly about myths surrounding sexuality in old age;
- counseling the elderly about normal changes with aging, and assisting them to re-adjust attitudes and expectations toward satisfying needs for sexual intimacy;
- providing and/or respecting the privacy needs for sexual expression [16].

REFERENCES

1. Masters WH, Johnson VE: *Human Sexual Inadequacy.* Boston: Little, Brown and Company. p. 316–334, 1970.
2. Masters WH, Johnson VE: *ibid.* p. 335–350, 1970.
3. Semmens JP, Semmens EC: Sexual function and the menopause. *Clinical Obstetrics and Gynecology* 27(3):717–723, 1984.
4. Pfeiffer E, Verwoerdt A: Sexual behaviour in aged men and women. *Arch Gen Psychiat* 19:753–758, 1968.
5. Verwoerdt A, Pfeiffer E: Sexual behavior in senescence: Patterns of sexual activity and interest. *Geriatrics* 24:137–153, 1969.
6. Brecher EM: *Love, Sex and Aging—A Consumers Union Report.* Boston: Little Brown and Company, 1984.
7. Mullens HG: *Love, Sexuality and Aging in Nursing Homes and Public Housing in Saskatchewan* (Senior Citizens' Provincial Council, Regina, Sask.), 1984.
8. Adams CG, Turner BF: Reported change in sexuality from young adults to old age. *The Journal of Sex Research* 21(2):126–141, 1985.
9. Hite S: *The Hite Report—A Nationwide Study of Female Sexuality.* New York: Dell Publishing Co., 1976.

PROPERTY OF WASHINGTON
SCHOOL OF PSYCHIATRY
LIBRARY

10. Martin CE: Factors affecting sexual functioning in 60–79-year-old married males. *Archives of Sexual Behavior* 10(5):399–420, 1981.
11. Comfort A (ed.): *Sexual Consequences of Disability.* Philadelphia: George F. Stickley Company, 1978.
12. *The Medical Letter on Drugs and Therapies* 29(744), July 17, 1987.
13. Wein AJ, Van Arsdalen KN: Drug-induced male sexual dysfunction. *Urologic Clinics of North America* 15(1): 23–31, 1988.
14. Kass MJ: Geriatric sexuality breakdown syndrome. *Int Journal Aging and Human Development* 13(1):71–77, 1981.
15. Urologic Clinics of North America 15(1), 1988.
16. Cowling WR, Campbell VG: Health concerns for aging men. *Nursing Clinics of North America* 21(1):75–83, March 1986.

FURTHER READING

Butler, RN, Myrna I: *Love and Sex After 40—A Guide for Men and Women in their Mid and Later Years.* New York: Harper and Row, 1986.

12 HYPERTENSION AND POSTURAL HYPOTENSION

CASE PRESENTATION

Mrs. K., an 82-year-old retired physician, comes for a routine check-up. She occasionally has mild dizzy spells but has never fallen. She lives alone; and apart from some mild memory loss, arthritis, and dry skin, she is well. She has been a widow for many years; her only child lives in New Guinea.

Her blood pressure today is 190/100 lying, 140/70 standing, and 170/95 sitting. You note that previous measures have been similar to this over the past few years. Electrocardiogram shows left ventricular hypertrophy. She has refused to take antihypertensive medications. She eats a low-salt diet.

You want to recommend an antihypertensive agent again to her; but you can't decide whether a diuretic, calcium channel blocker, or ACE inhibitor would be the drug of choice in these circumstances.

R. Clarnette
D.W. Molloy

Consider the following statements (true or false)

1. In the elderly, diminished aortic distensibility causes a narrowing of the pulse pressure.

2. In this patient, the lying blood pressure should be taken as the baseline since it is the highest blood pressure recorded. Treat the lying BP and ignore the standing BP.

3. Treatment of hypertension in the elderly results in a reduction in stroke and cardiovascular mortality.

4. Give a low dose thiazide diuretic, for example, hydrochlorothiazide 25 mg daily, and review in one week to repeat lying, standing, and sitting BP.

5. Before any treatment is undertaken, do screening blood work, ECG, *etc*. Give a test dose of drug, for example, captopril 6.25 or 12.5 mg, and monitor BP afterwards.

1. FALSE

In older patients systolic hypertension dominates the clinical picture [1]. Systolic hypertension is a better predictor of cardiovascular mortality from myocardial infarction, stroke, and heart failure than diastolic blood pressure [2]. Hypertension in the elderly has some specific characteristics that allow us to differentiate it from hypertension in the younger patient.

With aging there is decreased distensibility in the arterial system [3], which may be due to the presence of hypertension itself [4]. This causes a larger pulse pressure. There is also an increase in peripheral vascular resistance, decreased baroreceptor sensitivity, increased sympathetic nervous system activity, decreased plasma renin activity, and adrenergic receptor imbalance [5]. These factors increase the risk of postural hypotension in the elderly. Postural hypotension, defined as a systolic reduction of 20 mmHg or greater on standing upright, is a common manifestation of impaired blood pressure homeostasis in the elderly.

Of community-dwelling elderly, 20% to 30% have postural hypotension [6]. A decline in baroreceptor sensitivity plays an important role [7]. Hypertension also reduces baroreceptor sensitivity; and as a result, the heart is less responsive to adrenergic stimulation. This diminishes baroreceptor mediated cardioacceleration and vasoconstriction in response to a hypotensive challenge. The factors that increase the risk of hypertension and hypotension are listed as follows:

1. decreased cardiac output,
2. increased peripheral vascular resistance;
3. decreased baroreceptor sensitivity;
4. decreased beta adrenergic sensitivity;
5. decreased plasma volume,
6. decreased renin, increased catecholamines; and
7. decreased renal blood flow and function.

Drugs that decrease cardiac contractility can precipitate heart failure in the elderly. The frequency of concomitant problems such as diabetes mellitus, congestive heart failure, and the use of multiple medications for associated conditions, complicates the management of hypertension in this group. Patient compliance with the drug regimen also influences management. Beta-blockers and thiazide diuretics in particular should be used with caution in diabetic patients.

Mrs. K. has given a history of "dizzy spells." It would be important to establish if these spells were related to a change in posture. Is there a diurnal variation? There is marked intra-individual variability in postural blood pressure changes. When basal blood pressure is highest in the morning, the postural drop is greatest. Orthostatic hypotension in many elderly is related to hypertension. The goal of any treatment and the choice of agents used to treat hypertension, postural hypotension, and dizzy spells necessitates an assessment of risk from the hypertension and side effects of the treatment.

The effects of memory loss on compliance and the effects of drug therapy on memory must be taken into account with some hypotensive agents. Abrupt discontinuation may have adverse effects. Therefore any treatment must be simple to ensure compliance and monitored closely to avoid worsening the postural hypotension.

2. FALSE

Before one decides to treat hypertension in an elderly patient, it is necessary to consider the following: First, what level should be treated? A Canadian task force on hypertension in the elderly made the following recommendations:

1. Treatment indications for a 65–75-year-old patient:
   - diastolic greater than 100 mmHg;
   - diastolic greater than 90 mmHg with target organ damage and/or other diseases present, such as diabetes, congestive heart failure;
   - systolic greater than 200 mmHg (treatment may be of value); or
   - systolic greater than 180 mmHg (treatment may be of value if target organ damage is present).

2. Treatment indications for a patient over age 75:
   - diastolic greater than 120 mmHg (treatment may be of value);
   - diastolic greater than 100 mmHg (treatment may be of value in presence of target organ damage); or
   - systolic greater than 180 mmHg (treatment may be of value in the presence of target organ damage).

Second, which BP measurement should be treated: lying, sitting or standing? In this case the lying BP is 190/100. However, the standing BP is only 140/70. Any treatment may lower the lying BP, which is desirable.

But a further drop in standing BP may decrease cerebral blood flow and precipitate falls or confusion. It is reasonable to treat this woman's lying BP, but it is necessary to monitor the standing BP. If the lying BP is lowered and the standing BP falls, then treatment must be modified. Therefore, one treats both blood pressures.

3. TRUE

The estimated prevalence of hypertension in the elderly may be as high as 40%, depending on the definition of hypertension used. Recent reports, however, estimate it to be closer to 20% [8]. Elevated blood pressure, particularly a systolic above 190 mmHg, causes an unacceptable increase in the incidence of stroke in these patients. In the hypertension detection and follow-up program, there was a significant reduction in the incidence of stroke in elderly patients treated with stepped care [9].

More recently, the European working party on hypertension in the elderly (EWPHE) trial compared the effects of pharmacologic intervention on morbidity, mortality, and quality of life in elderly subjects with hypertension [10]. Admitted to this double-blind placebo controlled trial were 840 patients aged 60 and older (mean 72). Systolic BP ranged from 160 to 239 mmHg and diastolic BP from 90 to 119 mmHg. Patients were followed for up to seven years. They were treated with placebo or hydrochlorothiaze plus triamterene, with methyldopa added if needed. One half of the patients received placebo. Therapy lowered the mean systolic BP by about 20 mmHg and diastolic by 12 to 15 mmHg. However, in the very old patients, those aged 80 or more, there was no difference in cardiovascular mortality between placebo and active treatment. In patients aged over 80, mortality was actually less in the placebo group. It is worth noting that most of the patients in the over-80 group were female. Other studies have also demonstrated similar lack of treatment efficacy in women in younger age groups.

About 10% of the elderly over age 65 suffer from a dementing illness. There is an association between increased BP and changes in intellectual function. Hypertension may be associated with impaired response time, long- and short-term memory, attention, and visuospatial organization [11].

However, antihypertensive therapy (*e.g.*, beta-blockers), may have negative effects on mood, memory, and work performance. If the patient's memory loss and dizzy spells are caused by her hypertension, then treatment is indicated. However, if the dizzy spells occur at night or in the morning when she gets out of bed, then they may be related to postural hypotension; and treatment may be contraindicated.

A comprehensive history detailing the frequency, duration, associated features (*e.g.*, palpitations), and precipitating factors that promote these dizzy spells is essential. If an electrocardiogram shows any arrhythmia or block, then Holter monitoring is indicated. Does the patient have any symptoms associated with the fall in BP while rising in the office?

4. FALSE

Before any treatment is commenced, further assessment is necessary. In the elderly it is essential to maintain cerebral, coronary, and renal blood flow. Hypotensive agents associated with postural hypotension should be avoided. Choose a therapeutic agent that has been studied in the elderly and best suits that individual patient's profile. Nonpharmacologic prescriptions should be considered despite absence of data from randomized controlled trials confirming efficacy. The patient should be urged to reduce salt and alcohol consumption and to exercise regularly to increase fitness and promote weight loss if necessary.

Diuretics

The Joint National Committee of the National Heart, Lung, and Blood Institute recommended diuretics as initial therapy for the elderly hypertensive [12]. Diuretics have limitations in this group. Blood volume is decreased by diuretics. Diuretic-induced hypokalemia may predispose the patient to arrhythmia and sudden death [13]. In the elderly taking Digoxin, the risk of arrhythmia from diuretic-induced hypokalemia is best avoided. Diuretics increase glucose and uric acid levels and are best avoided in patients with gout and/or diabetes [14]. Diuretics also increase cholesterol levels, which may be of less concern in the very elderly. By lowering plasma volume, diuretics increase the risk of postural hypotension. Before any therapy is considered, this patient should have screening blood work that includes CBC, electrolytes, urea, creatinine, uric acid, thyroid function, B_{12}, and blood glucose. If there is any hypokalemia, hyperuricemia, or hyperglycemia, then an agent other than a diuretic should be considered.

Beta-Blockers

Beta-blockers have been widely used to control hypertension in the elderly. However, their associated properties make alternative agents more desirable. The elderly generally have low renin hypertension, and as a result beta-blockers may be less effective. Furthermore, beta-blockers lower cardiac output, increase peripheral vascular resistance, and lower heart rate, which can precipitate cardiac failure. Nonetheless, they may be useful in patients with hypertension and left ventricular hypertrophy and/or angina.

Methyldopa

This centrally acting agent provides effective antihypertensive therapy while preserving cerebral and renal blood flow. Postural hypotension, sedation, drowsiness, and depression make it less desirable in a patient with memory loss and documented postural hypotension [15].

Calcium Channel Antagonists

The calcium channel antagonists verapamil, diltiazem and nifedepine may be particularly effective in the elderly. They cause a reduction in blood pressure and peripheral vascular resistance while increasing renal blood flow, all desirable effects in the elderly [5]. Verapamil and, to a lesser extent, diltiazem affect atrio-ventricular node conduction and are best avoided in a patient taking digoxin. Nifedipine acts peripherally and may exacerbate this patient's postural hypotension and cause reflex tachycardia. The latter effect may be lessened with the prolonged-action preparation. These drugs are well tolerated, but constipation can be a problem with verapamil. Edema, palpitations, flushing, and headaches are a problem shared by all of these agents.

ACE Inhibitors

The two angiotensin converting enzyme (ACE) inhibitors available for use in hypertension are captopril and enalapril. Captopril has been studied in the elderly with hypertension. The mechanism of action of captopril is not solely renin-dependent [16]. Captopril lowers peripheral vascular resistance without increasing heart rate, decreasing cardiac output, or affecting baroreceptor response. Captopril preserves renal and cerebral blood flow. Captopril does not interfere with the sympathetic or central nervous system.

ACE inhibitors are useful in the hypertensive elderly with heart failure, chronic obstructive pulmonary disease, peripheral vascular disease, and hyperlipidemia. Liberatore and Botta [17] described 1400 hypertensive patients more than 60 years of age treated with captopril. The elderly tolerated captopril very well. Tuck *et al.* [18] used 25 to 50 mg of captopril twice daily in elderly patients with hypertension. The captopril was well tolerated, and only 5% had to discontinue the drug because of side effects. Captopril improved quality of life in the hypertensive patient, particularly a feeling of well-being [19].

Enalapril is a prodrug that requires hepatic activation which delays the onset of hypotensive effects [20]. Enalapril's longer half-life may cause prolonged hypotension. Captopril is usually administered twice daily to the elderly, but may even be administered once daily with the desired effect. Captopril 25, 50, or 100 mg once daily may be equally as effective as enalapril 10 to 20 mg once daily.

Hypotension can occur with all the ACE inhibitors. Use of diuretics or a low-salt diet exaggerate this effect. Renal function may deteriorate in patients with underlying renal artery stenosis [21].

5. TRUE

Before any treatment is commenced in this patient, perform the following screening investigations:
- CBC, B_{12}, ESR;
- electrolytes;
- urea, creatinine;
- uric acid;
- ECG, chest x-ray;
- blood sugar; and
- T3, T4, TSH.

Elevations in uric acid, glucose, or hypokalemia would contraindicate therapy with a thiazide. Hyperkalemia and significant renal impairment would contraindicate the use of ACE inhibitors.

Further investigation of the dizzy spells should include a detailed history (especially for syncope). Order Holter monitoring if there is any history of palpitations, syncope, or abnormality on resting ECG that suggests arrhythmia (see Chapter 10, Falls).

If the dizzy spells occur on standing or shortly afterwards, or if the patient was symptomatic on standing in the office, then postural hypotension is the likely cause of her dizziness. A screening Standardized

Mini-Mental State Examination will provide a measure of her cognitive function that may help to establish the degree of memory loss and predict potential compliance problems.

A test dose of 12.5 or 6.25 mg of captopril may be tried in the office if the screening blood work is negative. Get the patient to take the test dose about an hour before her next appointment. Take serial measures of lying, sitting, and standing BP within three to four hours. If postural hypotension is increased, then do not treat the hypertension. If the systolic BP is less and the postural hypotension is decreased, then continue with this dose for two or three weeks. Any increase in captopril should be done very cautiously. Follow electrolytes and renal function at each visit.

Before antihypertensive therapy is undertaken, causes of dizziness other than postural hypotension should be considered. Vertebrobasilar insufficiency may also present in this way and may be aggravated by a fall in BP. Aspirin may improve symptoms (*e.g.*, 325 mg po/day). Use of drugs such as prochlorperazine and meclizine are not recommended for dizziness due to these conditions. The anticholinergic activity of these drugs may precipitate delirium and worsen postural hypotension.

True vertigo should be considered since this usually indicates a peripheral vestibular lesion, for example, benign positional vertigo. Central vestibular lesions are less common, but may be investigated further with CT scanning. Aspirin may in fact be relatively contraindicated in the latter conditions because of the potential for ototoxicity.

Seizures can usually be differentiated from symptoms of cerebral hypoperfusion by taking a careful history. An EEG is necessary to rule out epilepsy, if there is a suspicion of seizures.

In this woman, whose dizziness is probably due to cerebral hypoperfusion, a single dose of aspirin may be useful and less harmful than a diuretic or a small dose of captopril. The efficacy of aspirin therapy in reducing cardiovascular morbidity and mortality is not known in the elderly as it is in middle-aged subjects. However, in this situation it is a reasonable alternative to hypotensive agents.

Before antihypertensive therapy is commenced, it is well to remember that antihypertensive therapy in the elderly decreases cardiovascular mortality but does not decrease mortality overall. There are no trials to show that treating hypertension in the very elderly—that is, those older than 75 years—decreases mortality. Accordingly, any treatment in this patient should be undertaken with the following in mind:

1. screening and blood work;
2. monitor specific symptoms, for example, dizziness;
3. monitor postural hypotension;
4. start with a very low dose and increase very slowly, and monitor carefully;
5. monitor compliance and cognitive function, mood, and behavior; and
6. get a community nurse to follow the patient's function; compliance; and lying, standing and sitting BP.

It seems unlikely and almost impossible to perform and take all of these precautions in the case of a forgetful 82-year-old living alone. If one is certain that one can give an antihypertensive safely to this patient (who does not want to take drugs for her problem) with the knowledge that no studies have shown benefit in this age group, then a very careful, controlled trial with a small dose of antihypertensive might be attempted. Otherwise 325 mg of enteric coated aspirin daily may be safer until we know more of the effects of therapy and the relationship between hypertension, postural hypotension, and falls in the very elderly. We would therefore not elect to treat this woman for hypertension under the present circumstances.

REFERENCES

1. Drizd T, Dannenberg AL, Engel A: *Blood Pressure Levels in Persons 18–74 Years of Age from 1976 to 1980 and Trends in Blood Pressure from 1960 to 1980 in the United States.* Hyattsville, Maryland: U.S. Dept. of Health and Human Services, 1986 DHHS Publication No. (PHS) 86–1684. (Vital Health Statistics Series, no. 11.)
2. Kannel WB, Wolf PA, Garrison RJ (eds.): *The Framingham Study: An Epidemiological Investigation of Cardiovascular Disease.* Section 34: Some risk factors related to the incidence of cardiovascular disease and death using pooled and repeated biennial measurements. Framingham Heart Study, 30-year follow up. Washington, D.C.: U.S. Dept. of Health and Human Services, NIH Publication No. 87–2703, 1987.
3. Gonza ER, Marble AE, Shaw A, *et al.*: Age related changes in the mechanics of the aorta and pulmonary artery of man. *J Applied Physiol* 36:407–411, 1974.
4. Carethers M, Blanchette PL: Pathophysiology of hypertension. *Clinics in Geriatric Medicine* 5:657–674, 1989.
5. Applegate WB: Hypertension in elderly patients. *Ann Int Med* 110:901–915, 1989.
6. Caird FI, Andrews GR, Kennedy RD: Effect of posture on blood pressure in the elderly. *Br Heart J* 35:527, 1973.

7. McGintry K, Laher M, Fitzgerald D, *et al.*: Baroreflex function in elderly hypertensives. *Hypertension* 5:763–766, 1983.
8. Vogt TM, Ireland CC, Black D, Camel G, Hughes G: Recruitment of elderly volunteers for multicenter clinical trial: The SHEP pilot study. *Controlled Clinical Trials* 7:118–133, 1986.
9. Five year findings of the hypertension detection follow-up program: Hypertension detection follow-up cooperative group. *JAMA* 242:2562–2571, 2572–2577, 1979.
10. Amery A, Biekenhager W, Brixko P, *et al.*: Mortality and morbidity results from the European working party on high blood pressure in the elderly trial. *Lancet* 2:1349–1354, 1985.
11. Solomon S, Hotchkiss E, Saravay SM, *et al.*: Impairment of memory function by antihypertensive medication. *Arch Gen Psychiatry* 40:1109–1112, 1983.
12. Report of the joint national committee on the detection, evaluation and treatment of high blood pressure. *JAMA* 237:255–261, 1977.
13. Whelton PK, Watson AJ: Diuretic induced hypokalemia and cardiac arrhythmias. *Am J Cardiol* 58:5A–10A, 1986.
14. Gavras G, Gavras I. Management of specific problems associated with hypertension. *In* Gavras G, Gavras I (eds.): *Hypertension in the Elderly*. Boston: John Wright PSG, 1983.
15. Croog SH, Levine S, Testa MA, *et al.*: The effects of antihypertensive therapy on the quality of life. *N Engl J Med* 314:1657–1664, 1986.
16. Williams GH: Converting enzyme inhibitors in the treatment of hypertension. *N Engl J Med* 319:1517–1526, 1988.
17. Liberatore SM, Botta G: Treatment of essential arterial hypertension with captopril: Outpatient drug supervision study with particular reference to elderly patients. *Cardiovascular Reviews and Reports* 7:29–43, 1980.
18. Tuck ML: Low dose captopril in mild to moderate geriatric hypertension. *J Am Ger Soc* 34:693–696, 1986.
19. Jenkins AC, Dreslinski GR, Tadros SS, *et al.*: Captopril in hypertension: Seven years later. *J Cardiovasc Pharmacol* 7:S96–S101, 1985.
20. Larmour I, Jackson B, Cubela R, *et al.*: Enalapril (MK-421) activation in humans: Importance of liver status. *Br J Clin Pharmacol* 19:701–704, 1985.
21. Hricik DE, Browning PJ, Kopelman AS, *et al.*: Captopril induced functional renal insufficiency in patients with bilateral renal artery stenosis or renal artery stenosis in a solitary kidney. *N Engl J Med* 308:373–381, 1983.

Part II

NERVOUS SYSTEM

13 | DEPRESSION

CASE PRESENTATION

Mr. Wallace, an active 78-year-old retired businessman, lives alone since his wife of 35 years died a year ago. His daughter is concerned because over the past two months he has become more withdrawn. He has not been looking after his home and has complained of feeling tense. He is more forgetful and is having trouble concentrating. He has given up reading, one of his favorite activities.

About two months ago he came to you with insomnia and a burning sensation in his stomach. He has had similar symptoms in the past. You prescribed cimetidine and a benzodiazepine hypnotic at night. He has been treated for hypertension with propranolol for many years. Otherwise, he has been well.

His daughter became alarmed recently when she returned from a trip and thought that he had "slowed down." He failed to brighten even when she brought her children over to visit. He mentioned at the time that he wondered if life was worth living. Mr. Wallace thinks there is a blockage in his bowels, and asks what tests you plan to do on him.

You wonder if he has depression from one of his medications, an underlying disease presenting as depression, or a major affective disorder that may respond to pharmacologic therapy.

D.W. Molloy
K. LeClair
E.A. Braun

Consider the following statements (true or false)

1. Depressive symptoms are the commonest psychiatric complaints in the elderly.

2. The first step in Mr. Wallace's assessment would be to establish a physical or cognitive cause for his dysphoria. Pay particular attention to his drug and alcohol use.

3. In the depressed elderly, a number of features predict a positive response to treatment with antidepressants.

4. Somatic delusions related to the gastrointestinal tract (individuals believe they have cancer or a blockage in their gut) are common in the depressed elderly.

5. The first step in the management of Mr. Wallace is to withdraw cimetidine, propranolol and the benzodiazepine hypnotic.

1. TRUE

Depressive symptoms are the most common psychiatric complaints in the elderly [1]. Gurland reported that the prevalence of depression was up to 10% in men and 15% in women over age 65 [2]. On formal psychiatric interview, 2% were found to be depressed.

With aging there may be an increase in some factors that cause depression, such as loss of

1. health from associated disease,
2. financial security,
3. social supports, and
4. cognitive function.

With aging, adaptations to changing roles must be made. Alterations in cerebral neurotransmitters and the neuroendocrine system may compromise the ability of the elderly to make these adaptations.

2. TRUE

In the elderly, always rule out physical causes for any behavioral or psychiatric symptoms first. Depression may occur with any chronic medical illness that significantly affects function or vitality or that causes pain. Certain physical illnesses—for example, cancer of the pancreas—are associated with symptoms and signs that present like a major affective disorder. Parkinson's disease often presents like depression because of decreased psychomotor activity and akinesia. There is also an increased incidence of depression in the Parkinson's population. This depression may be responsive to antidepressants. The medical conditions that are most often mistaken for depression are as follows:

1. *Neurologic diseases*, for example, Parkinson's syndrome, normal pressure hydrocephalus, Alzheimer's disease, and stroke;
2. *Cancer*, for example, of the pancreas, the brain, or bronchus;
3. *Metabolic/endocrine*, for example, hypothyroidism, B_{12} deficiency/anemia, hypercalcemia, adrenal insufficiency, and electrolyte imbalance;
4. *Chronic painful illness*; and
5. *Alcoholism*.

Patients with cognitive disorders, normal-pressure hydrocephalus (NPH), early Alzheimer's disease, strokes, and brain tumor may present as depression. Hypothyroidism may be mistaken for depression because of associated psychomotor retardation.

The possibility of alcoholism should always be considered in an elderly individual with depression. It may not be considered because of denial by the patient and family and a lack of vigilance on the part of the clinician. The sequelae of alcohol abuse, such as B_{12} deficiency, anemia, and metabolic disorders can also cause depression.

The use of drugs, both prescription and nonprescription, is highest in the elderly. Of all prescription drugs sold in the United States, 30% are used by the elderly, who make up only 10% of the population.

Almost 70% of the elderly regularly use nonprescription drugs. Drug toxicity is more common because of changing pharmacodynamics and pharmacokinetics in this group. Consider the influence of all pre-scription and nonprescription drugs used. Some drugs that can cause depression are listed below. This list is not complete, and a good rule of thumb is to suspect any medication as a possible cause of depression in the elderly.

1. *Antihypertensive drugs*, for example, propranolol, reserpine, methyldopa, hydralazine, clonidine, and guanethidine.
2. *Cardiovascular drugs*, for example, digitalis and procainamide.
3. *Neuroleptic drugs*, for example, fluphenazine and haloperidol.
4. *Psychoactive drugs*, for example, alcohol, benzodiazepine, and barbiturates.
5. *Anti-Parkinsonian drugs*, for example, L-Dopa and amantadine.
6. *Hormones*, for example, estrogen, progesterone, and cortico-steroids.
7. *Antibiotics*, for example, sulphonamides and gram negative agents.

Primary care physicians frequently miss depression in outpatients and inpatients [8–12]. Depressed medical patients are more likely to complain of somatic problems than of cognitive or affective symptoms. These complaints are often misdiagnosed and inappropriately treated without first identifying the cause [13]. In an elderly individual, when there is an acute deterioration of function without any obvious physical cause, consider depression.

The elderly differ from younger patients in the presentation of depression in that they are more likely to experience weight loss and less likely to report feelings of worthlessness and guilt.

3. TRUE

Presentation of Depression in the Elderly

Although there are no definitive tests or criteria, a number of factors have been identified that are related to a positive response to drug therapy in depression. Some characteristics of a depressive episode may facilitate the choice of an appropriate treatment for a depressed older adult. Persistent anhedonia (loss of interest or enjoyment in all activities that previously gave pleasure), lack of reactivity, diurnal variation in mood, early-morning wakening, weight loss (greater than 2.3 kg), and/or a history of a previous episode of depression suggests melancholic depression, which usually responds to antidepressant therapy.

Before antidepressant therapy is commenced it is important to consider three factors to establish the type of depression and the need and risk of treatment. They help in deciding if antidepressant treatment is indicated.

1. History
2. Symptom complex
3. Risk of disease and treatment benefit

1.   History

Establish the individual's and family history of psychiatric illness. If there is a family history of depression, particularly a bipolar illness, then that individual has an increased risk of depression. Inquire about any previous episodes of depression. Has that individual been treated by a psychiatrist in the past or admitted to an institution? Did the patient ever miss work for prolonged periods with a vague or undiagnosed illness?

Since the patient's own history is often unreliable, it is important to obtain an independent account from a family member or friend. If the patient had a previous episode of depression, obtain the old charts to establish the diagnosis, what medications were used, and the patient's response to them. A family or individual history of depression makes a major depressive disorder more likely.

A diagnosis of a major depressive disorder is likely in the presence of a severe loss of self-esteem. The diagnostic criteria for major depressive episodes are listed in Table 13-1. A life review is often negative and filled with inappropriate and delusional guilt. Suicidal thoughts, a sense of helplessness and hopelessness about the future, and feelings of lack of control or impossibility of recovery are also indicators of a major depressive disorder.

Table 13-1 Diagnostic Criteria for Major Depressive Episodes.

1. Dysphoric mood, depressed or sad mood, or loss of interest and pleasure in most usual activities.

2. Durations of at least two weeks, with four of the following symptoms present to a significant degree:
   - poor appetite or significant weight loss, or increased appetite or significant weight gain;
   - insomnia or hypersomnia;
   - loss of energy;
   - psychomotor agitation or retardation;
   - anhedonia (loss of interest or pleasure in usual activities), decreased libido;
   - feelings of self-reproach or inappropriate guilt;
   - diminished ability to think or concentrate; and
   - suicidal ideation.

3. Syndrome not superimposed on schizophrenia, schizophreniform disorder, or paranoid disorder.

4. None of the following dominating the clinical picture for more than three months after the onset of the depressive episode:
   - preoccupation with mood-incongruent delusion or hallucination;
   - marked formal thought disorder;
   - bizarre or grossly disorganized behavior.

Adapted from DSM III American Psychiatric Association, Third Edition, Washington 1982.

2. Symptom complex

Certain clinical features in the presentation of depression predict a positive response to antidepressant therapy. When physical or pharmacologic causes have been ruled out, search for these factors in the presentation. In deciding if antidepressant therapy is indicated, consider what change in overall function has occurred with the illness.

a. *Major affective disorder:* The DSM III criteria for a major affective disorder are listed in Table 13-1. A diagnosis of a major depressive disorder is likely in the presence of a severe loss of self-esteem. The diagnostic criteria for major depressive episodes that favor the use of antidepressants or ECT are
   - major affective disorder,
   - change in psychomotor activity and lack of reactivity,

- melancholic symptoms or pervasive mood change,
- diurnal variation in mood,
- guilt,
- delusions, and
- atypical presentations.

A life review is often negative and filled with inappropriate and delusional guilt. Suicidal thoughts, a sense of helplessness and hopelessness about the future, and feelings of lack of control or impossibility of recovery are also indicators of a major depressive disorder.

b. *Change in psychomotor activity and reactivity:* Depression may be associated with decreased activity—withdrawal, apathy, with a change in normal daily routines and function—or increased activity, with pacing, hand wringing, and anxiety.

Associated with this change in activity there is often a lack of reactivity. Mr. Wallace has slowed down. He is not taking care of his house and has stopped going on social outings. He failed to react to his daughter or grandchildren when they came to visit.

Elderly patients who are lonely usually respond to visitors and company. Mr. Wallace did not brighten up or react to his family's visit. This important feature in the history and examination of the change in psychomotor activity with a loss of reactivity increases the likelihood of a biologically responsive illness.

c. *Melancholic symptoms (pervasive mood change):* In primary depression, patients often describe their sadness or feeling as different from any others they have ever felt. A cardiac patient with angina often remarks that myocardial infarction pain had a different intensity and quality. In a similar fashion a depressed patient may describe this melancholia as being like a cloud or heaviness that cannot be lifted. It is described as a feeling different from usual sadness or grief that they have felt previously after a death or life tragedy. It often has a distinct quality that is overpowering.

d. *Diurnal variation:* The diurnal variation of the mood disturbance may be characteristic in depression. In depression the mood is often worse in the morning. Patients with physical illness often feel good after a night's rest and get tired later in the day. Depressed patients are often worse in the morning and get better as the day goes on. This characteristic diurnal variation supports depression. There may also be associated sleep disturbance or early-morning wakening.

e. *Pathologic guilt:* Patients with depression often ruminate about the past. They think of all the unpleasant events in their lives. Sad events that may have happened many years ago resurface, and the patient will often blame himself or herself for these events. Depressed patients' thoughts are filled with feelings of uselessness and guilt.

f. *Delusions:* Delusions are frequently missed. Elderly patients often feel ashamed or afraid of their delusions, and will not talk about them easily or spontaneously. They often have delusions of poverty. They believe that they have no money, or that their property or savings are gone. Delusions of persecution may be exhibited, where the patient may believe that she or he is being tortured or poisoned by family, health professionals, or neighbors.

Ask about delusions of nihilism. The patient may believe that parts of his or her body are missing, or that he or she is dead, or that he or she does not exist anymore. Depressed patients often believe that they deserve what is happening to them—they are being punished for wrongs that they have committed.

3. *Risk*

Before deciding to use antidepressants or ECT, compare the risk of the depression to the patient, and evaluate the risk/benefit of therapy.

Risk of Depression

1. *Physical function:* The depressed elderly often experience a deterioration in function. They fail to cope with their environment and may stop eating and lose weight. They may not take medications for other conditions and deteriorate physically. They may stop paying bills and shopping, abandon hobbies, and spend more time doing less and less. Mr. Wallace does not keep his house clean. He may well stop shopping and cooking for himself. Secondary physical illness will therefore intervene and may cause irreversible functional and physical disability.

2. *Quality of life:* Mr. Wallace displays apathy and anhedonia (loss of feeling of pleasure in acts that normally give pleasure). He has given up the hobbies that gave him pleasure. He has stopped reading and does not enjoy his family anymore. He clearly has had an acute deterioration in his quality of life. This is typical in depression and may be reversed by treatment.

3. *Suicide*: In any depressed elderly patient, establish what risk, if any, there is of suicide. The elderly are at increased risk of suicide compared

to the rest of the population. The risk of suicide rises sharply in depressed widowed males. Ask if he has thought about suicide, or if he has suicidal urges. The assessment of suicide risk is discussed in Chapter 14.

Risk of Treatment

The elderly have increased risk of adverse reactions to drugs. Tricyclic antidepressants are the drug of choice for the treatment of depression in the elderly. Become familiar with a few of these agents. Monitor closely for side effects to minimize the risk of serious injury. Side effects can often be reversed by decreasing the dose or by using a different agent.

Before tricyclic antidepressants are commenced, measure blood pressure lying and standing. Lay the patient on a couch or bed for about 10 or 15 minutes. Then measure the blood pressure. Leave the cuff on and stand the patient up. Measure the blood pressure immediately on standing, and again after about 2 minutes. Ask for any symptoms of weakness, dizziness, or lightheadedness.

Before therapy is considered, establish if the patient has prostatism, glaucoma, constipation, or dry mouth. If any of these is present, use tricyclics with great caution, monitoring carefully for worsening of symptoms. A baseline ECG should be done in the elderly to diagnose ischemia or conduction problems. If conduction problems are evident, close monitoring is probably advisable.

Of community-dwelling elderly, 20% to 30% have a postural drop greater than 20 mmHg. If Mr. Wallace has a significant postural drop, it may be necessary to discontinue his propranolol and see what effect if any this has on his postural hypotension.

4. TRUE

Delusions are common in depression. They may be differentiated from delusions in paraphrenia and dementia from their content and from the patient's reaction to them.

Delusions in Depression

With somatic delusions, the patient describes a physical complaint that has no apparent physical basis. These somatic complaints are often associated with the bowel. Patients believe that there is a blockage of the stomach or bowels, or that food is rotting inside. Mr. Wallace may not volunteer this information for fear that people will think he is going crazy. It is important to ask for these symptoms. Does he believe that he has a cancer in his bowels? A helpful question to ask is, "Sometimes, Mr. Wallace, people who are depressed feel that there is something wrong with them physically. Do you?" Symptoms of discomfort or pain are often nonspecific and poorly localized. Examination of the abdomen may reveal generalized tenderness without guarding or rebound. On the other hand, patients may complain of significant physical symptoms in the absence of any physical signs.

Delusions in Paraphrenia

Delusions in paraphrenia are different from those in depression. Here external agents are more likely to be involved. Patients believe that neighbors are plotting against them, listening in to their conversations, or trying to poison them. The delusions may be quite complex, well developed, and bizarre. These patients often complain about the delusions. They may feel that they do not deserve what is happening. As mentioned, patients with depression often feel that they deserve what is happening to them, because they are being punished for what they have done in the past.

Delusions in Dementia

In dementia, delusions are commonly simple paranoid feelings. Patients often believe that the neighbors or family are stealing money, taking things from them. These delusions have been found to occur early in dementia more in females and those with past psychiatric history. They may be the first sign of cognitive impairment. Therefore, it is important to investigate intellectual ability in these patients because they are often very socially appropriate. Do not mistake misperceptions in the environment in demented patients for hallucinations. Demented patients may believe that people they see on television are actually in the house. They often "hear voices" that are on the radio. Many demented patients talk back to the TV. This should not be mistaken for delusions or hallucinations and does not require treatment. Advise the family that these misperceptions are normal and do not require treatment.

Delusions will be missed unless one asks about them. If they occur in depression, neuroleptics may be required as an adjunct to tricyclic antidepressants. Depression in the elderly is also missed because it may have an atypical presentation.

Atypical Presentations of Depression in the Elderly

Dysphoric symptoms in some cases may be absent or denied.

Somatic complaints:

These are often referred to the bowel. They may be associated with anorexia and weight loss, suggesting gastrointestinal malignancy. These somatic complaints may be delusional in quality, and the presentation and interpretation may be distorted.

Pseudodementia:

This is a depression presenting as dementia. This type of depression usually presents with a loss of interest, attention, and concentration [4,16]. In a younger patient the change in attention, concentration, and memory are easily recognized as depression. In the elderly they are often inappropriately blamed on "senility." The loss in cognitive function is often patchy and inconsistent over a relatively short period of months. Alzheimer's disease usually presents with a progressive, gradual cognitive decline over a longer period of years. The cognitive difficulties precede the depressive features in Alzheimer's disease. In depression, the mood change may precede the cognitive loss.

The depressed patient is often very concerned and distressed by memory loss. He or she may refuse to do memory tests. He or she is likely to point out personal faults and have good insight into their losses. The demented patient often lacks insight into cognitive impairment and tries, when requested, to perform tasks. The qualitative signs help to differentiate dementia from depression. Alzheimer's patients frequently have near misses, confabulation, and perseveration. Table 13-1 illustrates some features that distinguish pseudodementia from dementia.

Late-onset neurosis:

Depression can often present like a neurosis or change in personality. Personality disorders do not occur for the first time in late life, unless there is a medical or psychiatric cause. Personality disorders are present since early life and represent a long-standing pattern of adaptation to the environment. Depressive disorders may present with changes in personality or neurotic symptoms such as dramatic, impulsive, manipulative behavior, or emotional lability.

Depression with confusion:

Some depressions in old age may be associated with a confusional state. This may be secondary to an underlying physical illness like hypothyroidism, poor nutrition, or metabolic disorders. These patients are at increased risk of suicide. The confusion may result from a nutritional, drug or electrolyte abnormality.

"It's just his age"—understandable depression:
In these cases the depression is overlooked because the symptoms and/or signs are attributed to an underlying chronic disease or advancing age. Chronic pain or disability can be associated with depression. Chronic disease is not an inevitable consequence of aging and must always be investigated and treated in spite of the person's age. Furthermore, chronic disease is frequently accompanied by an underlying depression that may worsen functions, and this may cause significant deterioration in the patient's quality of life. Treatment of concomitant depression may have dramatic results.

When elderly individuals lose interest in their hobbies or become quiet, passive, and withdrawn, suspect depression. These patients may benefit significantly from antidepressant therapy.

5. TRUE

The first step is to withdraw the medications that may be precipitating his depression. Gradually withdraw the sedative and cimetidine. Substitute an ACE inhibitor captopril, a thiazide diuretic, or a calcium channel blocker for propranolol if necessary. This alone may solve the problem. A decision tree for the management of depression is shown in Figure 13-1. If Mr. Wallace remains depressed after these medications have been withdrawn or substituted, then he may require treatment with a pharmacologic agent. Order B_{12}, electrolytes, urea, creatinine, CBC, thyroid function, ECG, chest x-ray, liver enzymes, and other tests as indicated.

Tricyclic antidepressants:
The tricyclics are the drugs of choice for treating major depression in late life. Agents with mild anticholinergic effects such as nortryptiline and desipramine have been used extensively in the elderly. Select each drug on the basis of its action and side effects.

Nortryptiline is sedating and is the agent of choice for any elderly depressed patient with sleep disturbance. Begin with 10 mg at night, and increase the dose by 10 mg about every week or two, until a response occurs or side effects limit further increases. Doses of 50 to 75 mg are usually sufficient. Many elderly respond to even lower doses.

Figure 13-1 Decision Tree to Use in Psychobiological Intervention in Elderly with Depression.

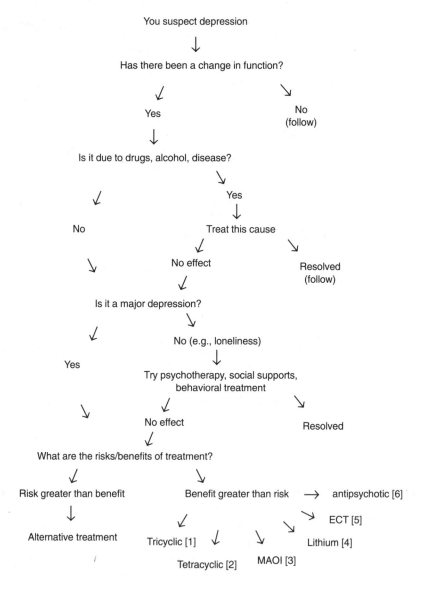

MONITOR FOR SIDE EFFECTS

Desipramine is less sedating and can be given during the day to patients with retarded depression. Both of these agents have minimal anticholinergic effects and cause less problems with orthostatic hypotension. Nonetheless, close monitoring is essential. Although doxepin has significant anticholinergic properties, it is well tolerated in the elderly, especially in those who benefit from its sedative effects at night.

Tricyclics may also cause delirium, constipation, urinary retention, and dry mouth. They may be contraindicated in elderly patients with bladder-outlet obstruction or established symptomatic postural hypotension.

Tetracyclic antidepressants:

Trazodone and maprotiline, two tetracyclic antidepressants, are useful in patients who cannot tolerate the anticholinergic effects of the tricyclics. Give 50 mg trazodone at night and increase by 50 mg increments, until 200 to 300 mg is given or until patients develop side effects. Patients frequently develop drowsiness or dizziness. These agents are not well tolerated in the elderly.

Lithium:

Lithium carbonate may be used in the elderly with bipolar illness or when they have failed to respond to tricyclics or tetracyclics. Blood levels of 4 to 6 meq/l may be adequate in the elderly.

Monoamine oxidase inhibitors (MAOI): MAOIs [tranylcypromine (parnate), phenelzine (nardil)] may be used in patients with refractory depression. Monitor for postural hypotension and use tyramine-free diets. Tricyclic antidepressants should have been discontinued for at least one week before MAOIs are commenced. MAOIs have significant interactions with other drugs. Avoid where there is poor compliance.

Psychostimulants:

Methylphenindate (Ritalin) 5 to 10 mg in the morning has been used to augment the tricyclics; and particularly in the withdrawn, apathetic, depressed elderly, it may be increased up to 10 mg three times per day.

Electroconvulsive therapy (ECT):

In older persons, particularly those with psychotic depression and those who are more likely to have troublesome limiting side effects with pharmacotherapy, ECT may be indicated. In refractory depression, where there is an acute suicidal risk or there is an acute physical deterioration from neglect or anorexia, ECT may be the treatment of choice.

Neuroleptics:

These are used in addition to tricyclics or other medications where there are delusions or hallucinations. Start with pimozide 2 mg, haloperidol 0.25 mg, or loxapine 5 mg at H.S. or BID. These doses can be increased gradually, depending on side effects or the individual's response to therapy.

REFERENCES

1. Blazer D, William CD: Epidemiology of dysphoria and depression in an elderly population. *Am J Psychiatry* 137:439–444, 1980.
2. Gurland B, Deal L, Cross P, .Golden R: The epidemiology of depression and dementia in the elderly: The use of multiple indicators of these conditions. *In* Cole JO, Barrett JE (eds.). *Psychopathology in the Aged.* New York: Raven Press, 1980.
3. Jarvik LF: Aging and depression: Some unanswered questions. *J Gerontol* 31:324–326, 1976.
4. Ban T: Chronic disease and depression in the geriatric population. *J Clin Psychiatry* 45:8–24, 1984.
5. Kitchell MA, Barnes RF, Vieth RC, *et al.*: Screening for depression in hospitalized geriatric medical patients. *J Am Geriatr Soc* 30:174–177, 1982.
6. Miller L: Towards a classification of aging behaviours. *Gerontologist* 19:283, 1979.

7. Derogatis LR, Morrow GR, Fettin BJ: The prevalence of psychiatric disorders among cancer patients. *JAMA* 249:751–757, 1983.
8. Moffic HS, Paykel ES: Depression in medical in-patients. *Br J Psychiatry* 126:346–353, 1975.
9. Nielson AC, Williams TA: Depression in ambulatory medical patients. *Arch Gen Psychiatry* 37:999–1004, 1980.
10. Seller RH, Blascovich J, Lenkei E: Influence of stereotypes in the diagnosis of depression by family practice residents. *J Fam Pract* 12:849–854, 1981.
11. Linn LS, Yager J: The effect of screening sensitization and feedback on notation of depression. *J Med Educ* 55:942–949, 1980.
12. Linn LS, Yager J: Recognition of depression and anxiety by primary physicians. *Psychosomatics* 25:593–595, 599–600, 1984.
13. Katon W: Depression: Relationship to somatization and chronic medical illness. *J Clin Psychiatry* 45:4–12, 1984.
14. Neshkes RE, Gerner R, Jarvik LF, *et al.*: Orthostatic effect of imipramine and doxepin in depressed geriatric outpatients. *J Clin Psychopharmacol* 5:102–106, 1985.
15. Roose SP, Glassman AH, Siris SG, *et al.*: Comparison of imipramine and nortriptyline induced orthostatic hypotension: A meaningful difference. *J Clin Psychopharmacol* 1:316–319, 1981.
16. Weingartner H, Cohen RM, Bunney WE, *et al.*: Memory-learning impairments in progressive dementia and depression [Letter]. *Am J Psychiatry* 139:135–136, 1982.

14 | SUICIDE

CASE PRESENTATION

A 78-year-old man, widowed for four months, complains of anxiety, insomnia, loss of appetite, and of a tightness in his abdomen that worsens at night. He lives alone and drinks heavily. Physical examination reveals nothing. You consider referral for a barium meal and gastroscopy. "Maybe it would be better if I were gone," he says. You ask if he feels depressed. He replies, "I have a gun at home, and one shot would solve all my problems." You consider prescribing antidepressants, referring him to Alcoholics Anonymous, or arranging an emergency psychiatric assessment.

G. Muir
K. LeClair
D.W. Molloy

Consider the following statements (true or false)

1. Suicide rates increase with advancing age, and elderly men commit suicide more often than elderly women.

2. Major depression is often a cause of suicide in the elderly.

3. Alcohol abuse is associated with increased risk of suicide in the elderly.

4. It is dangerous to ask depressed patients about suicidal intent. This may make them think about and commit suicide, even if they had not considered it previously.

5. Appropriate management of the suicidal patient would be to prescribe a tricyclic antidepressant and see him weekly for one month. If the depression has not responded, referral to a psychiatrist is warranted.

1. TRUE

Suicide rates increase with age, peaking at age 85 or over [1]. The risk in the general population is 12.5 per 100,000. It increases to 30 to 40 per 100,000 in patients over age 65, and 53 per 100,000 at age 85. These rates may be underestimated because suicide is not always recognized as a possible cause of sudden death in the elderly. Overdoses of paracetamol, barbiturates, ASA, and combinations of benzodiazepines and alcohol may be reported as respiratory or cardiac arrest, especially if a previous medical problem has been diagnosed.

The elderly commit 25% of all suicides even though they account for only 10% of the population [2]. The ratio of attempted suicides to completed suicides is lower, however, because the elderly are successful more often [3]. Suicide rates and risks are higher in elderly men than women, probably because men use more lethal methods, including firearms, self-inflicted stab wounds, and jumping from heights. Women use potentially less lethal methods, including drowning, drug overdose, and wrist-slashing. In subjects aged 60 to 65, men commit suicide four times more often than women. By age 85, the ratio increases to 12 to 1. In Canada, elderly white widowers are at greatest risk of committing suicide [4,5].

2. TRUE

Causes of suicide in the elderly may be less obvious than in younger patients. It may be a reaction to losses in aging [6]. Over 60% of successful suicides have had clinical depression [7–9]. Many suicides occur in the early morning or late at night, when depression is usually most severe. Many suicidal patients have disturbed sleep, anorexia, hypochondriasis, and feelings of guilt, hopelessness, and worthlessness. Patients with severe psychomotor retardation are at greatest risk because their energy levels increase following the introduction of antidepressant therapy before their mood improves. Antidepressants and other medications should be administered in sublethal doses and the patient monitored closely. Others will often see improvement in activity, sleep, and appetite early in the tricyclic treatment, yet the depressed person will continue to feel severely dysphoric.

A suicidal patient needs support. An unfounded belief that he or she has no support is dangerous and may cause him or her to feel abandoned. Tell the patient it is a good sign that others are seeing improvement and that the depression eventually will subside. Depressed patients younger than age 65 have an increased suicide risk (from 12.5 to 159 per 100,000) compared to the general population. In people over age 55, depression increases suicide risk to 551 per 100,000.

3. TRUE

Drug abuse, alcoholism, and increased alcohol intake increase the suicide risk. Recent bereavement and minor losses, such as the death of a pet, predispose to depression and suicide risk [10]. Even presumptive losses, such as retirement, moving out of the family home, separation from family and friends, and the loss or change of a job, may precipitate depression.

Physical illnesses, especially those associated with loss of independence or function, such as stroke, Parkinson's disease, dementia, chronic pain, blindness, or deafness, increase depression and suicide risk. Underlying physical illnesses were found in 35% to 85% of the elderly who attempted suicide. Severe and disabling illnesses are associated with poor recovery from depression and an increased suicide risk [11]. Risk factors are indicated in Table 14-1.

4. FALSE

Depressed patients often believe life is intolerable and hopeless, and that they are a burden to others. Death is the only apparent solution. Patients, however, may be terrified by their suicidal thoughts. Many are relieved when physicians discuss suicide because it often indicates an understanding of how miserable the patient feels.

Table 14-1 Predisposing Factors.

Older
Male
Single
Alcohol abuse
Chronic physical illness (i.e., myocardial infarction, stroke, Parkinson's
    disease, chronic pain, deafness, loss of independence due to disability
    or perceptual difficulties)
Depressive illness
Loss or threat of loss (i.e., bereavement, death of spouse, loss or change of
    job, retirement, change of environment)

Question the patient in a friendly, matter-of-fact tone, but seriously. Do not ask indirect questions, such as: "I know you wouldn't do it, but this is a routine question . . ." A direct form is preferable, such as: "Do you ever wish you were dead?" or "Have you ever considered suicide?" A definite denial usually indicates low risk. A hedging reply, such as, "Wouldn't anybody who has been through what I have?" requires investigation. Additional questioning determines whether a major psychiatric disorder, delusions, and/or hallucinations are present.

Since guilt is a frequent distorted thought in the elderly, it is important to investigate the degree of guilt and the point at which the patient feels he should be punished. A patient is at high risk if he hears voices encouraging him to kill himself. Delusions of poverty and nihilism are common. The feeling that nothing exists and death is irrelevant is common in patients with distorted thoughts. Lack of reactivity and sleep, severe sleep disturbances, psychomotor agitation, and vegetative signs are important variables that increase risk.

Questions should establish how long the individual has been thinking about suicide, how often (is it a daily event?), and if plans have been made. Were there recent attempts? Does he feel closer to doing it now than before? What stopped him before and have these factors changed? In the interview, consider whether you can engage the patient and make him understand the reality and seriousness of suicide, whether he can focus on hope for the future, and whether the engagement is strong enough that he will consider treatment.

Evaluate the patient's impulsivity and judgment. Has he developed a more positive outlook during the assessment? Evaluate the patient's social supports and their adequacy and availability. Determine whether the patient will contact these supports if he becomes overwhelmed. More than 75% of elderly patients see a physician before committing suicide [12]. Physicians often fail to recognize suicidal signals because they have not been trained to recognize them. Question every depressed elderly patient for suicidal ideation and intent.

5. FALSE

Miller reported that 60% of suicide victims gave verbal or behavioral clues days, weeks, and even months prior to suicide [2]. Be aware of the following indicators.

Direct verbal clues such as: "I'm going to kill myself," should always be taken seriously. Eighty percent of individuals who threaten suicide eventually kill themselves.

Indirect verbal clues, such as: "It would be better if I were gone," or "I'm tired of living," need to be investigated. Do not misinterpret obtuse clues such as: "Pretty soon I won't be around." They must be followed up.

Direct behavioral clues, such as a suicide attempt, indicate the patient is at high risk.

Indirect behavioral clues, such as buying a cemetery plot, making a will, buying a gun, stockpiling pills, and withdrawing from friends and relatives, may signify risk.

Attempt to determine whether the patient has been thinking about or has decided to commit suicide. Patients who think about it and have a plan are at great risk. All suicidal patients must be admitted immediately to an emergency psychiatric unit. The patient's safety cannot be guaranteed outside the unit because constant supervision and treatment are required. Admission will determine the seriousness of the threat.

Prescribing tricyclic antidepressants is inappropriate for this patient because he drinks heavily, lives alone, is recently widowed, owns a gun, and has expressed suicidal intent. He should have an immediate psychiatric assessment.

REFERENCES

1. Manton KG, Blazer DG, Woodbury MA: Suicide in middle age and later life: Sex and race specific life table and cohort analyses. *J Gerontol* 42:219, 1987.
2. Miller L: Toward a classification of aging behaviors. *Gerontologist* 19:283, 1979.
3. Sendbuehler JM, Goldstein SJ: Attempted suicide among the aged. *J Am Geriatr Soc* 25:245, 1977.
4. Gardner EA, Bahn AK, Mack M: Suicide and psychiatric care in the aged. *Arch Gen Psychiatr* 10:547, 1964.
5. Resnick HLP, Cantor JM: Suicide and aging. *J Am Geriatr Soc* 18:152, 1970.
6. Barter JT: *Suicide Among the American Indians: Two Workshops*. U.S. Dept. HEW, USG GPO, PHS Publication, Washington, 1903:9, 1969.
7. Roth M, Morrissey JD: Problems in the diagnosis and classification of mental disorders of old age. *J Ment Sci* 98:66, 1952.
8. O'Neil P, Robins E, Schmidt EH: A psychiatric study of attempted suicide in persons over sixty years of age. *Arch Gen Psychiatr* 75:275, 1956.
9. Barraclough B: Suicide in the elderly. In: Skay DW, Walk A (eds.): *Recent Developments in Psychogeriatrics*. Royal Medico-Psychological Association, Headley Brothers, Ashford, Kent, England, 1971.
10. Sainsbury P: Suicide in later life. *Gerontol Clin* 4:161, 1962.
11. Post F: The management and nature of depressive illnesses in late life. *Br J Psychiatr* 121:393, 1972.
12. Capstick A: Recognition of emotional disturbances and the prevention of suicide. *Br Med J* 1:1179, 1960.

15 GRIEF

CASE PRESENTATION

A 68-year-old woman presents to your office because of problems with pain and loss of function due to arthritis of her knees and hips. She is sad, tearful, and anxious. Since her husband's death six months ago, she has lost interest in life and feels it is not worth living. She admits to hallucinating and sees visions of her husband in the early morning. Her arthritis has worsened over the past three months. She has made frequent visits to you since her husband's death [1].

She is isolated in the community because of disagreements with her sister and children. Her husband was a heavy drinker who treated her badly, but she won't tolerate anyone saying anything negative about him. She might possibly have a psychotic depression.

D.W. Molloy
G. Muir
E.A. Braun

Consider the following statements (true or false)

1. Hallucinations of a dead spouse or parent are usually indicative of a psychotic depression.

2. There is an increase in physical illness and mortality in the newly bereaved.

3. Benzodiazepines and antidepressants are unnecessary in the treatment of most grief reactions.

4. Suicide is rare in the bereaved.

5. The bereaved frequently idealize the dead and alienate the living.

1. FALSE

In Canada, over one million individuals are currently widowed, of whom 63% of the widows and 70% of the widowers are over the age of 65. There are approximately four times as many women widowed as men [2].

Widowhood represents a negative change in physical health, mortality, and mental health status [3]. Coping involves complex psychosocial variables, social networks, income, and religious commitments. Many studies examining depression in the bereaved have found a high proportion of subjects depressed one year following their loss. One study found that 35% of widows were depressed shortly after their bereavement [4], but only 17% were still depressed one year later [5].

Hallucinations of the dead spouse are frequent in the bereaved, with estimates that up to 50% claim to have clearly seen their mate [2]. These visions may provide an element of comfort [6], and few patients are frightened by them. Many patients do not report hallucinations, as they fear people might think they are "losing their mind" [7].

Patients should be reassured of their sanity and that such hallucinations are quite common and will gradually disappear. Hallucinations should be treated only if they cause serious interference with activities of daily living or increase the risk of self-harm. Normal grief does not include psychotic depression or affective illness [8].

2. TRUE

An increase in physical illness and mortality in the first six months after bereavement is not unusual [9,10]. Bereavement is the deprivation caused by the death of a spouse. Grief, a normal part of bereavement, is the emotional suffering caused by this loss. Normal grief is accompanied by denial, anger, depression, then acceptance. Pathological grief may be delayed or chronic.

Younger widows reported an increase in headaches, weight loss, general aching, fatigue, and emotional symptoms. Widows compared with age-matched controls had an increase in physical symptoms [5]. Men had an increase in physical illness and higher mortality rates compared to married men of the same age in the first six months after the death of the spouse [9]. Women presented with more symptoms in the second year of bereavement, especially in the older age group [11].

Most studies failed to show an increase in major physical illness such as cancer [10,12].

3. TRUE

Most grief reactions do not require intervention. Benzodiazepines may be required in the early stages, especially if the widow is having difficulty sleeping or is having somatic symptoms related to anxiety, fear, or extreme agitation. A short-acting benzodiazepine such as alprazolam (Xanax) in a dose of up to 0.5 mg tid or oxazepam (Serax) 15 mg qhs may be helpful.

Support and counseling for patients is essential. The patient should be given the opportunity to discuss feelings. Hostility or anger toward siblings or children should be explored.

Antidepressants may be prescribed if the grief reaction is prolonged (six months) or associated with morbid thoughts and guilt feelings. Vegetative signs such as weight loss, anorexia, or severely depressed mood require treatment. When in doubt, it is wise to prescribe an antidepressant and monitor the response.

Nortriptyline 10 mg to 50 mg qhs, imipramine 25 mg to 50 mg qhs, or trazodone up to 150 mg qhs might be instituted. If psychosis as shown by paranoid delusions, suicidal thoughts, or thought disorders is present, an antipsychotic such as Mellaril, haloperidol, or pimozide in the smallest doses should be given. Start with a small dose at bedtime and monitor the response, increasing the dose slowly until the symptoms are controlled. In the elderly very small doses are effective. In extreme cases electroconvulsive therapy (ECT) may be required for morbid grief reactions with suicidal ideation or severe self-neglect [13].

4. FALSE

The relative suicide rate in the first year of bereavement is 2.5 Men are at higher risk than women. The peak age for women is around 55, while the risk increases throughout life for men. The absolute suicide rates are 60 to 80 per 100,000 for men and 5 to 20 per 100,000 for women.

Suicide rates appear to be highest in those who are bereaved as a result of a spouse's suicide [14]. The bereaved of those who have suffered long, chronic illness such as Alzheimer's disease, in the absence of social networks, are especially at risk [15]. Danger signs include denial of bereavement, inability to come to terms with grief, worsening symptoms over time, lack of social supports, and pre-existing illness. The aged widowed spouse is often at high risk due to a diminished ability to form new relationships [16].

5. TRUE

· There is a tendency for idealistic glorification of the dead spouse [17]. Battered wives, or wives who have had unsatisfactory relationships, often idealize their dead husband. This may cause alienation from other family members, who do not understand the process. The bereaved may feel that family members are interfering with the image of the dead and are trying to "come between them." This occurs particularly if there is denial of loss, or loss of contact with reality. It is important to explain this reaction to the patient and family, and attempt a reconciliation. The patient needs the family's support at this time.

REFERENCES

1. Cobb S, Bauer W, Whitney I: Environmental factors in rheumatoid arthritis. *JAMA* 113:668, 1939.
2. Tudiver F: The bereaved elderly: Can we help them? *Can Fam Phys* 32:2699, 1986.

3. Gallagher D, Thompson L, Peterson J: Psychosocial factors affecting adaptation to bereavement in the elderly. *Int J Aging & Human Development* 14(2):79, 1981.
4. Bornstein P, Clayton P, Halikas J, Maurice W, Robins E: The depression of widowhood after thirteen months. *Br J Psychiatry* 122(27):561, 1973.
5. Clayton P, Halikas J, Maurice W: The depression of widowhood. *Br J Psychiatry* 120:71, 1972.
6. Marris P: *Widows and their Families.* London: Routledge and Kegan Paul, 1958.
7. Granville-Grossman K: *Recent Advances in Clinical Psychiatry.* London: Churchill Press, 1971.
8. Lindemann E: Symptomatology and management of acute grief. *Am J Psychiatry* 101:141, 1944.
9. Young M, Benjamin B, Wallis C: The mortality of widowers. *Lancet* 2:545, 1963.
10. Clayton P: The clinical morbidity of the first year of bereavement: A review. *Compr Psychiatry* 14(2):151, 1973.
11. Heyman D, Gianturco D: Long term adaptation by the elderly to bereavement. *J Gerontol* 28(3):359, 1973.
12. Mor V, McHorney C, Sherwood S: Secondary morbidity among the recently bereaved. *Am J Psychiatry* 143:158, 1973.
13. Myerson A: Prolonged cases of grief reaction treated by electric shock. *N Engl J Med* 230(a):255, 1944.
14. Shepherd D, Barraclough B: The aftermath of suicide. *Br Med J* 2:600, 1974.
15. Fulton R, Gottesman D: Anticipatory grief: A psychosocial concept reconsidered. *Br Med J* 137:45, 1980.
16. Blau D: On widowhood. *J Geriatr Psych* 8(1):29, 1975.
17. Stern K, Williams G, Prados M: Grief reactions in later life. *American J Psych* 108:289, 1951.

16 | PAIN

CASE PRESENTATION

A 74-year-old widow comes to your office complaining of gradual onset of pain in her legs over the past three months. It has become progressively worse. It now keeps her awake at night, and she says that she has lost her appetite and is losing interest in hobbies and housework. She feels worn out all the time. The pain is burning, occurs at rest, and extends from her feet about half way up her shins.

She had a mild stroke about two years ago affecting the right side of her body, but has made a good functional recovery. She also has diabetes mellitus treated with diet only. There is little relief from acetaminophen (paracetamol) or aspirin. About a month ago you prescribed codeine for the pain. She says that it had no effect.

On examination there is no regional deficit from her stroke, but she complains of dysthesia when you touch her feet and lower legs. You consider using an opiate or a benzodiazepine at night to help her sleep.

E. Tunks
D.W. Molloy

Consider the following statements (true or false)

1. The risk and prevalence of "persistent" (chronic) pain increases with advancing age.

2. Codeine may not adequately alleviate this pain. Tricyclic antidepressants are useful for constant burning neuralgia. Carbamazepine should be used for jabbing or intermittent pain. Start a tricyclic antidepressant.

3. This woman most likely has a thalamic pain syndrome from her stroke.

4. This pain most likely represents peripheral neuropathy, secondary to diabetes mellitus.

5. The most likely cause of this woman's pain is a sympathetic dystrophy of the lower limbs. This condition is similar to shoulder–hand syndrome in the upper limbs.

1. TRUE

Crook, Rideout, and Browne [1] determined the age-specific rates for pain in the community. "Temporary pain" affected 5% of all adult age groups. The incidence did not increase with age. Chronic or "persistent" pain (defined as pain that is "often or usually present, and had occurred during the previous two weeks") affected 11% of the adult population surveyed. The age-specific rates for persistent pains were: 19.9% in the sixth decade, 25.0% in the seventh decade, 29.0% in the eighth decade, and 40.0% in those aged 80 or more. These figures indicate that although the elderly have the same frequency of temporary or shortlived painful conditions as the rest of the population, the risk of persistent pain rises significantly with age.

The elderly do not complain more. Sternbach reported that the elderly were less likely to complain of headaches, backaches, muscle pains, stomach pains, and dental pains. They were more likely to suffer from joint pains [2].

Pain in the Elderly Person

The physiology of pain in the elderly has been reviewed [3]. Studies of cutaneous pain thresholds suggest that thresholds are elevated in the elderly due to local cutaneous factors. This decrease in sensitivity to pain may result from end-organ receptor changes. There may also be slower reaction times in response to painful stimuli. The elderly discriminate less well between levels of painful stimulation and underestimated the degree of pain. The rate of "silent myocardial infarction" is higher in the elderly than in younger populations. This is due to decreased susceptibility to pain.

Clinical Problems Arising from Treatment

Several factors make the elderly more liable to experience problems due to drugs prescribed for pain control. Because many drugs such as nonsteroidal anti-inflammatory drugs (NSAIDs) are protein bound, the lower serum albumin in the elderly may increase the probability of toxicity. Prolonged metabolism in the liver, and reduced clearance, contribute to gradual accumulation. This is often seen with the benzodiazepines that cause drowsiness.

The elderly frequently take multiple prescriptions, which adds to the risk of drug interactions. For example, phenothiazines may interfere with opiate metabolism, and barbiturates may accelerate the metabolism of other drugs. Glaucoma can be aggravated by anticholinergics. Neuroleptics such as phenothiazines, and metoclopramide may provoke marked extrapyramidal reactions in the elderly. The elderly are more susceptible to memory dysfunction and confusion [5,6]. Withdrawal may also cause physical and cognitive problems.

This woman does not warrant an opiate at this time. Other measures should be tried first.

2. TRUE

Opiates

Opiates may cause a variety of problems. They may drop blood pressure, resulting in syncope. They can precipitate confusion, hallucinations, depression, constipation, urinary retention, respiratory depression, bradycardia, or tachycardia.

Meperidine is usually more protein-bound than morphine, and it tends to cause greater toxicity in the elderly. Meperidine is also somewhat anticholinergic; and during its metabolism, normeperidine is produced. If the patient is also taking other drugs such as phenothiazines or phenobarbital, this metabolite will accumulate, causing delirium, coma, or convulsions.

Tricyclic Antidepressants

Tricyclic antidepressants have some analgesic effects. Postherpetic neuralgia or diabetic neuropathy may be treated with imipramine or amitriptyline. Other tricyclic drugs with similar effect are doxepin and clomipramine. All of these antidepressants affect the re-uptake of serotonin, a neurotransmitter implicated in the mechanisms of pain control. This re-uptake inhibition increases the amount of the transmitter in the synaptic cleft, inhibiting "pain transmission" [7]. The steady burning quality of neuralgia seems to be particularly relieved by these drugs. The elderly are more prone to adverse effects such as negative inotropic effects, aggravation of glaucoma, hypotension, confusion, hallucinations, constipation, and urinary retention due to the anticholinergic effects of these agents. Agents such as nortryptiline may be used since the anticholinergic effects are less.

Starting doses should be low. In the very elderly it may be prudent to use a liquid preparation so that doses as little as 5 mg may be used initially, then gradually increased weekly or every two weeks [3]. Phenothiazines may potentiate the effects of tricyclics in relieving neuralgia, but may also add to the risk of Parkinsonian symptoms, hypotension, confusion, and many of the other side effects shared with the tricyclic antidepressants.

Anticonvulsants

Anticonvulsants have been used for many years in the treatment of certain neuralgias. Drugs like carbamazepine and phenytoin are particularly useful when the pain has an intermittent or jabbing quality, as in tic douloureux. Valproate and other anticonvulsants may have similar effects [8].

The most studied drug is carbamazepine. Its side effects include nausea, dizziness, confusion, loss of coordination, skin rashes, aggravation of heart failure, acute urinary retention, and bone marrow depression. To reduce adverse effects, carbamazepine should be introduced slowly, at 50 or 100 mg bid to start with, increases every three to five days by 100 or 200 mg to a final dose of about 200 mg bid or tid. The effective dose of valproate is about 250 mg tid.

Baclofen

Baclofen is an antispastic drug that also has some pain-relieving properties useful in treating neuralgias. Its primary application has been in the treatment of spinal cord injuries. Adverse effects in the elderly include chest pain, confusion, ataxia, weakness, nausea, urinary retention, and changes in intestinal motility. Effective doses for neuralgia vary from 40 to 80 mg per day, in divided doses.

NSAIDs

Apart from the propensity to cause GI distress and peptic ulceration, NSAIDs in the elderly can provoke salt and water retention. They may cause headache, which causes the patient to take even more medication. In the elderly, NSAIDs can cause confusion and depression. They may worsen symptoms of chronic obstructive lung disease.

One of the most important pharmacological treatments in the elderly is detoxification. All but essential medications for identified medical conditions should be discontinued. Although a few elderly persons benefit from psychotropic drugs for diagnosed psychiatric conditions, the majority function better without multiple prescriptions of sedatives, hypnotics, opiate analgesics, and antidepressants.

Transcutaneous Electrical Nerve Stimulation (TENS)

Transcutaneous electrical nerve stimulation has earned an important place as a noninvasive method of pain control [9]. The elderly may encounter problems in its use since demand pacemakers will shut off in the presence of electrical stimulation. There is, at least theoretically, the danger of interference in cardiac function if the stimulator is applied over the precordium. Application over the anterior neck can stimulate the carotid sinus and precipitously drop blood pressure. Some elderly may misinterpret directions in application, and as a result enough electroconductive medium might not be applied. Electrodes may be applied improperly, or patients may fall asleep with the electrodes attached, causing burns. TENS is best used where pain is localized or confined to a smaller area. It is unlikely that such generalized pain will respond to TENS.

Exercise programs may be used to improve stamina and a sense of well-being. It is important to obtain a cardiogram and, if necessary, a stress test, prior to beginning a progressive exercise program.

3. FALSE

Thalamic Pain Syndrome

This is actually part of a spectrum of central pain disorders and can be provoked by stroke or damage to parts of the spinothalamic (pain transmission) system or to some parts of the thalamus that subserve pain sensation [10].

The syndrome involves spontaneous deep aching involving one side of the body. There is a reduced ability to localize stimuli, such as unpleasant cutaneous dysesthesia provoked by repeated scratching or pinprick. There is usually some anesthesia to warm, cold, or sharp stimuli over the affected body side. The degree of damage to these brain structures determines the degree of anesthesia.

Sometimes the pain is described as a circumferential, squeezing feeling. Usually it is a steady pain, but it can have a jabbing component. Although the pain is often severe, it may be momentarily relieved by the application of hand pressure, or vibration, in the painful area. This pain is worse with fatigue and emotion, and especially with depression. Carbamazepine or phenytoin may be helpful, especially for the intermittent or jabbing features. Amitriptyline or doxepin are helpful in about half the cases, both for pain relief itself and also for the depression that often complicates the picture.

Although TENS might immediately relieve the pain, it does so only in the region in which it is applied. The relief usually lasts only until stimulation is stopped.

Because of the propensity of the pain aggravated by emotional tension, the pain may be relieved by helping the patient to become more active; try to provide some form of mental distraction or relaxation training.

4. TRUE

Diabetic Neuropathy

Several patterns of neuropathy may be encountered in diabetes mellitus. Pain is encountered in some cases of mononeuropathy and also in diffuse sensory polyneuropathy. Mononeuropathies may even present before the diabetic condition is diagnosed. Mononeuropathies usually occur in sites where there has been some degree of trauma. This accounts for the frequent occurrence of ulnar nerve lesions from pressure on the elbows. Symptoms include tingling and paresthesias in the nerve distribution, and painful dysesthesia that may involve burning.

Although one might hope for improvement with control of blood sugar, symptoms are not necessarily abated by improving diabetic control. The best management is conservation, protecting the nerve against further trauma. For severe pain, transcutaneous electric nerve stimulation and/or tricyclic antidepressant therapy may be effective.

Many polyneuropathies may pass unnoticed because they are limited to loss of cutaneous sensory acuity in the periphery. Painful polyneuropathies pose a significant problem, because the discomfort is relatively intractable. The major involvement is usually in the feet and ankles, and extends partway up the shins. There is a constant burning, formication, or tingling quality to the paresthesia, which strangely seems worst when resting. It may be somewhat relieved when the patient is active or distracted. As with other neuropathies, stimuli may provoke radiation of discomfort within the affected limb. Stimuli are poorly localized, and there is hypoesthesia to simple stimuli.

TENS often provides incomplete and transient relief. Amitriptyline, possibly in combination with a low dose of phenothiazine, relieves some patients [7]. Some reports suggest that phenytoin or carbamazepine may relieve pain in about 80% of sufferers [9], but that figure seems optimistic.

The best approach to any diabetic neuropathy is conservative (not operative). The blood sugar should be controlled, and then imipramine or amitriptyline may be used. Failing this, carbamazepine or phenytoin may be tried. For localized pain from a mononeuropathy, TENS may be helpful. Psychological techniques, such as relaxation therapy and activity programs, are also very important in palliation.

5. FALSE

Joint Pain After Stroke

As a late sequela of stroke, one may encounter pain that is aggravated by movement of the limb. Some joints are restricted in movement or "frozen." This is not a neurogenic pain problem but results from inadequate mobilization, causing pericapsulitis and contractures. The treatment is prevention, starting early mobilization and providing ongoing support to maintain mobility and function.

Shoulder–Hand Syndrome After Stroke

Stroke is one of the important causes of shoulder–hand syndrome, which is also called sympathetic dystrophy. The affected limb becomes painful with a deep ache, oversensitivity to stimuli, and often a burning sensation. With use, stimulation, or even emotional upset, the limb sweats, swells, turns cool, dusky, and painful. It results from overactivity of the sympathetic nervous system from the stroke and/or immobilization from weakness.

Sympathetic overactivity causes pain, which further interferes with the use of the limb. This creates a vicious cycle of pain, reduced and abnormal function, and more pain. Whatever the treatment, the intervention must be early and active. Stellate ganglion block, possibly followed by surgical or chemical sympathectomy, will reduce the pain and swelling in 75% of cases.

One may also consider using steroids. Start at a high dose and rapidly decline over about a week. Phenothiazines in low doses have also been used. An intervention should be combined with active mobilization and exercises to restore function. Without mobilization, sympathetic dystrophy becomes chronic.

Pain from Spasticity After Stroke

With upper motor neuron lesions, the resulting spasticity may lead to pain that may be felt both during clonic spasms and chronically in the limb and muscles of the trunk nearby. Diazepam or dantrolene sodium reduce painful flexor spasms and permit mobilization. Simultaneous active physical therapy is equally important to restore function and to prevent loss of mobility or the development of some other painful conditions mentioned above.

REFERENCES

1. Crook J, Rideout E, Browne G: The prevalence of pain complaints in a general population. *Pain* 18:299–314, 1984.
2. Sternbach RA: Survey of pain in the United States: The Nuprin pain report. *The Clinical Journal of Pain* 1:49–53, 1986.
3. Harkins SW, Kwentus J, Price DD: Pain and the elderly. In: *Advances in Pain Research and Therapy*, Vol. 7. C Benedetti, CR Chapman, G Moricca (eds.), New York: Raven Press, 1984, pp. 103–121.

4. Kwentus JA, Harkins SW, Lignon N, Silverman JJ: Current concepts of geriatric pain and its treatment. *Geriatrics* 40:48–57, 1985.
5. Molloy DW: Memory loss, confusion and disorientation in an elderly woman taking meclizine. *J Amer Geriatric Soc* 35(5):454, 1987.
6. Molloy DW, Brooymans MA: Anticholinergic medications and cognitive function in the elderly. *J Clin Exp Gerontology* (In press.)
7. Butler S: Present status of tricyclic antidepressants in chronic pain therapy. In: *Advances in Pain Research and Therapy*, Vol. 7. C Benedetti, CR Chapmans, G Moricca (eds.), New York: Raven Press, 1984, pp. 173–197.
8. Swerdlow M: Anticonvulsant drugs and chronic pain. *Clinical Neuropharmacology* 7:51–82, 1984.
9. Favale E, Leandri M: Neurophysiological foundations of peripheral electroanalgesia. In: *Advances in Pain Research and Therapy*, Vol. 7. C Benedetti, CR Chapman, G Moricca (eds.), New York: Raven Press, 1984, pp. 343–357.
10. Tasker RR: Deafferentation. In: *Textbook of Pain*. PD Wall, R Melzack (eds.), Edinburgh: Churchill-Livingston, 1984, pp. 119–132.

17 | INTRACRANIAL TUMORS

CASE PRESENTATION

A 75-year-old man has been brought to the emergency department because of increasing confusion. His wife informs you that he has been complaining of headaches and increasing right-side weakness for the past two months. On examination, he has hyperreflexia on the right side with a right extensor plantar response. You want to order an emergency head computerized tomography (CT) scan because you think he may have an intracranial tumor.

D.W. Molloy
J.D. Wells
D.E. Savelli
C.J. Patterson

Consider the following statements (true or false)

1. Intracranial tumors are uncommon in the elderly, and their incidence, particularly in the case of meningioma, decreases with age.

2. The most common presentation of malignant hemispheric tumor in the elderly is intellectual impairment with headache, vomiting, and/or papilledema.

3. The average history of meningioma is far greater than with malignant hemisphere tumors. The duration of onset reliably discriminates between benign and malignant tumors because the presenting symptom of a meningioma is very rarely acute.

4. Pituitary tumors in the elderly typically present with optic nerve involvement. Their presence can be confirmed by showing enlargement of the pituitary fossa on x-ray examination or CT scan.

1. FALSE

There is a progressive increase in the incidence of intracranial tumors, particularly meningiomas, with advancing age [1,2]. Intracranial tumors were previously thought to be uncommon in the elderly. Their presentation is typically nonspecific, and they are frequently confused with dementing illnesses or cerebrovascular disease [3–5]. Epidemiologic studies suggest that many intracranial tumors in the elderly are only diagnosed at autopsy [6]. Twomey reported that 0.4% of patients with a diagnosis of strokes were subsequently found at postmortem to have intracranial tumors [7].

2. FALSE

The most common presenting feature of a malignant hemispheric tumor is a progressive deficit—usually a hemiparesis. The onset is typically insidious and rarely acute. The next most common presentation is progressive intellectual deterioration. The history is that of a relatively rapid onset, usually less than six months, and may be associated with seizures. Features attributable to elevated intracranial pressure are uncommon in old age. Although headache, vomiting, and papilledema occur in up to 70% of younger patients with intracranial tumors, they are less frequent in the elderly. The infrequency of these classic symptoms makes the diagnosis more difficult in this group, and may account for the great number of misdiagnoses.

3. FALSE

Although meningiomas usually present with a gradually progressive neurologic deficit, associated with intellectual impairment and fluctuating symptoms, the duration of symptoms does not reliably discriminate between benign and malignant tumors. The average duration of symptoms is usually much greater with meningiomas than with malignant hemispheric tumors, but the duration of the complaint may be very short.

4. FALSE

Pituitary tumors increase in incidence with age and are commonly incidental findings in the elderly. They rarely cause symptoms and are usually picked up on straight skull x-ray or CT scan, while the patient is being investigated for another illness.

REFERENCES

1. Annegers JF, Schoenberg BS, Ozakaki H, *et al.*: Primary intracranial neoplasms in Rochester, Minnesota (1935–1977). In: Rose FC (ed.): *Clinical Neuro-Epidemiology*. Turnbridge Wells: Pitman Medical, 1980, p. 366.
2. Conney LM, Solitaire GB: Primary intracranial tumors. *Mod Geriatr* 4:234, 1974.
3. Daly D, Svein HJ, Yoss RE: Intermittent cerebral symptoms with meningiomas. *Arch Neurol* 5:287, 1961.
4. Friedman H, Odom GL: Expanding intracranial lesions in geriatric patients. *Geriatrics* 27:105, 1972.
5. Godfrey JG, Cairo FI: Intracranial tumors in the elderly: Diagnosis and treatment. *Age and Ageing* 13:152, 1984.
6. McLaurin RL, Helmer FA: Errors in diagnosis in intracranial tumours. *JAMA* 180:1011, 1962.
7. Twomey C: Brain tumours in the elderly. *Age and Ageing* 7:138, 1978.

18 | NORMAL-PRESSURE HYDROCEPHALUS

CASE PRESENTATION

An elderly man presents with his 84-year-old wife. He complains that she has "slowed down" in the past few months and has urinary incontinence that she does not notice. Her mental reactions are slow, she has trouble initiating walking, and her gait is flat-footed. She has mild memory impairment and is inattentive. You consider a diagnosis of normal-pressure hydrocephalus (NPH) due to her gait abnormality, incontinence, and cognitive impairment.

D.W. Molloy
C. Power

Consider the following statements (true or false)

1. NPH is a rare disorder, occurring in less than 0.5% of elderly demented patients.

2. Ataxia is the most common presenting complaint in NPH patients.

3. NPH patients may have spasticity of the lower limbs, hyperreflexia, and bilateral extensor plantar responses.

4. Computerized tomography (CT) scans of NPH patients usually show ventricular dilatation with sulcal atrophy.

5. Shunting is recommended for every NPH patient.

1. FALSE

NPH was first described by Hakim and Adams in 1965 [1]. Its prevalence in elderly demented patients may be as high as 2–5% [2]. Onset of idiopathic NPH occurs most frequently in patients in their late 50s [3].

Approximately 70% of cases of NPH are related to specific precipitating events such as subarachnoid hemorrhage, trauma, meningitis and previous surgery. These events may cause NPH by interrupting cerebrospinal fluid (CSF) circulation. Approximately 30% of cases of NPH are termed "idiopathic" because there is no obvious precipitating cause [4].

The normal circulation of CSF was first described by Pandy. CSF is produced in the choroid plexus of the lateral ventricles and flows through the third and fourth ventricles. From the fourth ventricle, it enters the cysterna magna and passes to the cerebral and spinal subarachnoid spaces. CSF is absorbed in the villi, saggital, and other venous sinuses [5].

NPH is a communicating hydrocephalus, as CSF circulation is not blocked from reaching the cerebral subarachnoid space. This is distinguished from obstructive hydrocephalus, which occurs when CSF flow is blocked within the ventricular system. It is unclear whether NPH results from the failure to absorb CSF or from dilatation of the ventricles due to a degenerative process that maintains normal CSF pressure but increases its force [1]. (See Figure 18-1.)

2. TRUE

NPH patients classically present with the triad of ataxia, incontinence and dementia; however, ataxia is the most common presenting complaint [6]. Patients may complain that their feet seem "glued" to the floor or that they are unable to initiate purposeful walking—"gait apraxia." Patients may have less control of their legs than of their arms. Complaints of rigidity in the lower limbs also are common.

Symptoms of dementia often are mild in early stages of NPH. Patients or family members may express concern over slowing of mental processes, apathy, or inattention. Establishing the duration of these symptoms is important, as details of trauma and previous cranial surgery or subarachnoid hemorrhage may correlate with the onset of symptoms and signs of NPH. If patients exhibit memory loss, obtain a history from the principal caregiver (spouse or family member). Patients with dementia often have poor insight or may give misleading or inaccurate histories.

Figure 18-1   Normal Cerebrospinal Fluid Flow.

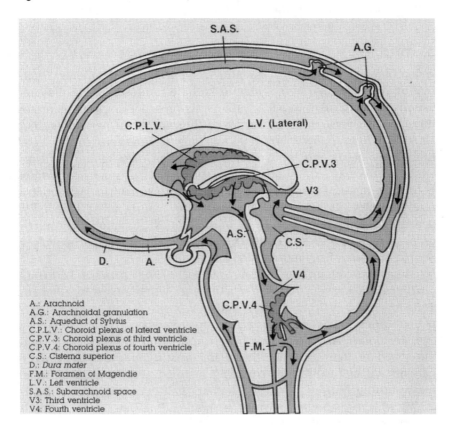

A.: Arachnoid
A.G.: Arachnoidal granulation
A.S.: Aqueduct of Sylvius
C.P.L.V.: Choroid plexus of lateral ventricle
C.P.V.3: Choroid plexus of third ventricle
C.P.V.4: Choroid plexus of fourth ventricle
C.S.: Cisterna superior
D.: *Dura mater*
F.M.: Foramen of Magendie
L.V.: Left ventricle
S.A.S.: Subarachnoid space
V3: Third ventricle
V4: Fourth ventricle

The slowing of mental processes in NPH patients is followed by overt cognitive impairment, memory loss, and disorientation. To confirm the presence of cognitive deficit, administer the Standardized Mini-Mental State Exam (SMMSE). This test may be administered by a nurse and takes approximately 10–15 minutes [7].

Common behavioral abnormalities in NPH patients include withdrawal, silence, and perseveration [8]. NPH may result in unexplained bladder and bowel incontinence. Urinary incontinence, however, is more common than fecal incontinence. Patients usually do not complain of incontinence, as they are unaware of the problem.

Although uncommon, a depressed level of consciousness or even akinetic mutism may be the predominant presenting feature of NPH.

3. TRUE

A neurologic examination is essential in suspected NPH patients. Examination of the cranial nerves should include fundoscopy. Papilledema usually is not present in NPH patients; its presence suggests increased intracranial pressure. Examination of the peripheral nervous system should include a power and tone assessment. Spasticity in the lower limbs may occur and is associated with brisk deep tendon reflexes. Patients also may exhibit bilateral extensor plantar responses (positive Babinski's sign). These findings usually are symmetric. Asymmetric findings often indicate previous stroke or tumor, rather than NPH. Sensory examination usually is normal in NPH patients. Primitive reflexes such as a grasp or snout reflex may be present, particularly if the patient has long-standing NPH and dementia.

A gait assessment is essential in suspected NPH patients. Look for a positive Romberg sign. Ask patients to stand with their feet together and arms extended in front of their body. A positive sign is indicated if patients are stable when their eyes are open and begin to fall when their eyes are closed. Ask the patient to walk approximately six meters—note the speed of their gait and the characteristic "magnetic feet." NPH patients will not exhibit the shuffling, stooped gait of parkinsonism or the waddling limp of the Trendelenburg gait. There is little point in asking elderly patients to walk "in tandem," as few normal elderly patients can accomplish this.

4. FALSE

Investigations should include a complete blood cell count (CBC), Venereal Disease Research Laboratory (VDRL) test, a chest x-ray, and electrolyte, blood sugar, calcium, B_{12} and T_3, and T_4 measurements. These tests may rule out potential treatable causes of dementia or ataxia. If tests are normal but symptoms and signs suggest NPH, patients should have a CT scan of the head. In NPH patients, CT scans may show ventricular dilatation and periventricular edema in the presence of normal sulci [9]. Patients with Alzheimer's disease may have significant atrophy of the sulci and dilatation of ventricles. If the CT scan is suggestive of NPH, consult a neurologist, geriatrician, or neurosurgeon. Specialists usually perform a radioactive iodinated serum albumin (RISA) scan in which RISA is injected into the intrathecal space. In NPH patients, reflux and stasis of RISA usually occurs in the ventricles, with delayed emptying through the venous sinuses [10].

During the RISA scan, a lumbar puncture is performed to facilitate the measurement of CSF pressure. An improvement in NPH following the removal of 50 cc of CSF indicates that the patient may respond to shunt therapy [11].

Electroencephalography (EEG) may be useful in diagnosing NPH. Unlike Alzheimer's disease, there may be normal background activity. Some tertiary care referral centers perform more sophisticated tests such as intracranial monitoring, infusion manometric testing, and central blood flow studies.

Diagnosing NPH depends on clinical findings and characteristic CT and RISA scan features. These tests do not predict the outcome of surgical therapies.

DIFFERENTIAL DIAGNOSIS

Parkinson's Disease

Obvious signs of Parkinson's disease include the presence of resting tremor, cogwheel rigidity, and bradykinesia. Patients with early-stage Parkinson's disease may present simply with gait abnormalities that may be difficult to distinguish from NPH [12]. Administering levodopa will help distinguish the two disorders. Levodopa may improve parkinsonian symptoms, but does not improve NPH symptoms.

Depression

Depression is common in the elderly and frequently is underdiagnosed. Depressed patients may present with agitation, slowing of mentation, loss of concentration, and a reduced attention span. Suspect depression in elderly patients with a personal or family history of depression, recent loss of a spouse or family member, diurnal variation, fluctation in performance, recent onset of depression, or an underlying mood change. If you suspect depression, refer your patient to a geriatric psychiatrist or geriatrician, or commence treatment.

Alzheimer's Disease

This may be difficult to distinguish from NPH. Word-finding difficulties that occur in Alzheimer's disease patients usually do not occur in NPH patients. Gait disorders and incontinence usually occur in later stages of Alzheimer's disease, if at all. Urinary incontinence rarely is a presenting feature of Alzheimer's disease. CT and RISA scans will help distinguish between these two conditions.

Multi-infarct Dementia

Multi-infarct dementia, resulting from multiple cerebral infarcts, may have protean manifestations and presentations and may mimic Parkinson's, Alzheimer's disease, or NPH. Patients may have a past history of hypertension, transient ischemic attacks, and myocardial infarction. Clinical examination may reveal carotid or femoral bruits, unilateral signs, peripheral vascular disease, or evidence of hypertension. Acute onset of signs and symptoms and evidence of multiple small strokes (as seen on a CT scan or with nuclear magnetic resonance imaging) help confirm the diagnosis. Patients also may exhibit spasticity in their upper limbs and positive Babinski signs in their lower limbs. Use of the Hachinski Ischemic Score may greatly facilitate the diagnosis (Table 18-1). A score of seven or more suggests multi-infarct dementia; a score of four or less suggests Alzheimer's dementia.

Drug Reactions

Neuroleptics such as haloperidol cause rigidity, ataxia, confusion, and parkinsonian side effects in the elderly. Sedatives such as benzodiazepines can precipitate dizziness, ataxia, and mental slowing. Before diagnosing NPH, discontinue these medications on a trial basis to determine their effects on the patient's condition.

Space-occupying Lesions

Patients with space-occupying lesions such as subdural hematomas may present with gait abnormality, dementia, or confusion. Patients at increased risk for subdural hematoma include those with a history of alcohol abuse, anticoagulant use, blood dyscrasia, seizures, or falls. CT scans may help distinguish subdural hematoma from NPH.

Elderly patients with tumors may present with cognitive impairment and ataxia. The presence of space-occupying lesions on a CT scan, lateralizing signs, and a history of seizure disorder usually confirms the

Table 18-1 Hachinski Ischemic Scale.

Feature	Point Value
Abrupt onset	2
Stepwise deterioration	1
Fluctuating course	2
Nocturnal confusion	1
Relative preservation of personality	1
Depression	1
Somatic complaints	1
Emotional incontinence	1
History or presence of hypertension	1
History of stroke	2
Evidence of atherosclerosis	1
Focal neurologic symptoms	2
Focal neurologic signs	2

Source: Hachinski VC, et al.: Cerebral bood flow in dementia. *Arch Neurol* 32:632, 1975.

presence of intracranial tumors. Before making the diagnosis of NPH, investigate for a family history of ataxia and ataxia caused by chronic alcohol abuse.

5. FALSE

Physicians face an ethical dilemma in referring NPH patients for treatment because the natural history of the disease is poorly understood. Surgical intervention such as shunting is associated with significant morbidity and mortality. The elderly frequently have associated medical conditions that increase the risks of general anesthesia. There are three types of shunts: ventriculoperitoneal, ventriculoatrial, and spinoperitoneal shunts. Ventriculoatrial and ventriculoperitoneal shunts are the most popular. They deliver more consistent performance postoperatively, although they may be associated with subdural collections and infection. Spinoperitoneal shunts have more shunt blockages, but result in fewer subdural collections and infection. A recent study showed that 20% of shunt recipients developed subdural collections, 8% developed seizures, and 3% developed infections. Shunts improved the condition of 64% of patients; had no effect on 27% of patients; and worsened the condition of 3% of patients [13]. Mortality rates from surgery vary from 5% to 12% [14].

Signs and symptoms of NPH may resolve immediately after surgery or up to eight months after surgery [15]. Ataxia usually is the first sign to improve. This may be followed by improvement in incontinence and dementia. Much of the research on NPH has attempted to determine which factors in the etiology and presentation of the disease predict a positive response to shunt therapy. Patients with a specific cause of NPH (such as trauma, subdural hematoma, meningitis, mild dementia, and prominent ataxia) and those with recent onset of their condition may respond better to shunting than idiopathic NPH patients. After being educated about their prognosis and surgical risks, patients and their families should make the final decision on whether to undergo shunting, as our understanding of the condition and the risks involved in surgery are limited. Do not recommend surgery if patients show no deterioration or very mild impairment with repeated follow-up.

REFERENCES

1. Hakim S, Adams RD: The special clinical problem of symptomatic hydrocephalus with normal cerebrospinal fluid pressure. Observations on cerebrospinal fluid hydrodynamics. *J Neurosurg Sci* 70:307, 1965.

2. Marsden CD, Harrison MJG: Correspondence: Presenile dementia. 1. *Br Med J* 3:50, 1972.
3. Terry R, Gershon S: Cerebrospinal fluid physiology and normal pressure hydrocephalus. *In* Katzman R (ed.), *Neurobiology of Aging.* New York: Raven Press, 1976, p. 142.
4. Katzman R: Normal pressure hydrocephalus in dementia. In: Wells CE, Davis FA: *Dementia,* Philadelphia, 1976, p. 142.
5. Dawson H, *et al.*: Mechanism of drainage of cerebrospinal fluid. *Brain* 96:329, 1973.
6. Fisher CM: Hydrocephalus as a cause of disturbances of gait in the elderly. *Neurology* (New York) 32:1358, 1982.
7. Molloy DW, Alemayehu E, Roberts R: A Standardized Mini-Mental State Examination (SMMSE): Its reliability compared to the traditional Mini-Mental State Examination (MMSE). *Am J Psych* 148:102–105, 1991.
8. Fisher CM: The clinical picture in occult hydrocephalus. *Clin Neurosurg* 24:270, 1977.
9. Adapon BD, *et al.*: Radiologic investigations of normal pressure hydrocephalus. *Radiolog Clin North Am* 12:353, 1974.
10. Richero G, *et al.*: RISA—ventriculography and RISA cisternography. *Neurology* 14:185, 1964.
11. Wikkelso C, *et al.*: Normal pressure hydrocephalus. Predictive value of the cerebral fluid tap-test. *Acta Scand Neurol* 73:566, 1986.
12. Sypert GW, *et al.*: Occult normal pressure hydrocephalus manifested by parkinsonism-dementia complex. *Neurology* 23:234, 1973.
13. Black FM, *et al.*: CSF shunts for dementia, incontinence and gait disturbance. *Clin Neurosurg* 32:632, 1985.
14. Pickard JD: Adult communicating hydrocephalus. *Br J Hosp Med* 27:35, 1982.
15. Myers JS, *et al.*: Evaluation of treatment of normal pressure hydrocephalus. *J Neurosurg* 62:513, 1985.

19 | SUBDURAL HEMATOMA

CASE PRESENTATION

An 82-year-old woman is brought to your office by her daughter, who complains her mother has become more confused than usual in the last two months, and also has been sleeping much more than usual. The patient is still taking anticoagulants for a deep venous thrombosis diagnosed three years previously. There is no history of recent falls. Her daughter, a registered nurse, asks if you think her mother may have a subdural hematoma (SDH).

D.W. Molloy
J.D. Wells
D.E. Savelli
C.J. Patterson

Consider the following statements (true or false)

1. The incidence of SDH increases with age.

2. In the majority of patients with SDH, the level of consciousness fluctuates.

3. Lateralizing neurologic signs occur characteristically on the ipsilateral side of the hematoma.

4. The majority of elderly persons with unilateral SDH show shift of the pineal gland on a plain radiograph of the skull.

5. Medical management of SDH with hyperosmolar fluids is preferable to surgery in the treatment of chronic SDH in the very elderly.

1. TRUE

The incidence of SDH increases with age, particularly in men. More than half will have no history of falls or head trauma. Falls may be minor or major and can be associated with alcohol intoxication or epilepsy. Patients taking anticoagulants or with blood dyscrasias are at increased risk. The clinical presentation is nonspecific, and almost two-thirds are missed [1].

2. FALSE

The most common sign is an alteration in the level of consciousness; fluctuation in consciousness is rare. Chronic SDH is one of the reversible causes of dementia and must be ruled out in all patients presenting with recent deterioration of mental function. When the level of consciousness fluctuates, seizures due to SDH should be included in the wide differential diagnosis of subacute delirium.

3. FALSE

Lateralizing neurologic signs are usually contralateral to the hematoma. In stroke, the hemiplegic signs are more marked than the impairment in the level of consciousness, while in SDH, the reverse is true. Headaches may occur, but other features of raised intracranial pressure such as nausea, vomiting, and papilledema are usually absent. Hemiparesis is a more common presentation of SDH in the elderly. Confusion often occurs before somnolence. Fifteen percent of SDHs are bilateral.

4. FALSE

Pineal shift, if present, is a useful sign. But pineal gland calcification is seen radiographically in only 60% of the elderly. The diagnosis of SDH is best established using computerized axial tomography (CAT) scans.

In the first week after a subdural has formed the lesion appears as a "hyperdense" region on the CAT scan. At this stage a fluid level is sometimes visible where the blood separates into serum or supernatant and red blood cells. At 7 to 10 days, the lesion may become "isodense" and may be missed. However, absence of sulci on the affected side may alert the radiologist to the diagnosis. After the isodense phase, the lesion liquifies, becomes "hypodense," and is usually visible on CAT scans.

5. FALSE

Surgery is the mainstay of treatment, and surgical and operative mortality is greatest in acute SDH [2]. Poor prognostic factors include advanced age, decreased level of consciousness, rapid change in clinical features, and hypertension [3,4]. Advanced age does not influence subsequent quality of life, if evacuation is successful. Hyperosmolar fluids (20% mannitol) may be used in the treatment of SDH, but because of increased risk of cardiac failure in the elderly, this age group does not tolerate hyperosmolar fluids as well as younger patients. The use of hyperosmolar fluids takes longer, delays rehabilitation, and does not cure the problem. Therefore, surgery is the treatment of choice in the elderly.

REFERENCES

1. Fogelholm K, Heiskanan O, Waltimo O: Chronic subdural hematomata in adults. *J Neurosurg* 42:43, 1975.
2. Jerris F, Schmidt K: Chronic subdural hematoma: Surgery or mannitol treatment? *J Neurosurg* 40:639, 1974.
3. Noltie K, Denham MJ: Subdural hematomata in the elderly. *Age and Ageing* 10:241, 1981.
4. Walker ME, Espir M, Shepard RH: Subdural hematomata: Presentation and diagnosis on medical wards. *Postgrad Med J* 44:785, 1968.

Part III

DRUGS

20 | DIGOXIN

CASE PRESENTATION

A 75-year-old man comes to your office complaining he has lost his appetite for the past two weeks and developed diarrhea with weakness. His son, who accompanies him, says his father is a little confused and disoriented. He has been treated with digoxin, 0.25 mg per day for congestive heart failure (CHF) for the last 15 years. Five years ago, a diagnosis of hypertension was made, and therapy with hydrochlorothiazide, 25 mg per day, was begun. Three years ago, he developed atrial fibrillation. On his previous visit to your office, you noted that he was free of CHF symptoms. His blood pressure was 135/85, ventricular rate 72 per min. Heart and lung examination were unremarkable. A chest x-ray taken one year ago was within normal limits.

Three weeks ago, while visiting his son in another city, he developed palpitations and mild shortness of breath. He visited an emergency room and was told that his atrial fibrillation was poorly controlled. He was started on quinidine (Biquin), 250 mg po, bid.

On examination today his heart rate is 52 per min, irregular; his blood pressure is 140/80. Examination of his heart, lungs and gastro-intestinal tract is unremarkable. Investigations that are immediately

R. Jaeschke
M. Sauvé
D.W. Molloy

available to you include serum sodium of 135 mEq/l, potassium of 3.2 mEq/l, urea 4.6 mEq/l. An ECG shows no p waves; narrow, regular QRS complexes at a rate of 50 per min, and multiple ventricular ectopic beats. Digoxin level will not be available for five days.

Consider the following statements (true or false)

1. Elderly people have an increased incidence of digoxin toxicity compared to younger people taking the drug.

2. The most likely cause of this man's nausea and weakness is hypokalemia.

3. The ECG changes are compatible with digoxin toxicity.

4. This patient should have quinidine and digoxin maintained at present doses until the serum digoxin is available.

5. Use of digoxin for CHF alone without atrial fibrillation was justified.

1. TRUE

Digitalis was the first known drug for the treatment of congestive heart failure (CHF). Digitalis enjoyed widespread use before the introduction of diuretics and vasodilators. In a recent study conducted on a representative sample of North American physicians, 37% used digoxin either alone or in combination with diuretics as an initial therapy for patients with CHF and sinus rhythm [1]. Unfortunately, digoxin has a narrow therapeutic window; and a large proportion of subjects on digoxin, from 5% to 25%, suffer from toxic side effects [2,3]. This incidence of digitalis toxicity is 2.5 times higher in patients over the age of 70 than in those under 65. Approximately 20% of elderly patients develop digitalis toxicity at some point during treatment.

The most important factors leading to digoxin intoxication in the elderly are impairment in renal clearance of the drug (accompanying the reduction in renal function) and change in drug distribution. The lean body mass reduction associated with aging reduces the volume of distribution of digoxin from about 500 l in middle age to 300 l in the elderly. Absorption and bio-availability of digoxin are not significantly altered by age.

Hypokalemia, hypomagnesemia, hypercalcemia, hypoxemia, and hypothyroidism predispose to digitalis toxicity and are more likely to occur in the elderly. Electrolyte abnormalities are often precipitated or exacerbated by the use of diuretics [4].

2. FALSE

Mild to moderate hypokalemia, with potassium depletion of less than 15% of total body potassium alone, does not result in significant symptoms for organ dysfunction. Loss of greater than 20% total body potassium (with serum levels of 3.0 mEq/l or less) is usually necessary to produce symptoms of muscle weakness, fatigue, and cramps. Hypokalemia, which is common in the elderly on diuretic therapy, may markedly exacerbate or even cause digoxin toxicity. Lack of potassium in the extracellular space enhances the action of digoxin and is the commonest precipitating cause of digoxin toxicity [3,4]. The common signs and symptoms of digoxin toxicity are presented as follows:

1. *Acute effects:* anorexia, nausea, vomiting, confusion (particularly in the elderly), and disorientation (particularly in the elderly).

2. *Chronic effects:* weight loss, cachexia, gynecomastia, delirium, depression, and yellow vision.

3. TRUE

Arrhythmia manifestations of toxicity include bradyarrhythmias, ventricular bigeminy, and atrial tachycardia with atrial block. Digitalis produces direct alteration in the electrical properties of the contractile cells of the heart and the specialized automatic cells. In the toxic range, there is increased automaticity and ectopic impulse activity. The most common arrhythmias associated with digoxin toxicity are

- premature ventricular beats,
- ventricular bigeminy,
- nonparoxysmal atrial tachycardia,
- sinus arrhythmia,
- junctional tachycardia,
- ventricular tachycardia,
- atrio-ventricular block, and
- sino-atrial block.

Digitalis also exerts action on the heart by altering the balance of the autonomic system, resulting in increased vagal tone. It prolongs the refractory period at the atrio-ventricular node, which slows the ventricular rate. Atrio-ventricular block of varying severity or variable atrio-ventricular block associated with nonparoxysmal atrial tachycardia may result.

Other electrical disturbances may include sinus arrhythmia, sinoatrial block, and sinus arrest. Digitalis-induced arrhythmias may precede subjective symptoms of digitalis toxicity in about one-half of these cases [4].

4. FALSE

The patient's presentation suggests symptomatic digoxin toxicity. Clinical manifestations of toxicity in the elderly differ significantly from those in younger patients. Among the elderly, central nervous system symptoms predominate rather than gastrointestinal symptoms such as anorexia. Symptomatology includes confusion, disorientation, and visual disturbances. It is even possible that the initial supraventricular arrhythmia that caused this patient's visit to the emergency room was an early manifestation of digitalis toxicity.

The administration of quinidine to a patient receiving digoxin raises the concentration of digoxin by reducing both the renal and nonrenal elimination of digoxin, and by reducing its volume of distribution. When quinidine therapy is initiated in patients receiving digoxin, serum digoxin concentrations must be carefully monitored and the digoxin dose reduced by one-half.

Other drugs implicated in triggering digoxin toxicity by increasing its level of effect are verapamil, amiodarone, spironolactone, beta blockers and others [5].

In this case one should not wait until the digoxin level becomes available, but assume until proven otherwise, that digoxin is responsible for the patient's recent problems. It would be appropriate to withdraw digoxin, replace potassium loss, monitor for cardiac arrhythmias, and use specific means as necessary to control rhythm or conduction disturbances, for example, pacemaker, phenytoin, lidocaine [6].

5. LIKELY FALSE

Our patient, while in sinus rhythm, spent 12 years on digoxin for his CHF. The value of this drug in patients with CHF and in sinus rhythm remains controversial. Recently, trials of digoxin have helped to clarify the situation. The two clear indications for digoxin are

1. atrial fibrillation with rates above 90 beats per minute, and
2. congestive heart failure with a dilated left ventricle and an S3 gallop rhythm.

Digoxin is of value as an adjunct to diuretics in improving symptoms and reducing frequency of acute exacerbations of CHF in patients with severe functional impairment (*i.e.*, dilation of the left ventricle on chest x-ray and presence of third heart sound [7,8]. Withdrawal of digoxin from patients well controlled on a combination of digoxin and diuretic has been practiced without any clinical consequences [9,10].

The introduction of vasodilators, mainly angiotensin converting enzyme inhibitors (captopril, enalapril), has decreased the need for digoxin in CHF patients. Vasodilators were shown not only to be more effective than digoxin in symptom control [11], but are also proven to reduce CHF-related mortality [12]. The usefulness of digoxin during the 12-year-long period when this patient was in sinus rhythm is at least of questionable value.

REFERENCES

1. Hlatky MA, Fleg JL, Hinton PC, *et al.*: Physician practice in the management of congestive heart failure. *JACC* 8:966–970, 1986.
2. Beller GA, Smith TW, Abelmann WH, Haber E, Hood WB, Jr.: Digitalis intoxication. A prospective study with serum level correlation. *NEJM* 284:989–997, 1971.
3. Smith TW: Digitalis. Mechanism of action and clinical use. *NEJM* 318:358–365, 1988.
4. Braunwald E: Heart failure. In *Harrison's Principles of Internal Medicine.* Braunwald E, Isselbacher KJ, Petersdorf RG, Wilson JD, Martin JB, Fauci AS (eds.). New York: McGraw-Hill Book Company, 1987, pp. 909–912.
5. Minson RB, McRitchie RJ: Digoxin in the 1980s. *Med J Australia* 147:403–408, 1987.
6. Doherty JE: Clinical use of digitalis glycosides. An update. *Cardiology* 72:225–254, 1985.
7. Guyatt GH, Sullivan MJJ, Fallen EL, *et al.*: A controlled trial of digoxin in congestive heart failure. *Am J Cardiology* 61:371–375, 1988.
8. Lee DC, Johnston RA, Bingham JB, *et al.*: Heart failure in outpatients. *NEJM* 306:699–705, 1982.
9. Taggart AJ, Johnson GD, McDevitt DG: Digoxin withdrawal after cardiac failure in patients with sinus rhythm. *J Cardiovasc Pharmacol* 5:229–234, 1983.
10. Flegg JL, Gottlieb SH, Lakatta EG: Is digoxin really important in treatment of compensated heart failure? A placebo-controlled crossover study in patients with sinus rhythm. *Am J Med* 73:244–250, 1982.
11. The captopril–digoxin multicentre research group. Comparative effects of therapy with captopril and digoxin in patients with mild to moderate heart failure. *JAMA* 259:539–544, 1988.
12. Mulrow CD, Mulrow JP, Linn WD, Aguilar C: Relative efficacy of vasodilator therapy in chronic congestive heart failure. Implications of randomized trials. *JAMA* 259:3422–3426, 1988.

21 | NONSTEROIDAL ANTI-INFLAMMATORY DRUGS

CASE PRESENTATION

Mrs. Rolland, an 84-year-old widow, comes to your office complaining of pain in the knees after walking short distances. She was seen by a rheumatologist two months ago. Osteoarthrosis (OA) of the knees was diagnosed, after a work-up that included x-rays and blood tests. She was given acetaminophen (paracetamol) 375 to 750 mg po to be taken every four hours as required; however, she has found little relief from them. She is allergic to codeine. She takes glibenclamide 5 mg daily for diabetes, and furosemide 40 mg daily for congestive heart failure and is well controlled on these medications. Urea and creatinine were taken three months ago and were found to be just above the upper limits of normal.

Clinical examination reveals varus deformity of both knees. Range of motion is diminished in both knees, and she complains of pain when the joints are moved. Heberden's nodes are evident bilaterally, and she has a trace of pedal edema.

She requests something stronger for her arthritis. You consider starting her on a nonsteroidal, anti-inflammatory drug (NSAID).

D.W. Molloy
L.E. Hart
W.E. DeCoteau

Consider the following statements (true or false)

1. NSAIDs are seldom effective in the treatment of osteoarthritis because the process in OA is one of joint failure rather than joint inflammation.

2. Full doses of acetyl salicylic acid (ASA) is a good choice in the treatment of OA when simple analgesia has failed. ASA is not only cheaper, but also less toxic and as effective as many of the newer NSAIDs.

3. If an NSAID is started, it may be necessary to halve the dose of glibenclamide. Salicylates may precipitate hypoglycemia in this patient.

4. Gastrointestinal hemorrhage is usually preceded by significant clinical symptoms such as dyspepsia.

After four weeks, Mrs. Rolland returns to your office to renew her prescription of the NSAID you prescribed. She brings you flowers and tomatoes from her garden. Her joint pains have almost completely resolved, but you note that her ankle edema is much worse.

5. You are reluctant to change the NSAID since it is so effective. It would be appropriate to increase her furosemide to 40 mg po bid.

1. FALSE

Osteoarthritis (OA) is the commonest of all joint diseases. This condition usually begins in middle age but often does not become evident until old age. It is characteristically confined to a few joints and does not usually spread to other joints like rheumatoid arthritis. However, there is a group, especially elderly women with Heberden's and Bouchard's nodes who have generalized polyarthritis. While we now know that there is a significant inflammatory component in most involved joints, it is not clear if this inflammation is primary or secondary to the degenerative process.

The synovial membrane of many patients with osteoarthritis shows marked inflammatory changes that are often indistinguishable from rheumatoid arthritis. Disruption of chondrocytes in the cartilage releases enzymes that may promote inflammation. All of these factors are evidence of an inflammatory process. This may explain why NSAIDs are often so effective in treating osteoarthritis. The NSAIDs are among the most frequently prescribed agents in current practice, and are used increasingly with elderly patients [1].

OA is usually mild, causing moderate pain. However, it can cause crippling disability at times, requiring joint replacement. Unless OA affects weight-bearing joints, such as the hip and knee, it does not seriously affect function.

By age 65, 80% of people complain of osteoarthritis [2]. A third of geriatric outpatients have OA [3]. In many of these people the arthritis is not clinically significant. Between the ages of 65 and 74, 87% of men and 74% of women had radiographic evidence of osteoarthritis [4].

In OA, morning stiffness is usually short-lived and may be easily relieved by motion, heat, and medication. OA is almost universal in the elderly and may even develop in patients with rheumatoid arthritis [5]. In the elderly, OA may be accompanied by peritendinitis or bursitis around the joints, which can give the impression that a polyarticular disease such as rheumatoid arthritis (RA) is present. Other conditions that need to be considered in the diagnosis of mono- or oligo-arthritis in the elderly include

- osteonecrosis (aseptic necrosis),
- pseudo gout (chondrocalcinosis),
- gout (sometimes superimposed on osteoarthritis),
- septic arthritis, and
- traumatic synovitis.

Mrs. Rolland takes a diuretic that might potentially cause hyper-uricemia. Measure her serum uric acid level, and keep this in mind as a potential cause of any exacerbation of her arthritis.

Clinically, patients with OA may have joint tenderness, decreased range of movement, pain with movement, and decreased muscle power around the affected joints [6]. All of these signs are fairly nonspecific and occur with many forms of arthritis in the elderly.

2. FALSE

Simple analgesics have traditionally been recommended for the treat-ment of OA. When symptoms persist despite optimal doses of a simple analgesic, it is reasonable to start the patient on an NSAID [7]. Many of the existing simple analgesics have disappointing effects in arthritis [8]. Codeine should be avoided where possible because its use can lead to addiction and abuse. Once a patient has started taking codeine, it is often impossible to get that patient off the drug. Codeine should be used with caution in the elderly because of its side effects, such as constipation and confusion.

Pentazocine is an excellent analgesic in many fields, but it is of little use in the treatment of joint pain. Stronger analgesics, such as morphine and its derivatives, have no place in the management of osteoarthritis because of the chronic nature of this disease [7].

Analgesics relieve pain but they rarely work as well as NSAIDs in the relief of arthritis. Analgesics have no effect on the inflammatory process, which may often make a significant contribution to the pain.

Aspirin and related drugs have been the cornerstone of treatment in rheumatic diseases for over 100 years. For optimal anti-inflammatory effects, a total daily dose of 3 to 6 g is usually required. At least one third of patients prove intolerant to these doses within one month of starting treatment. Treatment with aspirin is not more cost effective than therapy with nonsalicylate NSAIDs, if the cost of treating complications is included [9].

Most of the NSAIDs currently marketed are equally effective as anti-inflammatory agents and have fewer side effects than aspirin, par-ticularly on the gastrointestinal tract. There is often little significant difference in patient satisfaction between these agents [10].

The choice of a particular NSAID is empirical. It is not possible to predict which patient will respond best to any particular agent. Many patients, for unknown reasons, will show more obvious improvement on one drug than another; however, finding the agent that works best for any individual patient often requires trials with several preparations. When evaluating the efficacy of any of these agents, use only one drug at a time. There is nothing to be gained by combining NSAIDs. Side effects may be additive but anti-inflammatory effects are not.

Most of the NSAIDs produce their therapeutic effects within one week [7]. Therefore, when using NSAIDs, it is advisable to change the agents as often as necessary. The drug's final place in treatment should be determined by the patient's opinion of its benefits. In the elderly, it may take longer to assess a particular agent, since it is advisable to start with a low dose and increase the dose slowly. Continue to increase dosage until a clinical response is evident or side effects make it necessary to withdraw the drug. In the elderly, plasma binding, metabolic breakdown, and excretion rates are decreased [11–13].

3. TRUE

The NSAIDs are among the most frequently utilized agents in current practice, representing more than 4% of the total prescription market [1]. Use of NSAIDs increases with age. There is a seven-fold increase in the incidence of adverse drug reactions in those aged 70 to 79 compared to the 20 to 29 year olds [11]. Drug reactions have been implicated as the sole or contributing cause of hospitalization in over 10% of admissions to one geriatric medicine department [14]. The mechanism of NSAIDs' toxicity is described as follows.

1. Direct toxic effect:
   - gastric mucosa (ASA gastropathy),
   - inner ear (ASA tinnitus, deafness),
   - brain (indomethacin headache, dizziness),
   - liver (ASA decreases vitamin K production, causes cholestatic jaundice),
   - bone marrow depressant.
2. Results of prostaglandin inhibition:
   - damage to gastric mucosa—gastropathy (superficial ulcer, hemorrhage, deep ulcer, perforation),
   - decreased renal blood flow and renal medullary ischemia,
   - electrolyte disturbances (edema, hyperkalemia, and hyponatremia),

- decreased vasodilation of blood vessels (systemic hypertension, coronary spasm),
- decreased thromboxane activity in platelets with increased risk of hemorrhage,
- defective regulation of inflammatory response with increased production and/or release of (1) leucotrienes causing asthma, especially in association with nasal polyps; (2) leucotrienes, enzymes, and oxygen-free radicals with worsening of inflammation.
3. Drug interactions:
   - hypoglycemic effect (salicylates potentiate the effects of oral hypoglycemic agents),
   - diuretic,
   - saturate enzymes in liver involved in first pass metabolism resulting in increased bio availability of other drugs (ASA, indomethacin).
4. Miscellaneous:
   - hypersensitivity,
   - Stevens-Johnson syndrome

In general the NSAIDs are beneficial and are well tolerated in the elderly [15–18]. However, the elderly are especially at risk of developing side effects from NSAIDs. Reduced gastric acid may alter digestion and absorption. Fluid retention is increased, and central nervous system effects such as headache, dizziness, and confusion may be particularly troublesome. Up to 25% of the elderly develop CNS effects, especially headache and dizziness, with indomethacin. The need for simple dosage regimens is important, because the elderly are more likely to be taking numerous other drugs. Compliance decreases as more drugs are added.

Several important drug interactions may occur when treating the elderly with NSAIDs [10,19,20,21,22]. NSAIDs displace sulphonylurea hypoglycemic agents, oral anticoagulants, phenytoin, and sulphonamides from their protein binding sites. This increases the faction of free drug in plasma. Lithium levels may also be increased.

NSAIDs may interfere with diuretic-induced natriuresis and may interfere with the antihypertensive effects of various agents. Alcohol potentiates the gastrointestinal toxicity of salicylates. Mrs. Rolland should have the dose of glibenclamide halved when her NSAID is started, and her blood glucose levels should be monitored frequently to maintain control of her diabetes.

4. FALSE

Most NSAIDs block the synthesis of prostaglandins by inhibiting the membrane bound enzyme cyclooxygenase. Prostaglandins maintain the integrity of the gastric mucosal barrier. The inhibition of prostaglandin synthesis, even when administered by rectal suppository, accounts for many of the upper gastrointestinal side effects of the newer NSAIDs [22]. In addition, ASA is directly toxic to the gastric mucosa.

Although other NSAIDs are less toxic than aspirin, their most common side effects are on the upper gastrointestinal tract. Symptoms include dyspepsia, epigastric pain, indigestion, nausea, and vomiting. All the NSAIDs cause gastrointestinal lesions ranging from hyperemia to diffuse gastritis, superficial erosions, or ulcer crater formation [23].

The effects of 12 NSAIDs on the gastric mucosa was studied in 249 patients. The prevalence of endoscopically confirmed gastric lesions was 31% over a one-year period. While all the NSAIDs caused gastric damage, the greatest offender was aspirin [24]. There was a very poor correlation between subjective symptoms and endoscopic findings.

Anemia may result from slow gastrointestinal blood loss. The amount of blood loss is dose dependent. Studies of fecal blood loss in the elderly suggest that the elderly may not be more susceptible to gastrointestinal blood loss following the administration of NSAIDs.

The absence of symptoms does not rule out the possibility that significant gastrointestinal ulceration, hemorrhage, and/or perforation has occurred. Major life-threatening bleeds are common, especially in females who have been taking NSAIDs for months without any apparent gastrointestinal upset [25].

In order to avoid NSAID-induced gastropathy,

1. spend time educating the patient about the significance of dyspepsia or black stools. The patient may take this drug for life, so it is important to provide a warning not to take over-the-counter preparations such as aspirin or its derivatives for headaches, *etc.*, at the same time.
2. advise the patient to take the pills with milk or food and to drink a lot of water.

Practice Points

In practice, the choice between NSAIDs is largely empirical, because there is marked variation in response among different individuals. It is not possible to predict beforehand which patient will respond to a particular drug or who will get side effects. These simple rules should be followed:

1. Determine if the NSAID is really needed.
2. Do not add a second NSAID. (Anti-inflammatory effects are not additive, but the side effects often are.)
3. Start low and go slow with dosage.
4. Monitor all patients.
5. Be especially careful in the frail elderly with
   - congestive heart failure,
   - renal impairment,
   - hepatic impairment,
   - electrolyte abnormalities,
   - a history of gastrointestinal problems, or
   - hypoglycemic medications.
6. Give NSAIDs with milk or food, preferably early in the meal.
7. Consider a cytoprotective agent in patients with gastrointestinal problems.
8. Become very familiar with two or three NSAIDs.
9. Consider the addition of new drugs carefully.
10. Assume all drugs are toxic.
11. Start with half doses in older patients, especially with longer acting drugs.
12. Beware of new NSAIDs. They may not have been well studied in the elderly.
13. If in doubt, refer to a specialist.

Monitoring

Since NSAIDs are used so frequently, it is possible to become complacent when prescribing them. However, because of the risks of gastrointestinal, renal, hepatic, and hemopoietic effects, it is important to monitor for side effects. We recommend
   - CBC,
   - electrolytes,
   - urea, creatinine, and
   - liver enzymes,

either before an NSAID is started or before a change in dose is contemplated. These should be monitored monthly for the first few months and then every two to three months during maintenance therapy. Different patients may require different degrees of monitoring. Mrs. Rolland, because of the number of other complicating problems, should probably be followed up about every two or three weeks at the start. She should have blood work done at each visit. When and if she stabilizes on a maintenance dose, then it will be possible to lengthen the period between visits and blood work. Prospective trials of NSAIDs in 7000 patients reported 4.3% developed abnormal liver function test while taking NSAIDs [26].

Factors that increased the risk of hepatic dysfunction were
- congestive heart failure,
- advancing age of patient,
- patient on multiple drugs,
- duration of therapy, and
- presence of connective tissue disease, such as rheumatoid arthritis or systemic lupus.

Accordingly, liver function tests should be monitored, and the NSAID should be withdrawn if there is a significant elevation in liver enzymes, coagulation times, or bilirubin level. Slight elevations above the upper limit of normal can be followed fairly safely. If coagulation times are affected, the risk of gastrointestinal bleeding is further increased.

If Mrs. Rolland had these investigations done before the NSAID was started, it would have provided a valuable baseline. Now it will be very difficult to interpret an abnormal urea, creatinine, liver enzyme, or hemoglobin value. You may have to stop a very effective drug because you don't know what effects, if any, it had on a particular parameter.

Since these drugs are used frequently, it might be useful to recall each patient at regular intervals and check him or her. Plan this at the start and advise the patient why he or she must come back. If the patient understands the reasons for these precautions, compliance is likely to improve.

5. FALSE

Reversible depression of renal function is the most common renal complication of the NSAIDs. Although usually completely reversible within 24 to 72 hours following cessation of NSAID therapy, continued treatment can precipitate acute renal failure in some patients. NSAID renal toxicity is likely if there is an increase in serum creatinine, potassium, and body weight with a decrease in urine output.

Patients at increased risk for NSAID-induced renal insufficiency are those whose renal blood flow is being maintained by the action of vasodilatory prostaglandins and include those with

- reduced cardiac output such as that associated with congestive heart failure,
- renal ischemia due to low perfusion pressure,
- diuretic-induced hypovolemia,
- salt depletion,
- nephrotic syndrome,
- chronic renal failure, and
- hepatic disease with cirrhosis and ascites.

Mrs. Rolland is elderly and takes a diuretic for congestive heart failure. She also had renal impairment on routine renal function tests some months ago. Because of this, one should not ignore the finding of increased ankle edema. It may represent a significant deterioration in renal function.

If the furosemide is increased further at this point, it might decrease an already compromised renal blood flow and precipitate acute renal failure. Check her electrolytes, urea, creatinine, and CBC as soon as possible. You may even want to hold the NSAID until these results are available. In the elderly, there is a progressive decline in renal function, leading to an average decrease in GFR of 10 to 15 ml per min. per decade in individuals over 40 years of age. However, often this does not lead to an increase in baseline serum creatinine because creatinine production is lower due to loss of muscle mass with aging. Therefore, elderly patients can have normal serum creatinine in spite of a marked decrease in creatinine clearance. Poor renal reserve in the elderly increases their risk of NSAID toxicity. The Cockcroft-Gault equation can be used to estimate the true creatinine clearance [27].

$$Clearance \ = \ \frac{(140 - age) \times weight \ (kg)}{72 \times serum \ creatinine \ (mg/dl)}$$
$$(subtract \ 15\% \ in \ females)$$

Despite all of the potential problems with NSAIDs, they are very useful drugs in the treatment of arthritis [28]. Nonetheless, in the elderly, especially in those with other diseases and/or those taking other medications, NSAIDs must be used with caution.

REFERENCES

1. Baum C, Kennedy DL, Forbes MB: Utilization of nonsteroidal anti-inflammatory drugs. *Arthritis and Rheumatism* 28(6):686–692, 1985.
2. Kolodny AL, Klipper A: Final report on the cost of treating arthritic disease: Comparison between salicylates and nonsalicylate nonsteroidal anti-inflammatory drugs. *Seminars in Arthritis and Rheumatism* 14(3) (Supplement 1):20–24, 1985.
3. Brocklehurst JC: Geriatric services and the day hospital. *In* Brocklehurst JC (ed.): *Geriatric Medicine and Gerontology.* London and New York: Churchill Livingstone, 1978, p. 747.
4. Lawrence JS, De Graff R, Laine VA: Degenerative joint diseases in random samples of occupational groups. *In* Kellgren JH, Jeffrey MR, Ball J (eds.): *The Epidemiology of Chronic Rheumatism,* Vol. 1. Oxford: Blackwell Scientific, 1963, p. 98.
5. Ehrlich GE: Pathogenesis and treatment of osteoarthritis. *Comprehensive Ther* 5:36, 1979.
6. Ehrlich GE: Diagnosis and management of rheumatic diseases in older patients. *Journal American Geriatrics Society.* (Supplement to Vol. 30):S45–S51, 1982.
7. Mowat AG: Drug treatment of arthritis in the elderly. *Age and Ageing* 8 (Supplement), 1979.
8. Huskisson EC: Simple analgesics for arthritis. *Brit Med J* 4:196–200, 1974.
9. Kolodny AL, Klipper A: Final report on the cost of treating arthritic disease: Comparison between salicylates and nonsalicylate nonsteroidal anti-inflammatory drugs. *Seminars in Arthritis and Rheumatism* 14(3) (Supplement 1):20–24, 1985.
10. Schlegel SI, Paulus HE: Nonsteroidal and analgesic therapy in the elderly. *Clinics in Rheumatic Diseases* 12(1):245–273, April 1986.
11. Hurwitz N: Predisposing factors in adverse reactions to drugs. *British Medical Journal* 1:536–539, 1969.
12. Vestal RE: Drug use in the elderly: A review of problems and special considerations. *Drugs* 16:358–382, 1978.
13. Tandberg D: How to treat and prevent drug toxicity. *Geriatrics* 36(2) 64–73, 1981.

14. Williamson J, Choper JM: Adverse reactions to prescribed drugs in the elderly: A multicentre investigation. *Age and Ageing* 9:73–80, 1980.
15. Admani AK, Verma S: A study of sulindac versus ibuprofen in elderly patients with osteoarthritis. *Current Medical Research and Opinion* 8(5):315–320, 1983.
16. Gosh AJ, Rastogi AK: Symptomatic osteoarthritis in the elderly: A comparative study of sulindac and ibuprofen. *Current Medical Research and Opinion* 7 (Supplement):33–40, 1982.
17. Innes EH: Efficacy and tolerance of flurbiprofen in the elderly using liquid and tablet formulations. *Current Medical Research and Opinion* 5(1):122–128, 1977.
18. McMahon FG, Jain A, Onel A: Controlled evaluation of fenoprofen in geriatric patients with osteoarthritis. *Journal of Rheumatology* 3(2) (Supplement):76–82, 1976.
19. Hayes AH: Therapeutic implications of drug interactions with acetaminophen and aspirin. *Archives of Internal Medicine* 141:301–304, 1980.
20. Culpit GC: The use of nonprescription analgesics in an older population. *Journal of the American Geriatrics Society* 30(11) (Supplement):S76–S80, 1982.
21. Klotz U: Interactions of analgesics with other drugs. *American Journal of Medicine* 133–138, 1983.
22. Miller TA, Jacobson ED: Gastrointestinal cytoprotection by prostaglandins. *Gut* 20:75–87, 1979.
23. O'Brien WM: Pharmacology of nonsteroidal anti-inflammatory drugs: Practical review for clinicians. *American Journal of Medicine* 75 (Supplement):32–39, 1983.
24. Caruso I, Bianchi PG: Gastroscopic evaluation of anti-inflammatory agents. *British Medical Journal* 280:75–78, 1980.
25. Roth SH: Nonsteroidal anti-inflammatory drugs: Gastropathy, deaths, and medical practice. *Annals of Internal Medicine* 109:353–355, 1988.
26. Paulus HE: Government affairs: FDA arthritis advisory committee meeting. *Arthritis and Rheumatism* 25:1124, 1982.
27. Cockcroft DW, Gault MH: Prediction of creatinine clearance from serum creatinine. *Nephron* 16:31, 1976.
28. Pelletier JP, Martel-Pellitier J: The therapeutic effects of NSAIDs and corticosteroids in osteoarthritis: To be or not to be. *Jour of Rheumatology* 16:266, 1989.

22 | TRICYCLIC ANTIDEPRESSANTS

CASE PRESENTATION

Mrs. B., a 76-year-old female, presents eight months following the sudden death of her husband from myocardial infarction. She complains of insomnia for the past four months, with restlessness and early-morning wakening. She feels that she did not phone for an ambulance quickly enough when her husband complained of chest pain, which he felt was due to indigestion. Mrs. B. has experienced a loss of appetite, which she associates with the presence of occasional morning nausea and diarrhea, and disinterest in cooking and housekeeping, which she feels is due to no longer having anyone to look after. Over the past three months she has lost 7.5 kg. On direct inquiry, Mrs. B. does not admit to being depressed, but acknowledges that she does frequently feel "blue" and disappointed. She also agrees that she feels nervous and, particularly in the earlier part of the day, while thinking of her husband, she has brief, uncontrollable crying spells.

In review of her past history, Mrs. B. denies any history of depression but recalls that she had similar sleep problems and discouraged feelings during a two-year period following the accidental death of her son, 18 years previously. She also denies any family history of alcoholism or any psychiatric disorder.

J.S. Kennedy
M. Rodway-Norman

Past medical history, systemic inquiry, physical exam, and laboratory evaluation including EKG, SMAC, thyroid evaluation, and urinalysis are unremarkable.

Consider the following statements (true or false)

1. Untreated depression in the elderly has a good prognosis.

2. The tricyclics lengthen cardiac conduction time and should be used with caution in the presence of bundle branch block.

3. Nortriptyline is less likely to cause postural hypotension than amitriptyline or imipramine.

4. Anticholinergic effects of tricyclics may impair memory and cause or worsen confusion.

5. Nortriptyline has a "therapeutic window" that can usually be reached with doses of 10 to 40 mg in the elderly.

1. FALSE

Mrs. B. has sufficient symptomatology to justify the diagnosis of major depression. Depression within the geriatric population is a very common problem, presenting principally to the primary-care physician. This disorder is associated with significant morbidity and mortality within the elderly, with a reported one-year mortality of 11% for women and 19% for men [1]. Effective treatment, although often not simple, is available. Yet depression is suggested to be under-recognized and often, when recognized, undertreated or inappropriately treated [2]. Particularly in the elderly, depression left untreated or inadequately treated can result in a fatal outcome [3].

Before establishing a course of treatment, the physician should be reasonably sure that the patient does indeed suffer from a major affective disorder, depression. This is not always simple when assessing the older patient. Not only do some patients with a true depression deny dysphoric mood, but depression can present in an unusual fashion in the elderly, with the primary complaint being perceived cognitive impairment, anxiety, somatic concerns, or simply unease [4,5]. Nonetheless, reliance on the biological symptoms of depression (Table 22-1) serve as

Table 22-1   Symptoms and Signs of Depression.

Biological
1. Significant weight loss and/or decreased oral intake secondary to decreased appetite.
2. Fatigue or loss of energy, most pronounced in the morning.
3. Observed psychomotor agitation such as pacing, hand-wringing, or psychomotor retardation, (i.e., decreased spontaneous motor activity).
4. Disrupted sleep architecture, as manifested by initial, middle, or terminal insomnia.

Psychological
1. Depressed mood.
2. Feelings of guilt or worthlessness.
3. Impaired ability to think or concentrate.
4. Thoughts of death and/or suicidal ideation and/or intent.

Social
1. Significantly decreased interest in or participation in usual activities, for example, withdrawal from social engagements.

Source: *Diagnostic and Statistical Manual III-R.* Washington, D.C.: American Psychiatric Association, pp. 218–224, 1987.

Table 22-2   Rank-Ordered Antidepressant Receptor Binding.

1 = most binding; 7 = least binding

Antidepressant	Acetylcholine Muscarinic	Alpha-1 Adrenergic	Alpha-2 Adrenergic	Dopamine
Amitriptyline	1	3	3	3
Trimipramine	2	1	2	1
Doxepine	3	1	4	2
Imipramine	4	7	6	?
Nortriptyline	5	5	5	4
Desipramine	6	6	7	5
Trazodone	7	4	1	6

Source: Richelson E, Nelson A: *J Pharm and Exp Therapeutics* 230:(1), pp. 94–102, 1985.

a diagnostic aid, as well as a prognostic marker for those likely to respond to antidepressant therapy [6].

Treatment

Tricyclic antidepressants are the current choice of medication in the treatment of the nonpsychotic, nonsuicidal, depressed elderly patient. Because within-class differences in efficacy have not been demonstrated, the selection of an agent is based upon issues of safety and side-effect profile, which do vary within this class of medications [7]. The safety and side-effect profile of an agent is predicated by its effects on various neurochemical systems (Table 22-2), which in the elderly most relevantly are seen to involve important adrenergic influences on the cardiovascular system and cholinergic influences on the central and elements of the peripheral nervous system [8].

2. TRUE

Cardiac Effects

Concerns about detrimental inotropic effects, exacerbation of arrhythmias, and conduction defects arise in the use of tricyclic antidepressants in the elderly. Most reports of decreased ventricular performance have been associated with overdosages. At least one study has reported no impairment of left ventricular function using radionucleotide studies in patients within the therapeutic range [9]. Some tricyclics, such as imipramine, also have a quinidine-like action and, within a normal therapeutic range, suppress ectopic activity [10]. This effect may benefit patients with VPBs. Despite claims of the improved cardiovascular profile of some agents as compared to others, this has not been well established [11].

The tricyclics lengthen cardiac conduction time; this effect is of importance in the treatment of patients with conduction defects. Roose noted the aggravation of bundle branch block progressing to complete heart block in 3 out of 24 patients within the therapeutic range [12]. Pre-existing bundle branch disease demands extreme caution, and a P-R interval of greater than 0.20 is an indication for serial EKG monitoring as dosages are increased. If progression of the P-R interval is noted, the physician should consider discontinuing the medication and referral for alternative therapy such as ECT.

In summary, those patients with pre-existing cardiovascular disease demand a careful evaluation, but adverse effects are less than previously thought.

3. TRUE

Postural Hypotension

Postural hypotension is a common reason for terminating a trial of antidepressants within the elderly, and occurs much more frequently than in younger patients [13]. Severity of orthostatic hypotension is suggested to be greater with pre-existent cardiovascular disease [13], more likely to occur in the presence of other medications, and to present in the first six weeks of treatment, and is not readily predicted [14]. Orthostatic hypotension is unpleasant, if symptomatic, and has been associated with myocardial infarctions and falls [13,15]. It is therefore prudent to monitor serially an older patient's supine and standing blood pressure and take preventative steps to reduce its occurrence. It is good practice to advise adequate fluid and salt intake, and for the patient to rise slowly from a prone or sitting position. The physician should also reduce or eliminate other medications that also cause orthostatic hypotension. If clinically significant orthostatic hypotension persists, then Ted stockings worn during the day may help. In addition 50 to 250 µg of Florinef per day may be given [16].

In the prevention and management of postural hypotension, the antidepressant chosen is often the most important determinant of successful therapy. Nortriptyline has less postural hypotension than amitriptyline and imipramine [17], while desipramine may be better tolerated than imipramine, amitriptyline, doxepin, or trimipramine. Dosages should be increased slowly in a step-wise fashion, and be given as single dosages at night.

4. TRUE

CNS Anticholinergic Side Effects

Dry mouth (xerostomia), blurred vision, constipation, and urinary hesitancy may occur in any patient, as a result of peripheral muscarinic blockade; these problems are more frequent and often more serious for the elderly, aggravating pre-existing conditions, such as prostatic hypertrophy or slowed gut transit time, and leading to urinary retention or paralytic ileus [8]. These risks can be minimized by the use of agents with lesser anticholinergic activity (Table 22-2) [16]. Desipramine, nortriptyline, maprotiline, and trazodone exhibit a low anticholinergic profile. Anticholinergic side effects are not well correlated with dose, and, therefore, increasing the dose may not make them worse [8].

Central anticholinergic blockade, particularly in the elderly population, causes difficulties with memory. At even low dosages, an acute confusional state may occur, characterized by confusion (disorientation for person, place, and time), anxiety, and agitation. If severe, visual and auditory hallucinations, hyperpyrexia, myoclonus, convulsions and coma may ensue. Peripheral signs of anticholinergic toxicity, such as increased temperature, heart rate, and blood pressure, may be helpful in diagnosis but are not always present [16]. Selection of an agent such as nortriptyline, which has less anticholinergic activity than other tricyclics, may minimize this risk.

Sedation, a frequent side effect of tricyclics, may help insomnia. Unfortunately, sedative effects of tricyclics such as amitriptyline frequently extend into the day and produce excessive daytime drowsiness. The sedative effects of different tricyclic antidepressants vary widely, and the physician's choice of an agent can minimize unwanted daytime sedation. Secondary amines such as nortriptyline or desipramine are frequently effective in assisting sleep at night and show less propensity to produce daytime sedation [8].

If use of a sedating antidepressant is unavoidable, it is often helpful to recall that this side effect is most pronounced immediately after a dose increase and lessens during the first few weeks. Reassurance to a patient that this effect will diminish may enable the patient to tolerate sedation until it becomes less troublesome.

Dosage

A clinical impression that low doses are indicated within the older population is supported by physiologic considerations. Changes in distribution, metabolism, and elimination would all suggest lower doses be used within the elderly; and particularly for the tertiary amines, this appears to be true [19]. Studies indicate that for secondary amines (nortriptyline and desipramine) this may not hold [20]. The rule "start low, go slow" does not imply that under all circumstances dosages should end up low. Antidepressants should not be given in inadequate doses. If necessary, the medication chosen should be prescribed until limits imposed by side effects are reached, a usual adult dose is achieved, or response occurs.

5. TRUE

Serum Levels

Serum levels of the drug are useful in determining compliance, the presence of potentially toxic concentrations of drug, and the adequacy of a drug trial. Nortriptyline is the sole agent studied in the elderly which has been demonstrated to have a "therapeutic window" of 50 to 140 ng/ml [21]. The usual oral dose range required to reach this serum level is 10 to 40 mg, but some patients may require considerably larger dosages. Blood sampling should be done 7 to 10 days after a dose increase, in the morning, prior to the patient receiving a morning dose. Sampling at this time allows determination of the trough level, which, if in the therapeutic window, predicts an adequate clinical trial [11]. For all tricyclic antidepressants, serum levels on a given dose vary widely from individual to individual. Serum antidepressant levels are also useful in the identification of potentially toxic blood levels in asymptomatic individuals [21]. Should a patient develop symptoms and signs that might be manifestations of toxicity, a serum level may indicate high levels and thus serve as a justification to reduce dose further. The practitioner using serum levels has the advantage of ensuring that the difficulty lies with overdose and not with the selected agent. Similarly, a lack of response to a given agent after a three- to four-week length of time (at a therapeutic oral dosage) may be due to high clearance and resulting low serum levels, which serum levels will identify.

SUMMARY

Successful treatment of depression within the elderly population frequently requires the physician to adhere to a rational therapeutic plan that proceeds in a step-wise fashion and that starts with proper diagnosis. Use of the medication nortriptyline may be the first line of therapy due to its equivalent efficacy to other agents, lower side-effect profile, and available therapeutic window for efficacy monitoring.

Amitriptyline should be avoided; its role in therapy of depression on the elderly, if any, awaits further clarification because of its adverse side-effect profile.

REFERENCES

1. Murphy E: The prognosis of depression in old age. *Br J of Psychiatry* 142:111–119, 1983.
2. Keller MB, Kerman GL, Lavori PW, *et al.*: Treatment received by depressed patients. *JAMA* 248:1848–1855, 1982.
3. Murphy E, Smith R, Lindesay J, Slattery J: Increased mortality rates in late life depression. *Br J of Psychiatry 152:347–353, 1988.*
4. Leongotas A, Cooper T, Kim M, Hapworth W: The treatment of affective disorder in the elderly. *Psychopharmacology Bulletin* 19(2):226–236, 1988.
5. Bergman K: Neurosis and personality disorders in old age. *In* Isaccs AD, Post F (eds.), *Studies in Geriatric Psychiatry.* Chichester: Wiley, 41–75, 1978.
6. Klein DF: Endogenomorphic depression: A conceptual and terminologic revision. *Arch Gen Psychiatry* 31:442–454, 1974.
7. Jenike MA: *Handbook of Geriatric Psychopharmacology.* Littleton, MA: PSG Publishing, 1985.
8. Glassman AH, Carino JS, Roose SP: *Frontiers in Biochemical and Pharmacological Research in Depression.* E Usdin, *et al.* (eds.), New York: Raven Press, 1984.
9. Veith RC, Raskind, MA, Coldwell JH, *et al.*: Cardiovascular effects of tricyclic antidepressants in depressed patients with chronic heart disease. *New Engl J of Med* 306:954–959, 1982.
10. Giordina EGV, Bigger JT, Jr, Glassman AH, Paul JM, Kantor SJ: The electrocardiographic and antiarrhythmic effect of imipramine hydrochloride at therapeutic plasma levels. *Circulation* 60:1045–1052.
11. Luctins DJ. Review of clinical and animal studies composing the cardiovasculaar effects of doxepin and other tricyclic antidepressants. *Am J Psych* 140:1006–1009, 1983.

12. Roose Sp, Glassman AH, Siris S, Walsh BT, Wonding S, Bigger JT: Tricyclic antidepressants in depressed patients with cardiac conduction disease. *Arch Gen Psych* 44:273–275, 1987.
13. Muller DF, Londman N, Bellet S: The hypotensive effects of imipramine hydrochloride in patients with cardiovascular disease. *Clin Pharmacol Ther* 2:300–307, 1961.
14. Glassman AH, Walsh BT, Roose SP, Rosenfeld R, Bruno RL, Bigger JT, Jr, Giordina EGV: Factors related to orthostatic hypotension associated with tricyclic antidepressants. *J Clin Psych* 43:35–38, 1982.
15. Glassman AH, Bigger JT, Jr, Giordina EGV, Kanter SJ, Parel JM, Davies M: Clinical characteristics of imipramine-induced orthostatic hypotension. *Lancet* 1:468–472, 1979.
16. Pollack MH, Rosenbaum JF: Management of antidepressant-induced side-effects: A practical guide for the clinician. *J Clin Psych* 48(1) 3–8, 1987.
17. Roose SP, Glassman AH, Sinn SL, Walsh BT, Bruno RL, Wright LB: Comparison of imipramine and nortriptyline-induced orthostatic hypotension: of meaningful

difference. *J Clin Psychopharm* 1:316–319, 1981.

18. Van der Kolk BA, Shader RI, Grumblatter DJ: Autonomic effects of psychotropic drugs. *In* Lipton MA, DiMascio A, Killman KF (eds.), *Psychoharmacology: A Generation of Progress.* New York: Raven Press, 1978.

19. Preskorn SH, Mac DS: Plasma levels of amitriptyline: Effect of age and sex. *J Clin Psych* 46:276–277, 1985.

20. Kocsis JH, Hanin I, Bowden C, Brunswick D: Imipramine and amitriptyline plasma concentrations and clinical response in major depression. *Br J of Psych* 148:52–57, 1986.

21. Task Force on the Use of Laboratory Tests in Psychiatry. Tricyclic antidepressants–blood level developments and clinical outcome: an APA task force report. *Am J Psych* 142(2):155–162, 1985.

22. *Diagnostic and Statistical Manual III-R.* Washington, D.C.: American Psychiatric Association, pp. 218–224, 1987.

23 | HYPNOTICS

CASE PRESENTATION

A frail 80-year-old woman with a history of arthralgias, hypertension, constipation, and insomnia was brought by her family to the Emergency Department in a confused state. Her present medications included hydrochlorothiazide 25 mg daily, milk of magnesia 30 ml daily, acetaminophen 650 mg four times daily when needed, and flurazepam 15 to 30 mg at bedtime when needed. The family described a fairly recent onset of CNS symptoms, with a notable worsening in the last few days. The patient was admitted to the Geriatric Assessment Unit for observation. Forty-eight hours later the patient, now quite lucid, admitted that she had increased her flurazepam dose to 30 mg at bedtime for five nights prior to admission because her arthritic pain had worsened and she was having difficulty falling asleep. Flurazepam, which had been held since admission, was discontinued; and the patient was prescribed triazolam 0.25 mg at bedtime. Approximately one hour after her first dose, the patient became disoriented and agitated and attempted to leave the hospital. The patient was placed in bed with the siderails up and fell asleep approximately 30 minutes later. Upon awakening the following morning, the patient was unable to recall any events of the previous evening.

K.W. Hall
C. Sochasky

Consider the following statements (true or false)

1. The patient's presenting symptoms of somnolence and confusion were likely related to the flurazepam she was receiving as a bedtime hypnotic.

2. The elderly are susceptible to adverse effects of drugs because of physiologic changes, associated with aging, which alter the pharmacokinetic handling of drugs and the pharmacodynamic response to drugs.

3. The choice of triazolam as a replacement for flurazepam was a reasonable decision that can be justified in this patient on the basis of triazolam's different pharmacokinetic properties.

4. The syndrome of agitation, disorientation, and subsequent amnesia, which followed the first dose of triazolam, has been previously reported as an infrequent side effect of triazolam.

5. In the elderly, dependence and withdrawal reactions are more commonly encountered with benzodiazepines than with non-benzodiazepine sedative/hypnotics; therefore, other drugs such as chloral hydrate are preferred for use in these patients.

1. TRUE

In this particular case the patient's history of a recent increase in flurazepam dosage, and her improvement in CNS function following temporary discontinuation of the drug, strongly supports the implication of flurazepam as the cause of the recent CNS deterioration. Central nervous system depression is the most commonly encountered side effect of benzodiazepine therapy. In fact, it is the only adverse effect that studies have consistently documented to occur more frequently with benzodiazepines than with placebo controls [1]. The elderly are particularly susceptible to the CNS depressant effects of benzodiazepines, as demonstrated by a two-fold increase in adverse effects in those over 70 years of age as compared to those under 40 [2]. The typical adverse effects seen in the elderly—ataxia, sedation, slurred speech, confusion—are often regarded as symptoms of advancing age, and insufficient consideration may be given to drug-related causes of the CNS deterioration. The differentiation of drug intoxication from other causes of deteriorating cognitive function may require dosage reduction or temporary discontinuation of the suspected drug, followed by careful observation of the patient for signs of improvement.

The type of benzodiazepine the patient was receiving also supports the hypothesis that the patient's CNS depression was drug related. Flurazepam is classed as a long-acting benzodiazepine because its active metabolite, desmethylflurazepam, has a very long half-life of 50 to 100 hours, leading to drug accumulation with repeated doses. Accordingly the manufacturer recommends that the initial dose in the elderly should not exceed 15 mg, and most authors agree that flurazepam is rarely indicated in the elderly [3]. Flurazepam may be acceptable for the elderly patient who requires a hypnotic on a very infrequent basis, but otherwise this drug should be avoided.

2. TRUE

Aging is accompanied by many alterations in cellular function that are manifested as the physiologic changes of aging. Alterations in drug absorption, distribution, metabolism, and excretion are known to occur with aging [4]. Many underlying physiologic perturbations have been identified as contributing to these changes, including altered gastric pH, gastric emptying time, intestinal absorptive surface area, hepatic blood flow, hepatic cellular function, renal blood flow, renal tubular function, drug–protein binding, and ratio of body lipid to water content. There may also be changes in the pharmacodynamics of drug action in the elderly resulting from changes in drug receptor binding in the central nervous system, though such changes are difficult to quantify. The end result of these pharmacokinetic and pharmacodynamic changes is that the elderly usually are more susceptible to the adverse effects of these centrally acting psychoactive drugs [5]. It is therefore recommended that the starting dose be reduced to one-third or one-half that of the starting dose for younger adults and the patient's response be carefully observed before the dosage is increased further [3].

3. TRUE

Benzodiazepines vary in their pharmacokinetic properties (Table 23-1). The short-acting benzodiazepines are considered to be the drugs of choice for elderly patients who require hypnotics on a frequent basis [3,6]. Benzodiazepines with short half-lives of 8 hours or less result in fewer residual daytime sequelae, such as lethargy and confusion, than do the agents with longer half-lives. For example, triazolam with a half-life of 2 to 5 hours has been associated with fewer residual cognitive defects in the geriatric population than flurazepam, which has a half-life

Table 23-1 Benzodiazepines Used as Hypnotics.

Agent	Half-life (hr)	Onset of Action (hr)	Approximate Equivalent Oral Dose (mg)	Dosage Recommended in the Elderly
Long-acting				
Flurazepam	50–100	0.5–1	15	15 mg hs
Diazepam	20–100	0.5–1	5	2.5–5 mg hs
Intermediate-acting				
Lorazepam	10–20	1–2	1	1–2 mg hs
Temazepam	10–15	1–3	15	15 mg hs
Bromazepam	8–19	1–4	3	1.5 mg hs
Short-acting				
Triazolam	2–5	0.5–1	0.25	0.125–0.25 mg hs
Oxazepam	5–11	1–2	15	10–15 mg hs

of 50 to 100 hours [7]. Therefore, triazolam was, on the basis of its shorter half-life, a reasonable choice for this elderly patient who seemed to be suffering from flurazepam-related impairment of CNS function.

An alternative choice in the benzodiazepine class of drugs would have been oxazepam. Oxazepam, like triazolam, is a short-acting benzodiazepine with a half-life in the range of 5 to 11 hours. Oxazepam may, however, have a disadvantage in some elderly patients because of its slower onset of action, 1 to 2 hours, as compared to 1/2 to 1 hour for triazolam [8]. For patients receiving scheduled hypnotic therapy, this can be overcome by administering oxazepam approximately 1 hour before bedtime. Those patients who take a sleeping pill only when they have difficulty falling asleep may, however, find oxazepam to be too slow acting.

Equally important and often overlooked, as portrayed in this patient, is the recognition and elimination of other factors that may be contributing to the insomnia, such as pain, depression, or organic brain syndrome. More appropriate treatment with analgesics, antidepressants, or major tranquilizers can often eliminate or reduce the need for a hypnotic.

4. TRUE

Triazolam was a reasonable choice to replace flurazepam in this elderly patient, but there are several side effects associated with triazolam that the clinician should be aware of. There have been several reports of rather severe CNS dysfunction following triazolam, though the overall incidence of such a reaction is probably very low. In one report, two patients were reported to develop visual and tactile hallucinations with anterograde amnesia after ingesting triazolam [9]. In another report, five patients developed a syndrome characterized by reversible delirium, automatic movement, and anterograde amnesia [10].

Acute behavioral disturbances have also been reported for other benzodiazepines; but it appears that rapidly absorbed agents, like triazolam, are more likely to induce such a reaction than are more slowly absorbed, slower onset drugs such as oxazepam [11,12]. Though it is probably quite rare in occurrence, the clinician should be alert to the possibility that acute CNS dysfunction, such as that which occurred in our elderly patient, may be related to triazolam.

Rebound insomnia is a more commonly encountered side effect of short-acting hypnotics like triazolam. Since triazolam is rapidly eliminated, some patients experience early morning awakening due to a withdrawal phenomenon [6]. This rebound insomnia may be trouble-some for some patients, necessitating the use of a longer-acting agent.

5. FALSE

Dependence and withdrawal reactions have been reported to occur with benzodiazepine therapy, but the incidence and severity is much less than that attributed to the barbiturates and is probably also less than that seen with chloral hydrate [13]. Even when physical dependence has been reported with benzodiazepines, it has usually resulted from abuse of large doses of these drugs for prolonged periods of time. Furthermore, the withdrawal syndrome is usually less severe with benzodiazepines than with barbiturates, meprobamate, glutethimide, methyprylon, and other similar sedative/hypnotics [13]. With respect to benzodiazepines, the severity of withdrawal symptoms is greater with short-acting agents because longer-acting agents, which are slowly eliminated from the body, partly achieve their own withdrawal. It has been noted that despite the widespread use of benzodiazepines, the overall frequency and severity of dependence is gratifyingly low.

There are few circumstances where other hypnotic agents would be considered to be superior to benzodiazepines. Table 23-2 provides a comparative profile of the available hypnotics; the relative disadvantages of other drugs are evident. There is little or no justification for the use of barbiturates, methaqualone, glutethimide, or methyprylon except perhaps for a patient who has been taking these drugs for an extended period of time with minimal side effects.

Chloral hydrate is still considered by some clinicians to be an excellent choice for use in the elderly. It has a rapid onset of action, an intermediate duration of action, and is inexpensive. Its disadvantages include the frequent development of tolerance to its hypnotic effects when used on a chronic basis, its gastric irritant effect, and its potential to interact with other drugs such as warfarin.

Antihistamines, such as diphenhydramine or hydroxyzine, have been used as hypnotics. These drugs cause sedation and thus can be effective in reducing the time to fall asleep. They do not appear to be effective in maintaining sleep, however, and the anticholinergic side effects of these drugs generally prohibit their use in the elderly. These side effects include constipation, urinary retention, anticholinergic delirium, and general impairment of cognitive functioning.

In summary, benzodiazepines are considered by many clinicians to be the drug of choice in the elderly patient with insomnia. The available benzodiazepines vary in their onset and duration of action, and this provides a rationale for selection of different agents. In general the short-acting benzodiazepines are preferred for use as hypnotics, though the drawbacks of short-acting agents, such as rebound insomnia, also need to be recognized. Chloral hydrate represents a reasonable alternative to benzodiazepines in some patients. Its use should probably be restricted to patients with mild insomnia and those who require hypnotic medication on an infrequent basis.

REFERENCES

1. Greenblatt DJ, Shader RI, Divoli M, *et al.*: Adverse reactions to triazolam, flurazepam and placebo in controlled clinical trials. *J Clin Psychiatry* 45:192–195, 1984.
2. Boston Collaborative Drug Surveillance Program—Boston University Medical Center. Clinical depression of the central nervous system due to diazepam and chlordiazepoxide in relation to cigarette smoking and age. *NEJM* 288(6): 277–280, February 8, 1973.
3. Allen RM: Tranquilizers and sedative/hypnotics: Appropriate use in the elderly. *Geriatrics* 44:75–88, 1986.
4. Cohen JL: Pharmacokinetic changes in aging. *Am J Med* 80 (Suppl 5A) 31–38, 1986.
5. Reidenberg MM, Levy M, *et al.*: Relationship between diazepam dose, plasma level, age, and central nervous system depression. *Clin Pharmacol Ther* 23:371–374, 1978.
6. Fancourt G, Castelden M: The use of benzodiazepines with particular reference to the elderly. *Br J Hosp Med* 35(5): 321–326, 1986.
7. Carskadon MA, Seidel WF, Greenblatt DJ: Daytime carryover of triazolam and flurazepam in elderly insomniacs. *Sleep* 5:361–367, 1982.
8. Ban JA, Brown WJ, Da Silva T, *et al.*: Therapeutic monograph on anxiolytic-sedative drugs. *CMAJ* 124:1439–1446, 1981.
9. Einarson TR, Yoder ES: Triazolam psychosis—A syndrome? *Drug Intell Clin Pharm* 16:330, 1982.
10. Patterson JT: Triazolam syndrome in the elderly. *South Med J* 80(11): 1425–1426, (November) 1987.
11. Soldatos CR, Kales A, Boxler EO, *et al.*: Behavioral side effects of benzodiazepine hypnotics. *Clin Neuropharmacol* 8:S112–S117, 1983.
12. Rickels K, Schweizer E, Lucki I: Benzodiazepine side effects. In *Psychiatry: American Psychiatric Association Annual Review*, R Hales (ed.), Washington, D.C.: American Psychiatric Press, 1987.
13. Hollister LE: Psychiatric disorders. In *Avery's Drug Treatment: Principles and Practice of Clinical Pharmacology and Therapeutics*, 3rd Edition. M Speight (ed.), Auckland: ADIS Press Ltd., 1987.

Table 23-2 Attributes of Available Hypnotic Drugs.

Drug	Effectivenesss with short-term use	Effectiveness with long-term use	Residual day time sedation	Habituation, physical dependence	Comments
1. Flurazepam	Yes	Yes	Yes	Slight	Long acting, not usually recommended for elderly.
2. Triazolam	Yes	Yes	No	Slight	Very short acting, recommended for elderly. Disadvantage: rebound insomnia.
3. Oxazepam	Yes	Yes	No	Slight	Short acting, recommended for elderly. Disadvantage: slow onset.
4. Chloral hydrate	Yes	No	No	Yes	Recommended for elderly. Disadvantages: tolerance to hypnotic effects, ineffective in some patients, interaction with anticoagulants.
5. Barbiturates	Yes	No	Yes	Yes	Not recommended for elderly. Disadvantages: tolerance and addiction.
6. Methaqualone	Yes	No	Yes	Yes	Not recommended for elderly. Disadvantages: tolerance and addiction.
7. Glutethimide	Yes	No	Yes	Yes	Not recommended for elderly. Disadvantages: tolerance and addiction.
8. Methyprylon	Yes	No	Yes	Yes	Not recommended for elderly. Disadvantages: tolerance and addiction.
9. Diphenhydramine	Yes	No	No	No	Not recommended for elderly. Disadvantages: anticholinergic side effects.
10. Hydroxyzine	Yes	No	Yes	No	Not recommended for elderly. Disadvantages: anticholinergic side effects.

Part IV

INFECTIONS

24 | ASYMPTOMATIC BACTERIURIA

CASE PRESENTATION

A nurse in an acute care hospital calls you because an 84-year-old woman with a stroke has a positive urine culture. *Escherichia coli* was cultured from a mid-stream urine sample taken a few days before. The sample was taken when the staff noted the urine was dark and cloudy.

Mrs. R has been an inpatient for three months and is almost fully independent, continent, and does not have a urinary catheter in situ. Dysuria and hematuria are not present, although she has frequency which is long-standing. She is apyrexic, her white blood cell count is 6900, and she has a normal differential. Routine and microscopic urinalysis reveal 5 red blood cells and 10 white blood cells (WBCs) per high-power field. Bladder emptying is normal and the intravenous pyelogram performed recently was normal with no reflux or significant residual volume post-voiding. The *E. coli* is sensitive to cotrimoxazole and ampicillin.

L. Ramage
D.W. Molloy

Consider the following statements (true or false)

1. Asymptomatic bacteriuria occurs in approximately 20% to 25% of institutionalized elderly over the age of 70 years.
2. Appropriate management of the patient is to administer a 10- to 14-day course of cotrimoxazole.
3. One month later, the patient's urine becomes cloudy and foul-smelling. She is apyrexic and has persistent frequency. Results show 100 X 10^6 per liter of *Klebsiella pneumoniae*, resistant to ampicillin, cotrimoxazole, and nitrofurantoin, and sensitive to cephalothin, amikacin, and tobramycin. Appropriate management is to administer tobramycin for about two weeks.
4. Two months later, the patient develops a temperature of 37.8°C. Other causes for fever have been ruled out. Frequency is still persistent, and her urine remains cloudy, foul-smelling, and sensitive to tobramycin, amikacin, and cephalothin. A 10- to 14-day course of tobramycin or intravenous (IV) amikacin is worthwhile.
5. After two weeks of treatment, a repeat urine culture and sensitivity shows greater than 100 X 10^6 per liter of *Serratia marcescens* resistant to all antibiotics except amikacin. The patient has frequency, occasionally cloudy and foul urine, and a normal temperature. Appropriate management is amikacin IV for six weeks.

1. TRUE

Asymptomatic bacteriuria is common in the elderly. It may be defined as colony counts greater than 100,000 organisms per ml of urine without previous or current manifestations of infection, and the same results occurring in two consecutive samples [1].

Bacteriuria affects 6% of the elderly (2.4% of men and 9% of women over age 70) [2]. In institutions, bacteriuria affects 20% to 50% of patients over age 70. The rates may be as high as 68% in women and as low as 9% in men over age 68. Institutions such as hospitals, nursing homes, and long-term care facilities house patients who harbor many organisms and serve as reservoirs. The organisms are spread to other patients via the hands of hospital/nursing home personnel. Many institutionalized elderly have indwelling catheters, which increase the bacteriuric rate of the population [3–6].

2. FALSE

There is no apparent benefit in prompt antibiotic treatment of asymptomatic bacteriuria [3,7]. Antibiotics should be used only when the patient has a temperature, known ureterovesical reflux, gross hematuria, or specific symptoms related to the urinary tract that are recent in onset (including incontinence) and cannot be managed by simple basic measures [8–10]. Do not use antibiotics routinely in patients with asymptomatic bacteriuria.

Treatment involves initiating measures to increase the patient's fluid intake. Ensure that the patient is eating an adequate diet to promote proper nutrition. Evaluate patient-care practices. Does the patient use a bedpan? If so, encourage the use of a commode chair, which will facilitate bladder emptying. Observe the toilet habits of women. Teach them to wipe from front to back to reduce the risk of infection [11–15]. Incontinent patients should have a regular toilet program. Allow enough time to adjust and develop this as a habit. Evaluate the effectiveness of these measures once they are in place [6,16–17].

Anticholinergic agents administered in small doses may reduce incontinence, but may increase confusion in some patients and worsen their incontinence. Do not prescribe them at random unless urodynamic studies have been performed, because they may cause retention. Parasympathomimetic agents may help patients with retention or incomplete bladder emptying [17].

Indwelling catheters should be used as a last resort because they increase the risk of urinary tract infections (UTI). Almost all elderly patients develop UTI after catheters have been in place for 14 days or longer [11,12,15,17]. Consider using intermittent catheterization to increase blood supply to the bladder and reduce residual volumes of urine and overdistention of the bladder [6,17,18].

Intermittent catheterization does not reduce bacteriuria, but decreases the incidence of clinical UTI. Patients with asymptomatic bacteriuria managed on intermittent catheterization do not develop renal damage or septicemia at a different rate from those whose bacteriuria is treated. The administration of antibiotics increases the patient's risk of acquiring resistant organisms [7–10].

3. FALSE

It is common for bladder flora to change in a patient with bacteriuria, even if he or she has not received an antibiotic. Mrs. R's bladder flora changed from a sensitive *E. coli* to a more inherently resistant *Klebsiella pneumoniae*. The patient shows no signs or symptoms of infection that are recent in onset, and basic measures should be tried first before antibiotics are used [3,4,19,20].

The indiscriminate use of antibiotics causes superinfections with more resistant strains of bacteria. There is a strong likelihood that this patient had received antibiotics previously, which increased her risk for acquiring multiresistant organisms [5,8,9,21,22].

4. TRUE

The patient is symptomatic, and therefore should be treated. Other reasons for the increased temperature, such as pneumonia, have been ruled out. Draw blood cultures when temperature is elevated to rule out bacteremia.

Start therapy with ampicillin and tobramycin immediately prior to results of a urine culture, and continue with a strong antibiotic. In this case, tobramycin or amikacin IV should be given to cover the gram-negative organism *Klebsiella pneumoniae* [23].

Further investigations, such as cystoscopies and repeated urodynamic studies, may be warranted.

5. FALSE

Mrs. R's symptoms are not recent in onset, and management of the bacteriuria should involve following the simple, basic measures before the use of antimicrobial agents is instituted [9,24,25].

If Mrs. R's bacteriuria is left untreated, the multiresistant *Serratia marcescens* may disappear entirely on its own. It may take weeks or years for the bladder flora to change, or the patient may remain colonized with this multiresistant organism.

However, Mrs. R is a threat to other patients because she harbors an organism resistant to all aminoglycosides except amikacin. *Serratia marcescens* carries plasmids that have the ability to transfer intracellular information onto other microorganisms. Not only can *Serratia* be passed on to other patients, but the resistance pattern can be passed on to all of the sensitive organisms in other patients [22,24].

Staff must wash their hands following patient contact. Gloves must be worn when handling urine or any equipment or material that may be contaminated with urine. Any equipment (bed pan, urine measuring cups) used on Mrs. R that may be contaminated must be disinfected with a sodium hypochlorite solution (one part household bleach to nine parts water).

It is important to ensure Mrs. R is not in a room with patients who are catheterized or at high risk for acquiring infections. In some cases, moving the patient to a private room is the most appropriate solution [1,9,21,22,24–28].

REFERENCES

1. Center for Disease Control: Outline for surveillance and control of nosocomial infections. United States Department of Health and Human Services, Atlanta, 1972.
2. Nordenstam GR: Bacteriuria and mortality in an elderly population. *New Engl J Med* 314:18, 1986.
3. Nicolle LE, *et al.*: Bacteriuria in elderly institutionalized men. *New Engl J Med* 309:1420, 1983.
4. Boscia J, *et al.*: Epidemiology of bacteriuria in an elderly ambulatory population. *Am J Med* 80:208, 1986.
5. Warren JW, *et al.*: Antibiotic irrigation and catheter-associated urinary tract infections. *New Engl J Med* 299:540, 1978.
6. *The American Practitioners' Infection Control Curriculum for Infection Control Practice.* Dubuque, Iowa: Kendall/Hunt, 1983.
7. Maynard FM, Diokno AC: Urinary infections and complications during clean intermittent catheterization following spinal cord injury. *J Urology* 132:943, 1984.

8. Britt MR, *et al.*: Antimicrobial prophylaxis for catheter-associated bacteriuria. *Antimicrobial Agent Chemotherapy* 11:240, 1977.
9. Center for Disease Control. Epidemics of nosocomial urinary tract infections caused by multiresistant gram negative bacilli: Epidemiology and control. U.S. Department of Health and Human Services, Atlanta, 1976.
10. Lapides J, *et al.*: Follow-up on unsterile intermittent self-catheterization. *J Urol* 111:184, 1974.
11. Kunin CM: *Detection, Prevention, and Management of Urinary Tract Infections*, 3rd. ed. Philadelphia: Lea and Febiger, 1979.
12. Luckman J, Sorensen KC: *Medical/Surgical Nursing*. Philadelphia: WB Saunders, 1980, pp. 922–1018.
13. Miller PL: Problems of the urinary system. *In* Phipps WJ, Long BC, Woods NF: *Medical/Surgical Nursing: Concepts in Clinical Practice*. St. Louis: CV Mosby, 1979, pp. 1301–1345.
14. Smith DR: *General Urology*, 9th ed. Los Altos, California: Lang Medical Publishing, 1978.
15. Center for Disease Control. Guidelines for prevention of catheter-associated urinary tract infections. U.S. Department of Health and Human Services, Atlanta, 1981.
16. Axnick KJ, Yarbrough MG: *Infection Control: An Integrated Approach*. St. Louis: CV Mosby, 1983.
17. Nivinski J, Durham N, Miller PL: Management of the person with impaired elimination. *In* Phipps WJ, Long BC, Woods NF: *Medical/Surgical Nursing: Concepts in Clinical Practice*. St. Louis: CV Mosby, 1980, 1243.
18. Altshuler A, Meyer J, Butz M: Even children can learn self-catheterization. *Am J Nursing* 77:97, 1977.
19. Warren J, *et al.*: Fever, bacteremia and death as complications of bacteriuria in women with long-term urethral catheters. *J Infec Dis* 155:1151, 1987.
20. Boscia J, *et al.*: Therapy vs. no therapy for bacteriuria in elderly ambulatory non-hospitalized women. *JAMA* 257:1067, 1987.
21. Casewell MW, Pugh S, Dalton MT: Correlation of antibiotic usage with antibiotic policy in a urological ward. *J Hosp Infec Control* 2:55, 1981.
22. Mayer KH: The epidemiology of antibiotic resistance in hospitals. *J Antimicrobial Therapy* 18(supplement): C223, 1986.
23. Canadian Pharmaceutical Association: Compendium of Pharmaceuticals and Specialties. Canadian Pharmaceutical Association, 1987.
24. Simor A, Ramage L, Wilcox L, *et al.*: Molecular and epidemiologic study of multiresistant serratia marcescens infections in a spinal cord injury/stroke rehabilitation unit. *J Infection Control and Hospital Epidemiology* 1:27, 1988.
25. Center for Disease Control. National Nosocomial Infections Studies Report. Center for Disease Control, Atlanta, 1979.
26. Marrie TJ, *et al.*: Serratia marcescens—a marker for the infection control program. *J Infection Control and Hospital Epidemiology* 3:2, 1982.
27. Okuda T, *et al.*: Outbreak of nosocomial urinary tract infections caused by serratia marcescens. *J Clinical Microbiology* :691, 1982.
28. Schaberg DR, *et al.*: Nosocomial bacteriuria: A prospective study of case clustering in antimicrobial resistance. *Ann Int Med* 93:425, 1980.

25 | INFLUENZA VACCINATION

CASE PRESENTATION

A 77-year-old woman came to your office two days ago for her annual influenza vaccination. She was well and asymptomatic and taking digoxin 0.125 mg PO OD; hydrochlorothiazide 25 mg PO OD; slow K, one tablet PO BID; and THEO DUR (sustained release theophylline) 300 mg PO BID.

She returns today complaining of malaise, myalgia, nausea, vomiting and weakness. Her vital signs are heart rate 98 per min. regular, BP 120/70 mm Hg, temperature 38.1°C. Examination of heart and lungs is unremarkable.

G. Singh
D.W. Molloy

Consider the following statements (true or false)

1. Influenza vaccine should be administered annually to all people over 65 years of age. The risk of serious illness and death related to influenza is moderately increased even in healthy people in this age group.

2. This patient is most likely experiencing an allergic reaction to the influenza vaccination.

3. Increase the dose of patient's THEO DUR to one tablet TID for two or three days until her symptoms have resolved. Fever increases metabolism and may have caused a drop in the serum level of this drug.

4. Amantadine prophylaxis is 70% to 90% effective in preventing illness caused by Type A influenza but is not effective against Type B influenza.

5. Programs aimed at reducing the impact of influenza and increasing the vaccination rates should aim to vaccinate at least 80% of residents of long-term care facilities.

1. TRUE

It is convenient to divide the population into three groups according to who derives the greatest benefit from influenza vaccination [1].

High-Priority, High-Risk Group

The following group of people should always receive annual vaccinations because they are at greatest risk of influenza-related complications.

1. Adults with chronic or pulmonary disorders severe enough to require regular medical follow-up.
2. Residents of nursing homes or chronic care facilities. (These people generally have chronic medical conditions that put them at risk if they get influenza. The institutional environment also promotes spread of disease.)
3. Children with chronic pulmonary disorders or hemodynamically significant heart disease.

Medium-Priority, Medium-Risk Group

Annual vaccination is recommended for

1. people over 65 years of age;
2. an adult with chronic disease such as diabetes, renal disease, anemia, immunodeficiency, or immunosuppression; and
3. children with cancer, immunodeficiency, sickle cell disease, or those taking acetylsalicylic acid (acetylsalicylic acid increases the risk of developing Reye's syndrome).

Low-Priority, Low-Risk Group

This group includes contacts of those at high risk, that is,

1. health-care personnel who have contact with those at high risk; and
2. individuals who come into household contact with those at high risk (in this group one may consider homemakers, public health nurses, Victoria Order of Nurses).

Intramuscular injection in the deltoid muscle of adults and in the anterolateral thigh in infants and young children is the preferred route of administration.

2. FALSE

Fever, malaise, and myalgia occasionally occur within one to two days after vaccination. No significant excess risk of Guillain-Barre syndrome has been observed since 1976. Influenza vaccine does not predispose to Reye's syndrome and does not cause bronchospasm.

Allergic responses are rare and probably result from sensitivity to some vaccine component, most likely to egg protein, which is present in small quantities. Influenza vaccine should not be given to those with anaphylactic hypersensitivity to eggs manifested as hives, swelling of the mouth and throat, broncospasm, or hypotension.

This illness most likely represents a mild flu-like illness that has been precipitated by the vaccination. However, the possibility of drug toxicity has to be considered.

3. FALSE

Following influenza vaccination, the elimination and metabolism of drugs by cytochrome P-450 is decreased [2].

The usual side effects of the vaccine are manifested as mild flu-like symptoms. However, in this case, the patient has more serious side effects, and one must consider the possibility of theophylline [3] or digoxin toxicity. Both of these drugs have a narrow therapeutic index. Fever also causes an increase in the half-life of drugs that are metabolized by the liver [4]. Therefore, one might consider actually decreasing the dosages of these two medications for a few days until the patient's symptoms have resolved. It would not be appropriate to increase the dose of either of these medications at this time.

It would be interesting to check the serum levels of these drugs for future reference. However, it is likely that by the time the levels are available, the acute illness will have resolved. If this patient has normal renal function and no history of seizures, amantadine 100 mg daily may be given and continued for two days after symptoms have resolved.

4. TRUE

Amantadine is 70% to 90% effective in preventing illness caused by Type A influenza viruses but is ineffective against Type B strains. Amantadine prophylaxis should not replace vaccination. Amantadine may be used to control outbreaks in institutions.

1. During an outbreak, it should be given to all residents whether they have been vaccinated or not. A substantial proportion of elderly people have low antibody levels in spite of vaccination and are unprotected [5].
2. It should be given to high-risk groups during outbreaks if vaccine cannot be given or is contraindicated.
3. It can be given as an adjunct to vaccination in high-risk groups when vaccination is given after exposure. It is usually given for about two weeks in these cases.
4. It may supplement vaccination in immunosuppressed patients.

Amantadine decreases the severity and shortens the duration of influenza A [6]. The drug should be given within 24 to 48 hours of the onset of illness and continued until two days after its resolution. The usual dose is 200 mg daily in healthy adults. Persons over 65 years of age are at increased risk of toxicity because of decreased renal function. In this age group, 100 mg daily is recommended.

The common side effects associated with its use include insomnia, difficulty concentrating, lightheadedness, and irritability. Amantadine is excreted unchanged by the kidneys. People with impaired renal function should receive less. The dosage must also be decreased in patients with a seizure disorder.

5. TRUE

In spite of the fact that the influenza vaccination has been recommended for all our elderly patients, at present, only a small percentage of elderly outpatients and institutionalized elderly are vaccinated [7]. Despite physicians' strong belief in the vaccine, all methods of reminders to physicians have failed to increase their use of the influenza vaccine [8]. Only about 20% of those at high risk presently receive influenza vaccine.

Strategies to increase this coverage should include increasing the availability of the vaccine, informing the providers and recipients, and disseminating practical guidelines for vaccination programs. People at high risk under medical care should be routinely vaccinated in the autumn. Programs should aim to vaccinate 80% of residents of long-term-care facilities and of adults and children at high risk. In the future, it may be necessary to legislate that all consenting residents of chronic-care institutions receive influenza vaccination routinely on an annual basis.

REFERENCES

1. National Advisory Committee on Immunization: Statement on influenza vaccination for the 1988–1989 season. *CMAJ* 139:313–315, 1988.
2. Renton EW, *et al.*: Decreased elimination of theophylline after influenza vaccination. *CMAJ* 123:288, 1980.
3. Zwillich CW, *et al.*: Theophylline-induced seizures in adults: Correlation with serum concentration. *Ann Intern Med* 82:784–787, 1973.
4. Elin RJ, *et al.*: Effects of etiocholanolone-induced fever on plasma antipyrine half-lives and metabolic clearance. *Clin Pharm and Therap* 17:447, 1975.
5. Levine M, Beattie LB, McLean DM: Comparison of one- and two-dose regimens of influenza vaccine for elderly men. *CMAJ* 137:722–726, 1987.
6. Little JW, Hall WJ, Douglas RG, Jr, Hyde RW, Speers DM: Amantadine effects on peripheral airway abnormalities in influenza: A study in 15 students with natural influenza A infection. *Ann Intern Med* 85:177–182, 1976.
7. Patriaca PA, Weber JA, Parker RA, Hall WN, *et al.*: Efficacy of influenza vaccine in nursing homes. *JAMA* 253(8):1136–1139, 1985.
8. Stetia V, Serventi I, Lorenz P: Factors affecting the use of influenza vaccine in the institutionalized elderly. *J Amer Geriatrics Soc* 33:856, 1985.

26 | PNEUMONIA

CASE PRESENTATION

The daughter of an 84-year-old male patient telephones. Her father, an active, independent man, has taken to his bed for the last 24 hours and has become confused and disoriented. His daughter is concerned because he had an episode of urinary incontinence during the night. The patient suffers from Parkinson's disease and mild congestive heart failure. He takes levodopa 100/10 four times daily, and hydrochlorothiazide 25 mg daily. He takes no over-the-counter medications and does not abuse alcohol.

On examination you find he is more confused, disoriented, and drowsy than usual. His heart rate is 92 beats per minute and regular, blood pressure 110/60 mm Hg, respirations 24 per minute, and oral temperature 37.1°C. The only significant findings are cogwheel rigidity, pill rolling tremor, rhonchi, and decreased air entry to the right base. Cardiovascular, gastrointestinal, and neurologic examinations provide unremarkable results.

S. Shoham
D. Hogan
R.A. Fox
D.W. Molloy

Consider the following statements (true or false)

1. The absence of productive cough, tachycardia, fever, tachypnea, crepitations, and bronchial breathing does not rule out pneumonia as a cause of this man's confusion.

2. An easy method of obtaining the causative organism in elderly patients is from sputum cultures, obtained from expectorated sputum. Sputum samples yield the causative organism in 50% of cases.

3. A normal leukocyte count and chest x-ray at this time would not rule out pneumonia in this patient.

4. Pneumonia in the elderly, whether community- or hospital-acquired, can be attributed to the same organisms as similarly acquired pneumonias in younger patients.

5. *Streptococcus pneumoniae* is still one of the most common pathogens in bacterial pneumonia in the elderly. Prescribe penicillin empirically until culture reports are available.

1. TRUE

Pneumonia is an infection involving the respiratory bronchioles, alveo-
lar ducts, sacs, and alveoli. It usually is visualized radiologically as a
parenchymal infiltrate [1]. Clinically, pneumonia may be diagnosed in
the presence of an illness compatible with pneumonia in the presence
of a new pulmonary opacity on chest radiograph at the time of presentation or appearing within the following 48 hours.

When confronted with any elderly patient in an acute confusional
state, entertain a differential diagnosis that includes infection. Sir William Osler cautioned physicians that in the elderly, "the physical signs
(of pneumonia) are ill-defined and changeable" [2]. Infection or pneu-

Table 26-1 Prevalence of Symptoms and Signs of Pneumonia (%).

	Age (years)	
	<65	*>65*
Symptoms		
Fever	40	45
Chills	55	27
Rigors	18	6
Pleuritic chest pain	48	30
Cough	82	73
Productive cough	66	54
Anorexia	63	73
Myalgia	40	23
Arthralgia	24	14
Headache	34	23
Vomiting	32	22
Signs		
Temperature <37°C	26	57
Rales	79	77
Rhonchi	46	51
Consolidation	36	49
Nuchal rigidity	5	5
Confusion	16	19
Stupor	21	22
Respiratory failure		
Mechanical ventilation	25	20

Source: Marrie TJ, Haldane EV, Faulkner RS, *et al.*: Community-acquired pneumonia requiring hospitalization. Is it different in the elderly? *J Amer Geriatr Soc* 33:671, 1985.

monia may present in the elderly with no signs except a change in mental status. The elderly may not develop tachycardia or fever in response to pneumonia, and may be too confused to report dyspnea or change in sputum production.

Marrie *et al.* reported the presentation, investigations, clinical features, treatment, and outcome of 138 patients admitted to a hospital with community-acquired pneumonia [3]. They found the clinical presentation was different in the elderly compared to that of younger subjects. Elderly patients complained less frequently of chills, rigors, and myalgia. Fewer elderly subjects complained of cough, and only 50% of elderly patients with pneumonia had a productive cough. Almost 60% of the elderly had a temperature less than 37°C, and less than 50% had signs of consolidation on clinical examination. Table 26-1 shows the symptoms and signs of community-acquired pneumonia in younger and elderly subjects [3].

Lower respiratory tract infections occur more frequently and have a higher mortality in the elderly [4]. Ishii found that pneumonia was the most common cause of death in 5106 post mortem studies of people aged 80 years or more [5]. Since the mortality rate of pneumonia in patients aged 70 years or more has been reported to range from 25% to 43%, this man should be admitted to the hospital for monitoring and treatment [3,6,7].

2. FALSE

Elderly patients frequently are incapable of expectorating lower respiratory tract secretions that may aid in establishing a diagnosis. They may misunderstand directions and swallow their sputum, or provide saliva as sputum for culture. In the confused elderly, it may be impossible to get an adequate sputum specimen for culture. Even if a sputum sample is obtained, the culture may be contaminated by oropharyngeal organisms, oral debris, or saliva.

Marrie *et al.* reported that only 55% of patients with pneumonia were able to give sputum samples. The sample yielded the causative organism in 38% of those cultured. Overall, however, sputum yielded the causative organism in only 21% of cases. Still, sputum culture had a better diagnostic yield than blood culture (11.6%), throat washings (2.3%), or open lung biopsy (22%).

Gram stains may provide immediate results and should be performed on every patient with pneumonia. Some pneumonias, especially those caused by *S. pneumoniae*, can be diagnosed accurately with a gram stain. If the sputum specimen has less than 10 epithelial cells, more than 25 white blood cells per low-power field, and more than 10 organisms per oil immersion field, then a diagnosis of *S. pneumoniae* may be made with 65% sensitivity and 85% specificity [8].

Transtracheal aspiration eliminates oropharyngeal contamination, but is contraindicated in patients with bleeding disorders, or in confused hypoxic or agitated patients. Complications include mediastinal emphysema, local infection, bleeding, and death.

Tracheal suction may provide lower respiratory tract sputum or culture; however, this procedure may provoke arrhythmias and even cardiac arrest in the elderly.

If sputum is not available, blood cultures may be the only effective way to establish the diagnosis and allow for definitive antimicrobial therapy. As noted, however, the yield from blood cultures is low. Nasal swabs, throat washings, or sputum may be sent for viral culture. Counter immunoelectrophoresis (CIEP) is used to detect pneumococcal antigen in respiratory secretions. CIEP may give false negative results and a high rate of false positive results.

Direct immunofluorescent staining of sputum for *Legionella pneumophila* may provide an immediate diagnosis. Serum antibody determinations of *L. pneumophila*, viruses, and *Mycoplasma pneumoniae* may also be performed. They take up to one month to complete, however, and do not usually assist in the early diagnosis.

3. TRUE

Up to 20% of elderly patients with pneumonia may have a normal or depressed leukocyte count. In others, the leukocyte count may show only slight elevation with immature polymorphonuclear neutrophils in the peripheral blood. Many patients may have metabolic abnormalities, including raised urea, creatinine, serum glucose, hyponatremia, or hyperphosphatemia.

In the absence of other clinical signs, arterial blood gases may reveal a significant hypoxemia, accounting for confusion or delirium.

In this patient, chest x-ray revealed an infiltrate in the right lower lobe. X-rays may appear normal for the first 24 to 48 hours of pneumonia in the elderly. Pneumonic infiltrates in the elderly may be obscured by cardiac failure or emphysema. Chest x-rays may be difficult to interpret because of technically poor films performed on uncooperative or confused patients. A normal chest x-ray with a normal leukocyte count would not necessarily exclude a diagnosis of pneumonia. If the diagnosis is suspected, the chest x-ray should be repeated two or three days later.

4. FALSE

Bacterial pneumonia most likely results from aspiration of oropharyngeal contents. The elderly may be at increased risk because of abnormalities in swallowing, epiglottic function, esophageal motility, and decline in immune function. A number of chronic diseases such as diabetes mellitus and malnutrition are found more frequently in the elderly, and may predispose them to infection and pneumonia. The pathogenic mechanisms that predispose the elderly to infections are not completely understood.

The prevalence of oropharyngeal colonization with *S. pneumoniae* does not increase with age [9]. The prevalence of oropharyngeal colonization with *Staphylococcus aureus* and aerobic gram-negative bacilli increases with advancing age, particularly in residents of nursing homes or in chronically debilitated elderly (Table 26-2)[10].

In the preantibiotic era, acute bacterial pneumonia almost invariably

Table 26-2 Pathogens in Pneumonia in the Elderly (in order of frequency).

Community
    Pneumococcus
    Hemophilus influenzae
    Klebsiella pneumoniae
    Staphylococcus aureus
    Escherichia coli
    Enterobacter

Nursing home
    Klebsiella pneumonia
    Pneumococcus
    Staphylococcus aureus
    Escherichia coli
    Hemophilus influenzae

Hospital
    Pseudomonas
    Gram-negative bacilli
    Staphylococcus aureus

was caused by *S. pneumoniae*. It remains the most frequent cause of bacterial pneumonia in the elderly, but its prevalence has decreased significantly [11]. Currently it is responsible for about 50% of pneumonia in the elderly. Almost 50% of community and 90% of nursing home bacterial pneumonias in the elderly are caused by *Klebsiella pneumoniae, Hemophilus influenzae, S. aureus*, or *Escherichia coli*. The mortality of aged patients with acute bacterial pneumonia depends on the offending organism. *S. pneumoniae* has a 20% mortality, *S. aureus* and *H. influenzae* have a 30% to 40% mortality, while aerobic gram-negative bacilli have a 70% to 80% mortality [12]. Pneumonia in patients over 65 has a higher mortality rate than in younger patients (25% to 48% versus 10%) and is more likely to be of unknown cause (48% versus 11%).

5. FALSE

Because of the frequency of nonpneumococcal pneumonia in the elderly, penicillin alone does not provide sufficient coverage for the patient while gram stains or culture results are pending. Patients with community-acquired pneumonia should be treated with a first- or second-generation cephalosporin. Cefamandole 500 mg to 2 g intravenously may be the best empirical choice at present. Patients in nursing homes or hospitals who acquire pneumonia should receive an aminoglycoside with a B. lactamase-resistant cephalosporin, or penicillinase-resistant penicillin. When prescribing antibiotics such as aminoglycosides for the elderly, it is important to take into account reductions in creatinine clearance that occur with advancing age, and modify doses accordingly.

REFERENCES

1. Ralph ED: Infections of the lower respiratory tract. *In* Mandell LA (ed.), *Essentials of Infectious Diseases.* Boston: Blackwell Scientific Publications, 1985, p. 175.
2. Osler W (ed.): *The Principles and Practice of Medicine,* 1st ed. New York: D. Appleton, 1892.
3. Marrie TJ, Haldane EV, Faulkner RS, *et al.*: Community-acquired pneumonia requiring hospitalization. Is it different in the elderly? *J Am Geriatr Soc* 33:671, 1985.
4. Ecright JR, Rytel MW: Bacterial pneumonia in the elderly. *J Am Geriatr Soc* 28:220, 1980.
5. Ishii T, Hosoda Y, Maeda K: Cause of death in extreme old age: A pathologic study of 5106 elderly persons 80 years of age and over. *Ageing* 9:81, 1980.
6. Mufson MA, Chang V, Gill V, *et al.*: The role of viruses, mycoplasmas, and bacteria in acute pneumoniae in civilian adults. *Am J Epidemiol* 86:526, 1967.
7. Sullivan RJ, Doudle WR, Marine WM, *et al.*: Adult pneumonia in a general hospital: Etiology and risk factors. *Arch Intern Med* 129:935, 1972.
8. Murray PR, Washington JA: III Microscopic and bacteriologic analysis in experienced sputum. *Mayo Clinic Proc* 50:339, 1975.
9. Foy HJ, Wentworth B, Kenny GE, *et al.*: Pneumococcal isolations from patients with pneumonia and control subjects in a prepared medical group. *Am Rev Respir Dis* 111:595, 1975.
10. Valenti WM, Randeck RG, Bentley DW, *et al.*; Factors predisposing to oropharyngeal colonization from negative bacilli in the aged. *New Engl J Med* 298:1108, 1978.
11. Garb JL, Brown RB, Tuthill RW: Differences in etiology of pneumonias in nursing homes and community patients. *JAMA* 240:2169, 1978.
12. Esposito AL: Bacterial pneumonia in the elderly. *In* Pennington JE (ed.): *Respiratory Infections: Diagnosis and Management.* New York: Raven Press, 1983.

27 | HERPES ZOSTER

CASE PRESENTATION

Mrs. A., an active 79-year-old widow, developed a painful rash over her right lower chest area in January. A week later, she came to you and you diagnosed herpes zoster in the T8 dermatomal distribution. She was treated with acetaminophen (paracetamol) and calamine lotion.

The burning sensation and pain persisted. While on vacation in another city in February, she was taken to her daughter's family doctor, who prescribed topical acyclovir.

The rash resolved after three months, but the pain persisted so you started her on Tegretol (carbamazepine) 200 mg PO BID. The pain is constant and burning in character, worsened by touching. She has been taking carbamazepine regularly for three months now. She comes to your office today with insomnia and persistent agonizing pain, which is constant and intolerable. You consider increasing the carbamazepine, giving her a prescription for codeine, or referring her to a local pain clinic.

D.W. Molloy
A. Cranney

Consider the following statements (true or false)

1. With advancing age, the incidence and severity of herpes zoster increases.

2. With *acute* herpes zoster, the erythema and/or vesicles usually precede the pain by days or weeks.

3. Oral acyclovir modifies the course of acute herpes zoster. It reduces pain and shortens the duration of rash, if administered within 72 hours of the onset of the rash.

4. Post-herpetic neuralgia is more common and more severe in the elderly.

5. It would be appropriate to refer this patient to the local pain clinic, before you give a prescription for codeine.

1. TRUE

Herpes zoster (shingles) is an acute infection caused by the reactivation of latent varicella zoster virus in the sensory ganglia. Herpes zoster, a DNA virus, remains dormant in the dorsal root ganglia for many years following an episode of varicella (chicken pox). Following reactivation, it migrates along sensory nerves, causing skin eruptions in a dermatomal pattern.

The incidence and severity of herpes zoster increases with age [1–6]. The prevalence in adults is about 1.3:1000, and is equal in both sexes. More than 60% of patients with herpes zoster are aged over 45 years. The incidence in persons aged over 80 is 10:1000 per year [3].

Of patients with herpes zoster, 5% have a recurrence [7], and almost half of these patients have eruptions at the site of the original infection [8]. Bilateral zoster occurs in less than 1% of patients.

The incidence of zoster is higher in patients with cancer, especially hematological or reticuloendothelial malignancies, and in those receiving immunosuppressive therapy [9,10,11].

Loss of cell-mediated immunity to varicella zoster is primarily responsible for reactivation of herpes zoster [7].

Normal, otherwise healthy, elderly presenting with herpes zoster do not require a work-up for malignancy [12].

2. FALSE

The hallmark of herpes zoster is the rash. Pain or itch typically precede the appearance of the characteristic rash by several days [6,13]. The rash usually erupts over a 4 to 14-day period, first appearing as red papules over an erythematous base with central vesicles. At first the fluid in the vesicles is clear. It becomes cloudy in about 3 or 4 days. In contrast to herpes simplex, where the vesicles are uniform, the vesicles occur in clusters and vary in size.

Clusters may occur in patchy clumps or cover the entire dermatome. Crusting occurs in 5 to 10 days, and healing usually occurs within a month. In severe cases, however, they may become gangrenous on a background of secondary cellulitis. The vesicles are usually confined to one or two dermatomes, but a few can spread across the mid-line.

If five or more lesions appear beyond two dermatomes of the primary eruption, then the patient has "disseminated disease." Of patients with herpes zoster associated with malignant disease, 20% to 30% have disseminated herpes [7].

Of cases of zoster, 60% to 70% occur in the thoracic dermatomes, 10% to 15% in trigeminal, 12% to 17% in lumbosacral, and 10% in the cervical dermatomes [1,9,14]. The incidence of trigeminal involvement increases with age.

The diagnosis of herpes zoster is usually clinical. The Tzanck prep shows large intranuclear inclusions but does not differentiate between zoster and simplex. Counterimmunoelectrophoresis, culture, immuno-fluorescent staining, electron microscopy, gel effusion, or convalescent antibody titers confirm the diagnosis.

Herpes zoster usually begins with pain, paresthesia, and/or dys-thesiae in the affected dermatome(s), followed in a few days by the vesicular eruption. Some patients have severe pain in the prevesicular and vesicular phase, and others do not. Older patients are more likely to have pain in the acute stages than younger patients. Only about 20% of patients experience pain after the development of the rash [6].

Although it has been suggested that the occurrence of herpes zoster might indicate an occult malignancy or immunodeficiencies in the elderly, there is little evidence to support this. Extensive diagnostic work-up is not warranted in patients who develop segmental herpes zoster [5].

3. TRUE

Treatment of herpes zoster should include analgesics and antiviral agents. During the acute eruption, calamine lotion may be used to dry the lesions and an anesthetic spray may afford some temporary relief.

Acyclovir, an antiviral agent, modifies the severity of the infection [15]. Oral acyclovir given as 800 mg five times daily for seven days started within 72 hours of the onset of rash reduces the number and size of the vesicles, decreases new lesion formation, increases healing, and reduces acute pain and the need for analgesics [16]. Doses may require modification in patients with renal impairment. The most frequent adverse effects include headache, nausea and vomiting, diarrhea, skin rash, vertigo, and arthralgia. During oral use, overdose is unlikely be-cause of incomplete bioavailability from the gastrointestinal tract. Intra-venous acyclovir, 30 mg/kg/day is the drug of choice for immunologically compromised patients with herpes zoster and is recommended for patients with ophthalmic involvement [17].

4. TRUE

Post-herpetic neuralgia is defined as pain that persists after the rash has healed, or at least longer than one month [18]. Scarring is usually present and is pigmented in the early stages. Later it becomes pale, white, or silvery. The scars themselves are anesthetic but the skin area is often hyperesthetic. Because of this increased sensitivity to tactile stimuli, the patient often finds it difficult to have contact between clothing and skin.

Post-herpetic neuralgia occurs in 20% of all age groups, with an incidence of greater than 50% in those over 70 years. Pain persists for at least 1 year in 4% of patients under 20 years and in about 50% of those over 70 years. It is characterized by unrelenting aching, burning, or intractable itch [19]. The pain is frequently accompanied by depression. Depression is often accompanied by vegetative signs such as sleep disturbance, anorexia, lassitude, and diminished libido.

Post-herpetic neuralgia is more common after ophthalmic herpes zoster than it is after spinal segmental involvement. The pain syndrome is usually characterized by a constant burning and aching with superimposed shocks and jabs and is rarely throbbing or cramping. Patients usually describe the pain as agonizing and disruptive of daily routines and activities. Although pain fluctuates, it is usually present to some degree. There are no pain-free intervals. Although the vesicular eruption may not have covered the entire dermatome, the pain usually does. It is typically a unilateral stripe from the dorsal to the ventral mid-line.

5. TRUE

The treatment of post-herpetic neuralgia is a formidable task. There are many anecdotal reports of pharmacologic, anesthetic, and surgical therapies that have been successful in the treatment of this condition; but few treatments have withstood the test of properly controlled clinical trials [18].

Recently advocated pharmacologic treatments have focused on psychotropic and anticonvulsant drugs. Several series of cases have reported improvement with the use of tricyclic antidepressants either alone or in combination with a neuroleptic or anticonvulsants [19,20,21]. Amitryptyline at a medium dose of 75 mg (25 to 137.5 mg) caused significant improvement in the pain from post-herpetic neuralgia [20]. Carbamazepine is particularly effective in the treatment of lancinating or shooting pain [21]. Although anesthetic techniques have been often used to treat post-herpetic neuralgia, evidence of their success is limited to anecdotal series without proper controls and follow-up [22,23,24].

Neuroaugmentative approaches provide afferent stimulation in an attempt to augment and activate endogenous pain-modulating systems [24,25,26]. These include counterirritation, transcutaneous nerve stimulation (TENS), acupuncture, dorsal column stimulation, and deep brain stimulation. Counterirritation (rubbing affected skin) after application of a vapocoolant spray can be a useful technique [24]. TENS may afford moderate to complete pain relief by using a stimulator as needed [26].

Surgical procedures have been directed at every level from skin to cortex, including neurectomy, rhizotomy, sympathectomy, mesencephozatomy, mesencephalotomy, topectomy, lobotomy, leukotomy, and others [27]. Surgery is generally not an appropriate treatment of this problem, and it is important to protect patients from destructive surgery that may even make the problem worse.

The only surgical procedure with any merit is that of dorsal root entry zone lesions, in which radio frequency current makes a lesion in the dorsal horn area at multiple levels [28,29]. The response rate is about 50% in these patients.

Since this patient does not report shooting or lancinating pain but a constant burning pain, amitryptiline alone or combined with a neuroleptic should be tried. Counterirritation (rubbing affected skin) and/or TENS should also be tried. It would be appropriate to refer this woman to a pain clinic for advice and follow-up. It would not be appropriate to prescribe codeine or any narcotic analgesics until these other measures have been properly tested. Capsaicin cream shows some promise in the treatment of post-herpetic neuralgia [30]. Capsaicin depletes substance P, a member of a group of peptides called tachykins. Substance P is found in the nerve terminals in the skin and is a neurotransmitter involved in transmission of pain. The use of this substance will require further study with properly controlled trials before it can be recommended.

REFERENCES

1. Burgoon CF, Burgoon JS, Baldridge GD: The natural history of herpes zoster. *JAMA* 164:265–269, 1957.
2. Demorgas JM, Kierland RR: The outcome of patients with herpes zoster. *Arch Dermatol* 75:193–196, 1957.
3. Hope-Simpson RE: The nature of herpes zoster: A long term study and a new hypothesis. *Proc R Soc Lond [Biol]* 58:9–20, 1965.
4. Molin GJ: Aspects of the natural history of herpes zoster. *Acta Derm Venereol* (Stockh) 49:569–572, 1969.
5. Ragozzino MW, Melton LJ, Kurland LT, *et al.*: Population based study of herpes zoster and its sequelae. *Medicine* (Baltimore) 61:310–316, 1982.
6. Rogers RS, Tindall JP: Geriatric herpes zoster. *J Am Geriatr Soc* 19:495–503, 1971.
7. Reuler JB, Chang MK: Herpes zoster: Epidemiology, clinical features, and management. *South Med J* 77:1149–1156, 1984.
8. Portenoy RK, Duma C, Foley KM: Acute herpetic and postherpetic neuralgia: Clinical review and current management. *Ann Neurol* 20:651–664, 1986.
9. Mazur M, Dolin R: Herpes zoster at the NIH: A twenty year history. *Am J Med* 65:738–744, 1978.
10. Reboul F, Donaldson SS, Kaplan HS: Herpes zoster and varicella infection in children with Hodgkin's disease: An analysis of contributing factors. *Cancer* 41:95–99, 1978.
11. Rifkind D: The activation of varicella-zoster virus infection by immunosuppressive therapy. *J Lab Clin Med* 68:463–474, 1966.
12. Beaver T: Herpes zoster in the elderly. *Clinical Report on Aging* 2:3–8, 1988.
13. Juel-Jensen BE, MacCallum FO: *Herpes Simplex, Varicella and Zoster.* Philadelphia: Lippincott, 1972, pp. 127–132.
14. Brown GR: Herpes zoster: Correlation of age, sex, distribution, neuralgia and associated disorders. *South Med J* 69:576–578, 1976.
15. Balfour HH Jr, Bean B, Laskin OL, Ambinder R: Fetal acyclovir halts progression of herpes zoster in immunocompromised patients. *New Engl J Med* 308:1448–1453, 1983.

16. McKendrick MW, *et al.*: Oral acyclovir in acute herpes zoster. *Br Med J* 293:1529–1532, 1986.
17. Lass JH: Herpes zoster: Protecting older patients' vision. *Geriatrics* 39:79–94, 1984.
18. Loeser JD: Herpes zoster and postherpetic neuralgia pain. 29:149–164, 1986.
19. Woodforde JM, Dwyer B, McEwen BW, De Wilde FW, Bleasel K, Conneley TJ Jr, Ho CY: Treatment of post-herpetic neuralgia. *Med J Aust* 2:869–872, 1965.
20. Watson CPN, Evan RJ, Reed K, *et al.*: Amitriptyline *vs.* placebo in postherpetic neuralgia. *Neurology* 32:671–673, 1982.
21. Table A: Relief of postherpetic neuralgia with psychotropic drugs. *J Neurosurg* 39:235–239, 1973.
22. Colding A: The effect of sympathetic blocks on herpes zoster. *Acta Anaesthesiol Scand* 13:133–141, 1969.
23. Masud KZ, Forster KJ: Sympathetic block in herpes zoster. *Am Fam Physician* 12(Nov.):142–143, 1975.
24. Taverner D: Alleviation of post-herpetic neuralgia. *Lancet* 2:671–673, 1960.
25. Todd EM, Crue BL, Vergadamo M: Conservative treatment of post-herpetic neuralgia. *Bull Los Angeles Neurol Soc* 30:148, 1965.
26. Nathan PW, Wall PD: Treatment of post-herpetic neuralgia by prolonged electrical stimulation. *Br Med J* 3:645–647, 1974.
27. Portenoy RK, Duma C, Foley KM: Acute herpetic and post-herpetic neuralgia: Clinical review and current management. *Ann Neurol* 20:651–664, 1986.
28. Nashold BS: Current status of the DREZ operation: 1984. *Neurosurgery* 15:942–944, 1984.
29. Richter HP, Seitz K: Dorsal root entry zone lesions for the control of deafferentation pain: Experience in ten patients. *Neurosurgery* 15:956–959, 1984.
30. Purohit A, Watson P, Ross DR, *et al.*: Therapeutic advances in the management of post-herpetic neuralgia. *Geriatric Medicine Today* 7(6):20–40, 1988.

Part V

RHEUMATIC DISEASES

28 OSTEOARTHRITIS

CASE PRESENTATION

A 77-year-old woman presents with a five-month history of severe pain in the left hip, low back, right shoulder, and neck. She has had a long history of osteoarthritis dating back 25 years, when she presented with pain and stiffness in the fingers (distal and proximal interphalangeal joints), base of both thumbs, knees, great toes, and lower back. She was treated with aspirin and physiotherapy. After a few years the pain, for the most part, regressed. There was persistence of nodal deformities of hands, poor mobility of the thumbs, bilateral bunions, and occasional back discomfort. About two years ago she developed an aching pain in the buttocks, thighs, and calves. This was usually brought on by walking several blocks and was relieved after five to ten minutes of rest.

Eleven years ago the patient had a right mastectomy for carcinoma of the breast. She had regular follow-ups with no evidence of recurrence. A bone scan six months previously was apparently normal.

As was mentioned, the patient's pain returned rather abruptly about five months previously. It was often worse at night, and sleep became difficult without sedation. On examination the most painful areas were in the neck, right shoulder, low back, and lateral aspect of the left hip.

The laboratory investigations revealed a slight normochromic and normocytic anemia, a very high erythrocyte sedimentation rate at 105 mm per hour, and no monoclonal protein in serum or urine.

W.E. DeCoteau
L.E. Hart
D.W. Molloy

Radiographs of the spine, pelvis, and chest were obtained from another hospital, where they were ordered two months previously by a rheumatologist. These revealed marked degenerative change with obvious narrowing of the disc space at L5-S1.

After admission she had her nonsteroidal anti-inflammatory drug (NSAID) changed from ibuprofen to sulindac with minimal improvement. It was thought she might have a left trochanteric bursitis, but there was little pain relief with ultrasound and a local corticosteroid injection.

Consider the following statements (true or false)

1. The economic cost and disability produced by rheumatoid arthritis is much greater than that of osteoarthritis.
2. Osteoarthritis is characterized by the gradual loss of articular cartilage and remodeling of subchondral bone, with little inflammatory response.
3. Osteoarthritis is a heterogenous disorder that can involve both spinal and peripheral joints, including those that do not bear weight.
4. The patient's leg symptoms that come on with exercise are likely due to neurogenic claudication.
5. The recent attack of pain is likely due to exacerbation of osteoarthritis. Therefore, it would be reasonable to persist with physiotherapy and NSAID treatment without performing further investigations.

259

1. FALSE

The enormous socioeconomic burden produced by osteoarthritis in the United States has recently been summarized by Dieppe [1]. Osteoarthritis (OA) accounts for 140 million physician visits per year (13.6% of all visits to family physicians); 68 million days of lost work, which does not include those who are past working age; and 100,000 hip or knee operations per year. In comparison, rheumatoid arthritis accounted for 3.5 million physician visits and 2.2 million lost days of work. There are more cases of severe disability caused by osteoarthritis than by stroke, other circulatory disease, rheumatoid arthritis, and multiple sclerosis in the over-65 population. Although sufferers of OA outnumber all other causes of physical disability in the elderly, there has been much less research interest given to OA, and they have been called by Badeley "the forgotten disabled" [2].

A recent nursing home study revealed that 23% of residents had arthritis (usually osteoarthritis) and that it was the primary reason for admission in 15% [3].

2. FALSE

The events leading to the final common pathway of cartilage breakdown in OA appear to be [4]

1. abnormal stress (*i.e.*, excessive impact loading, trauma, or developmental abnormality) acting on normal cartilage, or
2. normal stress acting on abnormal cartilage modified by inflammation, crystal deposition, aging, immune mechanisms.

The hyaline cartilage covering subchondral bone at synovial joints is remarkably well adapted for weight bearing in that it contains no pain fibers, is durable, is almost frictionless, and is compressible. This hyaline cartilage is made up of chondrocytes (less than 0.1% of volume), which produce and maintain matrix. The matrix is composed of (a) collagen framework aligned to withstand force on weight-bearing yet reduce friction, and (b) large negatively charged molecules called proteoglycans that bind large quantities of water, which allows for a waterbed-like cushioning effect during weight bearing [5].

Osteoarthritis is also characterized by the formation of new bone around joint margins. This osteophytosis is poorly understood but is thought to also be part of the repair process. A variety of growth factors including insulin-derived growth factor (IDGF), formerly called somatomedin, and platelet-derived growth factor act individually or in concert to promote the proliferation of chondrocytes in the degenerating cartilage, leading to the formation of osteophytes at the articular margin. The IDGF effect probably accounts for the pronounced osteophytosis often seen in acromegaly and diabetes mellitus [6].

Recently it has been noted that the chondrocytes of cartilage and the synovial membrane in OA produce a significant inflammatory response in many cases. In OA, molecules with inflammatory properties, such as interleukin-1 (IL-1)[7], prostaglandin E-2, and phospholipase A-2 [8], all have the ability to cause cartilage breakdown by digesting collagen and/or proteoglycan. Some of the so-called chondroprotective actions of certain NSAIDs appear to be due to inhibition of the inflammatory molecules [8]. Chondrocytes also have the ability to repair damaged cartilage, but eventually in some cases the repair mechanism becomes overwhelmed and cartilage breakdown occurs [6].

3. TRUE

Osteoarthritis is a slowly evolving articular disease characterized by the gradual development of joint pain, stiffness, and limitation of motion [9]. OA exhibits the following general clinical profile:

1. It tends to worsen with advancing age. Prevalence rate increased from 4 per 100 among persons 18 to 24 years of age, to 85 per 100 at age 75 to 79 years. Of the latter group, 3% had moderate or severe disease, while under age 45 nearly all cases were mild [9].

2. The cardinal symptom of OA is pain, which at first occurs after joint use and is relieved by rest. As the disease progresses, pain may occur with minimal motion or even at rest. In advanced cases, pain may awaken the patient from sleep. Stiffness on wakening in the morning and after periods of inactivity during the day is common, but of short duration, usually less than 15 minutes.

3. On examination there is often local tenderness, crepitus, or mild joint enlargement with firm consistency from proliferation of bone and/or synovitis. As the disease advances there is loss of joint motion and even gross deformity. Joint effusion is usually not prominent, and synovial fluid yields a low cell count of predominantly mononuclear cells.

4. Joints that are commonly involved include the distal interphalangeal (DIP), proximal interphalangeal (PIP), first carpometacarpal (CMC), hip, knee, first metatarsal phalangeal (MTP), and lower lumbar and cervical spine. Metacarpal phalangeal (MCP), carpal, elbow, shoulder, and ankle joints are rarely involved unless trauma or calcium crystal deposition is present.

5. Rheumatoid factor is often absent; and the erythrocyte sedimentation rate tends to be normal or slightly elevated.

6. X-ray changes in involved joints tend to mirror the pathologic process. In mild cases there is often no x-ray change; more advanced cases demonstrate loss of joint space due to erosion of cartilage and evidence of repair, that is, marginal osteophytosis, increased thickening of subchondral bone, and major remodeling of joint surfaces.

Specific Joint Involvement in OA

1. *Hands and feet.* One of the most common manifestations of primary OA are Heberden's nodes, which represent cartilaginous and bony enlargement of the DIP joints of the fingers. They are more common in women and tend to run in families. They often develop insidiously with little pain but can appear rapidly with acute signs of inflammation. Bouchard's nodes are a similar type of involvement in PIP joints. Degenerative change involving the first CMC joint is often present with pain, localized tenderness, and limited motion. The OA process also commonly takes place at the first metatarsal phalangeal (MTP) joint of the foot.

   The distribution of arthritis in the hands and feet is useful in distinguishing rheumatoid arthritis (RA) from OA. MCP involvement is the rule in RA but rarely occurs in uncomplicated OA. Heberden's nodes do not occur in RA. PIP involvement occurs with both. Multiple MTP joints are involved in RA.

2. *Monarticular disease usually involves the knee or hip.* The main symptom of OA of the hip is insidious pain followed by a characteristic limp (antalgic gait). Hip pain is usually felt in the groin or anteromedial aspect of the thigh and occasionally over the trochanteric area. However, pain in the latter region is more often due to trochanteric bursitis, which is often successfully treated by a local corticosteroid injection. Occasionally hip pain will be referred to the knee via the obturator nerve. The

knee joint is frequently affected by primary OA, with involvement of one or more of the three compartments. The medial compartment is more apt to be involved in uncomplicated OA, especially if the patient is obese. Isolated patellofemoral disease suggests calcium pyrophosphate deposition disease, while isolated lateral compartment involvement suggests hydroxyapatite deposition disease [9]. Anserine bursitis is a common cause of knee pain that can be confused with OA.

3. *Osteoarthritis of the spine can involve diarthrodial or apophyseal joints and the synchondrosis or intervertebral discs.* The term spinal osteoarthritis describes changes in the apophyseal joints. Spinal osteophytosis or spondylosis deformans occurs as a result of degeneration of the annulus fibrosis portion of the intervertebral disc. The anterior longitudinal ligament becomes stressed, and traction osteophytes develop. A possible variant of spondylosis deformans is diffuse idiopathic skeletal hyperostosis (DISH), a term used to describe the condition of flowing ossification occurring along the anterolateral aspect of at least four contiguous vertebral bodies. It is often asymptomatic, but spinal stiffness can be prominent in the condition and has to be differentiated from ankylosing spondylitis. It is more common in males with glucose intolerance [9].

4. *Generalized osteoarthritis (GOA) is defined as involving three or more extraspinal locations.* An intense inflammatory response often heralds its onset at menopause. It has been said the hip is less frequently involved than hands, feet, or knees in GOA [10]. Another study found that 80% of those requiring operation for either hip or knee OA had polyarticular arthritis, although it was often quiescent in other regions [11]. As a result, an intrinsic tissue defect rather than a mechanical or aging process was postulated as the etiopathogenetic factor in GOA.

4. TRUE

The patient probably has lumbar spinal stenosis, which is a syndrome resulting from pressure on the spinal cord or cauda equina by a narrow spinal canal due to degenerative change [12]. There is hypertrophy of the ligamentum flavum, apophyseal joints, and vertebral body. The cardinal symptom of spinal stenosis is neurogenic claudication manifest by a feeling of discomfort or weakness in the buttocks, thighs, and calves brought on by standing or walking and relieved by sitting, lying down, or adopting a stooped position. (Such patients can often comfortably ride an exercise bicycle for a considerable length of time.) Paresthesias in the lower extremities are common, and the electromyograph (EMG) of affected muscles is often abnormal. The peripheral pulses are usually palpable unless there is co-existing peripheral vascular disease. In vascular claudication, leg pain is provoked by walking but relieved by standing. The pulses are generally not palpable, and the EMG to the muscles of the lower extremity is normal.

A similar type of bony overgrowth can occur in the lower cervical spine with the production of a cervical spondylotic myelopathy characterized by a spastic gait, hyperreflexia in the lower limbs, and Babinski's signs. There may be upper and/or lower motor neuron signs in the upper extremities, depending on the site of compression. Neck pain can be absent, but restricted neck motion is usual. The myelopathy must be distinguished from amyotrophic lateral sclerosis and subacute combined degeneration due to deficiency of vitamin B_{12} [12].

5. FALSE

The patient had gone for some years without much pain in her joints. Therefore, the abrupt onset of pain in a patient with a previous history of breast cancer makes metastatic malignancy a definite possibility [13]. In this case, a repeat bone scan revealed multiple areas of metastases involving mainly her sites of pain. Therefore, it is imperative that physicians be alert for a second process causing pain in a patient with obvious osteoarthritis. Osteoarthritis in no way protects a person from developing either primary or metastatic malignancy to the bones. Moreover, it is not unusual to see other arthritic conditions such as polymyalgia rheumatica [14] or crystal deposition disease [15] superimposed on osteoarthritis.

The treatment of osteoarthritis has been well outlined by Brandt [16], who suggests that patients with OA are all very different, and optimum management should not be based on a "cookbook" approach. Instead, the management of the pain will depend on the cause of the pain in a particular patient: Is the pain due to synovitis or tendonitis, peri-articular muscle spasm, defective mechanics (joint instability or postural abnormality), or endstage joint disease? Is the pain persistent or episodic? What are the expectations of the patient?

The main approaches utilized in effective treatment of OA are (1) drug therapy (analgesics, anti-inflammatory agents, local corticosteroids); (2) reduction of joint loading; (3) education and physical therapy; (4) orthopedic surgery.

Simple analgesics such as acetaminophen or NSAIDs on demand can be effective in controlling mild, episodic disease. When persistent pain due to synovitis is present, regular NSAID treatment can be effective, providing the cartilage damage is not too advanced. There has been a suggestion, based on clinical observation plus lab and animal experimentation, that some NSAIDs cause cartilage damage while others are "chrondro protective." However, well-designed human clinical trials are needed to answer the question as to whether NSAIDs are harmful or protective to cartilage [16]. The same applies to the efficacy of non-NSAID "cartilage promoting compounds" like glycosaminoglycan peptide (Rumalon) and glycosamine sulfate polypeptide (Arteparon).

Local corticosteroids are very useful in treating localized tender pericapsular sites and conditions such as tendonitis or bursitis, but they are potentially hazardous when given by intra-articular injection. Corticosteroids can cause direct cartilage injury, and the amelioration of pain from their use may lead to overuse of the joint with further cartilage damage. Moreover, studies have shown that they may be no more effective than injection of local anesthetic without corticosteroid [16].

Reduction of joint loading can be accomplished by attempting to have the patient alter her or his lifestyle so as to protect the damaged joint(s) and/or take regular periods of rest. Poor body mechanics, such as the excessively lordotic lumbar spine or pronated foot, can be compensated for by supports. A cane (which should be held in the contralateral hand) is helpful if knee or hip involvement is unilateral. If involvement is bilateral, a walker is more helpful.

Weight reduction is also helpful in improving function, but there is no evidence, except for medial compartment disease of the knee, where obesity *per se* might be a cause of osteoarthritis.

Physical therapy is an indispensable part of the treatment plan for most patients with OA. This involves the use of heat or cold plus a therapeutic exercise program tailored to the individual.

Orthopedic surgery can be extremely helpful for patients with advanced disease who have intractable pain or markedly impaired function. Tibial or femoral osteotomy can produce excellent pain relief in selected cases by altering loading stresses. In advanced disease total joint arthroplasty can be very effective, while arthrodesis can be useful if carried out on non-weight-bearing joints. Unfortunately, many frail elderly patients who would benefit from total joint arthroplasty in terms of pain relief and improvement of function cannot undergo the procedure because of other serious health problems that accumulate with age [16].

REFERENCES

1. Dieppe PA: Update on crystal associated arthropathies and osteoarthritis. Section VI, *Biennial Review of Rheumatic Diseases*. Atlanta, Georgia: American Rheumatism Association, 1988.
2. Badeley L: The prevalence and severity of major disabling conditions. *Int J Epidemiol* 7:145, 1978.
3. Guccione AA, Meenan RF, Anderson JJ: Arthritis in nursing home residents. *Arthritis and Rheum* 32:1546, 1989.
4. Howell DS: Etiopathogenesis of osteoarthritis in arthritis and allied conditions. *In* McCarty DJ (ed.), *Arthritis and Allied Conditions*. Chapter 101. 11th ed. Lea and Febiger, pp. 1595–1604, 1989.
5. Fujii K, Tajiri K, Kajiwara T, *et al.*: The role of cytobines in chondrocyte mediated cartilage degradation. *J Rheumatol* 16(suppl. 18):28, 1989.

6. Hamerman D: The biology of osteoarthritis. *N Engl J Med* 320:1322, 1989.

7. Pelletier JP, Martel-Pelletier J: Evidence for the involvement of interleukin-1 in human osteoarthritic cartilage degradation: Protective effect of NSAID. *J Rheumatol* 16(suppl. 18):19, 1989.

8. Vignon E, Mathieu P, Louisot P, *et al.*: Phospholipase A2 activity in human osteoarthritic cartilage. *J Rheumatol* 16(suppl. 18):35, 1989.

9. Moskowitz RW: Clinical and laboratory findings in osteoarthritis. *In* McCarty DJ (ed.), *Arthritis and Allied Conditions.* Chapter 102. 11th ed. Lea and Febiger, pp. 1605–1630, 1989.

10. Davis MA: The epidemiology of osteoarthritis. *Clinics in Geriatric Medicine (Rheumatic Disorders)* 4:241, 1988.

11. Cooke TD: The polyarticular features of osteoarthritis requiring hip and knee surgery. *J Rheumatol* 10:288, 1983.

12. O'Duffy JD: Spinal stenosis. *In* McCarty DJ (ed.), *Arthritis and Allied Conditions.* Chapter 93. 11th ed. Lea and Febiger, pp. 1464–1472, 1989.

13. Svarra CJ, Nortin MH: Back pain. *Clinics in Geriatric Medicine (Rheumatic Disorders)* 4:395, 1988.

14. Koji I, Shighikawa K, Nishioka J, *et al.*: *Ann Rheum Dis* 46:908, 1987.

15. Doherty M, Dieppe P: Crystal deposition disease in the elderly. *Clinics in Rheumatic Disease (Arthritis in the Elderly)* 12:97, 1986.

16. Brandt KD: Treatment of osteoarthritis. *In* McCarty DJ (ed.), *Arthritis and Allied Conditions.* Chapter 103. 11th ed. Lea and Febiger, pp. 1631–1644, 1989.

29 | INFLAMMATORY POLYARTHRITIS

CASE PRESENTATION

A 71-year-old man presents with a three-month history of progressive joint pain and muscle stiffness. Previous to this he was completely asymptomatic. His pain and stiffness are much worse in the mornings and persist for several hours. On clinical examination, he looks surprisingly well. However, movement of the shoulders (especially abduction) is markedly restricted and very painful. You notice mild atrophy of both deltoid muscles. There is considerable synovial thickening, tenderness, and stress pain of both wrists and, to a lesser extent, of the metacarpal and proximal interphalangeal joints of the hands. In the lower extremities there is evidence of moderate synovitis of his knees but no abnormality of the feet and ankles. His hemoglobin is slightly decreased at 10.8 g per cent. The white cell count and differential are normal, but his platelet count is elevated at 660,000 per cubic millimeter. The erythrocyte sedimentation rate is 65 mm per hour, and the rheumatoid factor is negative. The patient has been treated with nonsteroidal anti-inflammatory drugs that have failed to relieve his symptoms.

L.E. Hart
D.W. Molloy
W.E. DeCoteau

Consider the following statements (true or false)

1. Shoulder synovitis is a common presentation of several forms of arthritis in the elderly.

2. Systemic lupus erythematosus (SLE) is unlikely in view of the man's relatively advanced age.

3. In the presence of apparent inflammation, osteoarthritis is also unlikely.

4. The patient is rheumatoid factor (RF)–negative; but if RF were present, the diagnosis of rheumatoid arthritis would be secured.

5. Rather than immediately proceeding to disease-modifying antirheumatic drugs (DMARDs) in this patient, it would be appropriate to start him on low-dose prednisone.

1. TRUE

A common cause of bilateral synovitis of the shoulders in an elderly person is polymyalgia rheumatica (PMR). However, it is important to realize that several other rheumatic diseases present with shoulder synovitis and features that can be confused with PMR. Late-onset rheumatoid arthritis (RA) and acute exacerbations in established classical RA in an elderly person might present in this way [1]. In addition, the occasional case of systemic lupus erythematosus (SLE) can present with a PMR-like picture [2]. Moreover, patients with bilateral synovitis of the shoulders can develop disease atrophy and secondary weakness of the shoulder girdle muscles that may be misdiagnosed as polymyositis. However, unlike true polymyositis, these patients will not have high serum levels of muscle enzymes, abnormal EMG studies, or evidence of inflammation on muscle biopsy. An underlying malignancy can also present with a syndrome that is similar to PMR.

In recent years it has been noted that many elderly patients develop a syndrome that is characterized by bilateral shoulder synovitis plus inflammation in other joint regions. The feet are rarely involved. These patients frequently are rheumatoid factor–negative, have a high erythrocyte sedimentation rate (ESR), a low hemoglobin level, and an elevated platelet count. For all practical purposes, they closely resemble patients with PMR in both their presentation and response to treatment. However, they differ from patients with PMR in that their disease has extended beyond the shoulder and pelvic girdles. It is appropriate to label this syndrome as idiopathic inflammatory arthritis of the elderly [3].

2. FALSE

SLE should be definitively ruled out in this patient, since more cases of spontaneous lupus are being recognized with late onset in both men and women [4,5]. It is also very important to consider drug-induced lupus in an elderly person presenting with arthritis, since several of the drugs that are often given to the elderly can produce this problem [6]. Among the more commonly prescribed are procainamide (Pronestyl) and hydralazine (Apresoline). Therefore, any elderly patient who presents with a polyarthritis and who is on medications that may be implicated in causing SLE should have an antinuclear antibody (ANA) test performed. The presence of ANA is not specific for SLE but a negative ANA would considerably weaken a diagnosis of either spontaneous or drug-induced lupus in this patient. Recently, a new test for procainamide-induced lupus has been developed and shows great promise. Apparently patients who are about to develop symptomatic procainamide-induced lupus have an antibody to histone [7].

3. FALSE

It has recently been shown that there is quite a profound synovitis in many cases of osteoarthritis [8]. Immune factors probably play a role in this condition, with animal studies demonstrating an immune response to cartilage proteoglycan [9]. Inflammatory osteoarthritis is a well-described entity that occurs mainly in elderly females and involves particularly the distal interphalangeal joints (Heberden's nodes), the proximal interphalangeal joints (Bouchard's nodes), and the first carpometacarpal joints [10]. The great toes are also frequently involved in this syndrome. The pattern of joint distribution should not be confused with that of RA or SLE except when metacarpophalangeal joints are involved with an osteoarthritic process.

The idiopathic polyarthritis syndrome described in Question 1 can be superimposed on well-established OA. When this occurs, the easily recognized OA often obscures the inflammatory problem that often has to be addressed as a separate issue [11].

4. FALSE

While it is true that up to 90% of patients with definite RA who possess the characteristic erosions on x-ray examinations will have rheumatoid factor, the auto-antibody is found in other disease states as well [12]. These include other forms of connective tissue disease such as SLE, scleroderma, and related conditions such as the CREST syndrome and mixed connective tissue disease. Primary Sjögren's syndrome can be associated with a low-grade form of synovitis that mimics RA and invariably is found with high serum titers of rheumatoid factor [12]. It needs also to be realized that about 5% of normal elderly persons have rheumatoid factor, and this certainly can obscure the correct diagnosis in these patients [13].

5. TRUE

Patients with idiopathic inflammatory polyarthritis usually improve after NSAIDs are started, but, like PMR, they often respond very dramatically to low-dose corticosteroids. However, it must be pointed out that some of these patients develop classical RA. Unfortunately. we do not have a simple marker to identify such cases. However, a recent study has reported that 21 of 22 cases with older onset. seropositive, erosive RA had the typical "RA" HLA phenotype—DR4 (Dw14 and Dw4) and DR1—while only 9 of 18 cases with seronegative, nonerosive inflammatory arthritis had such a phenotype [14]. An incidence rate of 15% (in the latter group) approximates what might be expected in the general population. The dramatic difference in the frequency of this marker in these two populations with rheumatoid arthritis suggests that HLA typing may help to differentiate between the two.

All patients with inflammatory polyarthritis should be followed closely to monitor their response and toxicity to corticosteroids. If there is a poor clinical response to corticosteroids or if the case develops into a more typical rheumatoid syndrome, consider DMARD therapy. It should also be emphasized that some cases of idiopathic inflammatory polyarthritis can be associated with temporal arteritis, with its attendant complications [15] (see Chapter 35, Giant Cell Arteritis).

REFERENCES

1. Healey LA, Sheets P: The relation of polymyalgia rheumatica to rheumatoid arthritis. *J Rheumatol* 15:750, 1988.
2. Hutton CW, Maddison PJ: Systemic lupus erythematosus presenting as polymyalgia rheumatica in the elderly. *Ann Rheum Dis* 45:641, 1986.
3. Healey LA: Late onset rheumatoid arthritis *versus* polymyalgia rheumatica: Making the diagnosis. *Geriatrics* 43:69, 1988.
4. Hashimoto M, Tsuda H, Hirano T, *et al.*: Differences in clinical and immunological findings of systemic lupus erythematosus related to age. *J Rheum* 14:497, 1987.
5. Bell D: SLE in the elderly—Is it really SLE or systemic Sjögren's syndrome (editorial). *J Rheum* 14:723, 1987.
6. Hess E: Drug-related lupus (editorial). *N Eng J Med* 318:1460, 1988.
7. Totoritis MC, Tan E, McNally E, *et al.*: Association of antibody to histone complex H2A-2B with symptomatic procaine-induced lupus. *N Eng J Med* 318:1431, 1988.
8. Altman RD, Gray R: Inflammation in osteoarthritis. *Clin Rheum Dis* 11:353, 1985.
9. Cohen IR, Holoshitz J, van Edel W, *et al.*: T-cell clones in adjuvant arthritis. *Arthritis Rheum* 28:841, 1985.
10. Hochberg M: Osteoarthritis: Pathophysiology, clinical features, management. *Hospital Practice*, December 1984.
11. Inoue K, Schichikawa K, Nishioka J, *et al.*: Older age onset rheumatoid arthritis with or without osteoarthritis. *Ann Rheum Dis* 46:908, 1987.
12. Healey LA: Rheumatoid arthritis in the elderly. *Clin Rheum Dis* 12:173, 1986.
13. Morgan SH, Hughes GRV: The laboratory investigation of rheumatic and connective tissue diseases. *Clin Allergy and Immun* 5:513, 1985.
14. Nepom GT, Byers P, Seyfried C, *et al.*: HLA genes associated with rheumatoid arthritis: Identification of susceptibility alleles using specific oligonucleotide probes. *Arthritis Rheum* 32:15–21, 1989.
15. Ginsburg WW, Cohen M, Hall S, *et al.*: Seronegative polyarthritis in giant cell arteritis. *Arthritis Rheum* 28:1362, 1985.

30 CRYSTAL-RELATED ARTHROPATHY

CASE PRESENTATION

A 76-year-old female has recently been diagnosed as having calcium pyrophosphate dihydrate deposition (CPPD) disease. Her problem started 15 years ago with painful knees. She was thought to have osteoarthritis and was treated with salicylate on demand. The pain progressed and became severe on weight bearing and even at rest. The knees were frequently swollen, and flexion contractures developed. For the past five years she has had discomfort in her shoulders, ankles, wrists, and knuckles. Seronegative rheumatoid arthritis was diagnosed. She was treated with injectable gold salts and nonsteroidal anti-inflammatory agents without effect.

On two occasions over the past three years, she developed acute pain, swelling, and redness over the right wrist. The first episode was thought to be infectious, but antibiotics were stopped when synovial fluid cultures were negative. One year later she developed another episode, which was thought to be due to gout or pseudogout. This episode responded to intravenous colchicine after salicylate treatment failed.

Apart from pain and immobility from the arthritis, her health is generally good. She takes a thiazide for borderline hypertension.

W.E. DeCoteau
L.E. Hart
D.W. Molloy

About three months ago a rheumatologist diagnosed CPPD on the basis of her clinical picture and radiologic studies showing severe degenerative changes. These findings were predominantly in the knees, ankles, shoulders, wrists, and metacarpophalangeal joints. There were flecks of calcium in the right triangular ligament of the wrist. Routine hematology and biochemistry, including calcium and phosphorus, are normal. Serum uric acid is slightly increased. She asks you for a prescription for something in case she has another acute episode of inflammation and pain.

Consider the following statements (true or false)

1. A pseudogout syndrome is the commonest articular manifestation of symptomatic CPPD.

2. Chondrocalcinosis must be present on routine x-ray to diagnose any form of the CPPD syndrome.

3. Hyperparathyroidism is an important underlying cause of CPPD.

4. Urate gout is rarely found in elderly females.

5. The syndrome known as "Milwaukee" shoulder is an example of hydroxyapatite crystals producing destructive arthropathy.

1. FALSE

The first recognized cases of calcium pyrophosphate deposition (CPPD) arthritis were acute and monoarticular, involving the knee. Calcification was noted in cartilage structures, and CPPD crystals rather than monosodium urate (MSU) were noted in the synovial fluid of the affected joint. The knee, rather than the great toe, was most commonly involved. The process resembled gout, but was not gout. Hence the name pseudogout [1].

Later it was noted that CPPD crystals affected the musculo-skeletal system in several different ways [2]. Resnick described a chronic degenerative arthritis associated with CPPD crystals, which he called pyrophosphate arthropathy [3]. In one large study of 105 consecutive cases of CPPD, 29 persons had the pseudogout syndrome. These were often younger males. Seventy-six had chronic polyarthritis of the pyrophosphate type. This group was composed of predominantly elderly females, 8 of whom were originally mislabeled as rheumatoid arthritics [4].

Unlike classical rheumatoid arthritis, persons with the pseudo-rheumatoid state of CPPD do not have positive rheumatoid factor or articular erosions, and they respond poorly to disease-modifying antirheumatic drugs (DMARDs).

The acute pseudogout syndrome often responds to nonsteroidal anti-inflammatory drugs (NSAIDs) and/or mere aspiration of fluid from an inflamed joint. Intra-articular corticosteroid can also be helpful [5]. Oral colchicine can also be utilized, but almost invariably produces severe diarrhea and/or abdominal cramps before the joint inflammation abates. Intravenous colchicine, in a dose of 1 to 2 mg, often controls the acute inflammation and does not produce bowel disturbance. However, the drug must be used with caution since intravenous colchicine can produce a severe chemical phlebitis if the colchicine goes outside the vein. Bone marrow suppression is also a worry. Therefore, the drug must be used cautiously and very sparingly, especially in the elderly [6].

The treatment of chronic pyrophosphate arthropathy resembles that of osteoarthritis—analgesics and NSAIDs, weight reduction, physiotherapy, walking aids, and joint replacement in selected cases. Intra-articular steroid can also be helpful. Recently, intra-articular yttrium has shown promise for treatment of inflamed joints that have not responded to the above measures [5]. However, yttrium should be used only by specialists who are familiar with its use.

2. FALSE

CPPD deposition occurs in cartilaginous structures, especially those composed of fibrocartilage, such as menisci of the knee and the triangular ligament of the wrist. It occurs less commonly in the hyaline cartilage of joints.

CPPD deposition is frequently asymptomatic, but it can be associated with any or all of the arthritic syndromes [7]. In many cases of pyrophosphate arthropathy, no calcification of cartilage is detected by routine x-ray examination [3]. In the absence of calcification, CPPD may be suspected by the presence of one or more of the following features:

1. degenerative arthritis in joints not usually involved in primary osteoarthritis, that is, shoulder, elbow, metacarpal-phalangeal joints, and/or ankle;
2. unusual intra-articular distribution of arthritis compared to osteoarthritis, that is, patellofemoral and/or radiocarpal joints;
3. presence of loose bodies, calcification of ligaments, bursae, synovial membrane, or joint capsule of affected joints;
4. extensive subchondral cyst formation; and
5. hypertrophic new bone formation, especially at the patellofemoral joint [3].

With crystal release into the synovial fluid, there is an inflammatory response. The presentation of the syndrome results from the pattern of inflammation, crystal release, and deposition. An acute short-lived release of crystals into one joint causes a pseudogout picture. A more persistent release of crystals into several joints mimics rheumatoid arthritis [5]. The deposition of crystals in cartilage can also be associated with severe degenerative disease, but it is still not established if the crystals damage cartilage and lead to degeneration or if the degeneration occurs first and is followed by crystal deposition [7].

3. TRUE

Hyperparathyroidism with hypercalcemia is responsible for some cases and should always be sought in CPPD. Rule out other persistent hypercalcemic states such as idiopathic hypercalciuria with hypercalcemia. Other known causes of CPPD relate to the presence of excessive pyrophosphate, which results from either excessive production of pyrophosphate by damaged cartilage or from decreased destruction of pyrophosphate because of a deficiency of pyrophosphatase enzyme activity [7].

Changes can also occur within the cartilage matrix that leads to the deposition and growth of calcium pyrophosphate dihydrate crystals [8]. Presumably, matrix abnormality is the mechanism in the hereditary form of CPPD. This is a very important cause of CPPD in some communities [7].

An example of how prior cartilage injury can lead to CPPD is suggested by Doherty. He found in a long-term follow-up of unilateral knee miniscetomy patients that there was a much higher incidence of CPPD in the operated than in the non-operated knee (20% *versus* 4%) [5].

4. FALSE

Urate gout is extremely rare in premenopausal females, possibly due to (a) normally lower plasma uric acid levels in these females [9] and (b) stabilization of the lysosomes of inflammatory cells by estrogen [10]. With menopause, the plasma level of uric acid in women increases, while estrogen is not available to stabilize lysosomes. An even more important factor appears to be the frequent use, or perhaps misuse, of thiazide diuretics in elderly females [11]. Thiazide can commonly lead to the development of three gout syndromes:

1. typical monoarticular gout of great toe or ankle;
2. polyarthritis of small joints that resembles rheumatoid arthritis [12]; and
3. tophaceous gout as a first manifestation of disease. The tophi tend to occur in finger joints already affected with osteoarthritis (for example, Heberden's nodes) [11].

Physicians should become sensitized to the atypical features of thiazide-induced gout of the elderly (especially females) and prescribe thiazides in this age group only when absolutely indicated.

An attack of acute gout can usually be brought under control quickly by any of the NSAIDs (except salicylate). NSAIDs can also be used to control the development of urate gout induced by thiazides where the thiazides cannot be discontinued for medical reasons. The NSAIDs are also preferred over oral colchicine because of colchicine's severe bowel toxicity at high dose (*i.e.*, 1 mg per hour for several doses). Intravenous colchicine is very useful in cases that are severe, especially if NSAID gastropathy is present (see Question 1).

Gout attacks may be precipitated by abrupt increases or decreases of plasma uric acid levels [13]. Alcohol and excessive ingestion of food of high purine content are known to increase uric acid, as is salicylate in low dosage (less than 2 g per 24 hours). At this level salicylates interfere with renal tubular secretion of uric acid. Therefore, salicylates are not good agents to use to treat gout. Conversely, the abrupt lowering of uric acid by the xanthine oxidize–inhibiting agent, allopurinol, can also precipitate gout in some persons. This apparent paradoxical effect of allopurinol tends to occur when the drug is given to individuals with an abnormally high uric acid pool (*i.e.*, tophaceous gout). Allopurinol-induced gout can usually be prevented by the concomitant administration of an NSAID and/or low-dose oral colchicine (*i.e.*, 0.5 mg two to three times per day). After several months, when the body pool of uric acid has been lowered, small-dose allopurinol will prevent gout [13].

However, allopurinol should be used with caution in the elderly and especially those with poor renal function. Rash, hepatitis, and bone marrow suppression are not common but should be kept in mind. A fatal hypersensitivity syndrome consisting of fever, exfoliative rash, hepatitis, and renal failure occurring one to six weeks after beginning allopurinol therapy has been described and is more common in the elderly with poor renal function [14].

5. TRUE

A form of rapidly progressive, destructive, degenerative arthritis of large joints found in association with the presence of hydroxyapatite crystals in synovial fluid was described a few years ago by McCarty as "Milwaukee" shoulder [15]. He postulated that the crystals activated the production of collagenase in the shoulder joint. There was subsequent injury and digestion of the rotator cuff, as well as damage to joint cartilage and subchondral bone. The early cases were elderly females. Males can also develop the problem. The process can occur in the knee and/or shoulder.

Recently it has been suggested that Milwaukee shoulder is probably the same process that has been called cuff-tear arthropathy by an American orthopedist, epaule senile hemorrhagique by the French, and apatite-associated destructive arthropathy by the British [11].

Apatite crystals can also deposit in tendons and cause an acute inflammatory response (*i.e.*, calcific tendonitis).   Apatite and CPPD crystals can deposit in degenerative hip cartilage and may be responsible for some of the inflammation seen in some cases of osteoarthritis of the hip [11].

REFERENCES

1. McCarty DJ, *et al.*: The significance of calcium phosphate crystals in synovial fluid of arthritis patients: "The pseudogout syndrome". *Ann Int Med* 56:711–737, 1962.
2. McCarty DJ: Calcium pyrophosphate dihydrate deposition disease (CPPD). *Arth Rheum* 19(suppl.):275–286, 1976.
3. Resnick D, *et al*: Clinical, radiologic and pathologic abnormalities in CPPD. *Radiology* 122:1–15, 1977.
4. Dieppe PA, *et al*: Pyrophosphate arthropathy: A clinical and radiologic study of 105 cases. *Ann Rheum Dis* 41(suppl.):371–376, 1982.
5. Doherty M: Pyrophosphate arthropathy—Recent clinical advances. *Ann Rheum Dis* 42(suppl.):38–43, 1983.
6. Spillberg I, McLain D, Simchowitz L, *et al.*: Colchicine and pseudogout. *Arthritis and Rheumatism* 23:1062, 1980.

7. Ryan LM, McCarty DJ: Calcium pyrophosphate crystal deposition disease. *In Arthritis and Allied Disorders* 10th ed. Ch. 94, pp. 1515–1545. Philadelphia: Lea and Febiger, 1986.

8. Pritzker K, Cheng PT, Rerlund RC: Calcium pyrophosphate crystal deposition in hyaline cartilage. Ultrastructural analysis and implications for pathogenesis. *J of Rheum* 15:825–835, 1988.

9. Calkins E, Papdemetrian T, Challa H: Musculo-skeletal disease in the elderly. *In The Practice of Geriatrics.* Ch. 36, p. 386. E Calkins, P Davis, A Ford (eds.). Saunders, 1986.

10. Weissman G: The molecular basis of acute gout. *Hospital Practice* 7:43, 1971.

11. Doherty M, Dieppe P: Crystal deposition disease in the elderly. *Clinics in Rheumatic Diseases* 12:97–113, 1986.

12. Curran JJ, Renold F, Jamieson TW: Clinical manifestations of acute polyarticular gout in female patients. *Arth and Rheum* 31:R31, 1988.

13. Wortman RL: Management of hyperuricemia. *In Arthritis and Allied Disorders.* Ch. 29, pp. 1481–1505. 10th ed. Philadelphia: Lea and Febiger, 1985.

14. Campbell SM: Gout: How prevention, diagnosis and treatment differ in the elderly. *Geriatrics* 43:71, 1988.

15. McCarty DJ, Halvorson P: Basic calcium phosphate (apatite) crystal deposition disease. *In Arthritis and Allied Disorders.* 10th ed. Ch. 29, pp. 1547–1564. Philadelphia: Lea and Febiger, 1986.

31 | BACK PAIN AND OSTEOPOROSIS

CASE PRESENTATION

A 68-year-old Caucasian female presents with severe mid-back pain. This pain came on three weeks ago after she bent down to pick up a shopping bag. The pain is aggravated by activity and is resolved by lying quietly. She has noticed that over the years she has lost almost two inches in height and has become more stooped over.

She had menopause spontaneously at age 48 years. She has no children and is a nonsmoker who drinks alcohol occasionally. She was an elite athlete as a young woman and represented her country in the 1948 Olympics.

Five years ago she had a lumpectomy for Stage I breast cancer. This was followed by a course of local radiation therapy. She takes 500 mg of calcium per day and hydrochlorothiazide 25 mg daily for mild hypertension.

On examination she is a tiny woman (5 feet tall and 95 lbs) in moderate distress. She has an obvious dowager's hump. There is considerable local tenderness in the region of T12 with marked associated muscle spasm. She has a scar from previous surgery on the right breast. Otherwise, physical examination is unremarkable.

Routine laboratory investigations, including complete blood count, creatinine, calcium, phosphorus, and alkaline phosphatase, are normal. You consider the possibility that she has a fractured spine

W.E. DeCoteau
L.E. Hart
D.W. Molloy
J.D. Adachi

and wonder about the use of estrogen, cyclic etidronate, or sodium fluoride.

Consider the following statements (true or false)

1. It is unlikely that this woman has an osteoporotic crush fracture because of the trivial nature of her trauma.

2. Even if a lateral x-ray of the thoracolumbar spine reveals anterior wedging of several lower thoracic and upper lumbar vertebrae with a collapse fracture of T12, it would be reasonable to investigate further with a technetium bone scan.

3. Multiple myeloma would be ruled out by the absence of osteolytic lesions on bone survey, normal calcium levels, and a normal serum protein electrophoresis.

4. Estrogen therapy is the most potent therapeutic approach to the prevention of bone loss.

5. Cyclic etidronate shows excellent promise as a bone-protective agent in the treatment of patients with vertebral osteoporosis.

6. Sodium fluoride shows promise as a bone-protective agent in the treatment of patients with vertebral osteoporosis. However, there is concern that it may increase the incidence of peripheral hip fractures in such patients.

1. FALSE

A crush fracture as a result of vertebral osteoporosis could account for the woman's back pain, even though she experienced only minimal trauma. Osteoporosis is characterized by reduced bone mass which sufficiently compromises the skeleton such that fractures may occur with minimal or trivial trauma [1].

There are several reasons for suspecting osteoporosis in this woman. She had lost significant height and had a dorsal kyphosis. Secondly, she also possessed important genetic and acquired risk factors commonly seen in persons who develop primary osteoporosis. The risk factors for osteoporosis are

- sex (female),
- white or asiatic,
- diet (low lifelong calcium intake),
- early menopause (oophorectomy),
- amenorrhea of young females (elite athlete or anorexia nervosa),
- multiparity,
- sedentary lifestyle,
- alcohol abuse,
- cigarette smoking,
- high caffeine intake (coffee, cola drinks),
- high phosphorus intake, and
- high protein intake.

This patient is a white female of small stature, which indicates diminished bone mass at maturity. In comparison black, Latino, and even large-framed white females tend to have a greater bone mass and are less likely to develop osteoporosis. She had a normal menopause but conceivably could have had transient functional hypogonadism due to her athletic endeavors as a young woman. Total bone mass before maturity may also be increased by an adequate calcium intake and regular weight-bearing exercise [2]. Skeletal mass increases until about 30 years, followed by a period of stabilization; age-related bone loss occurs in both sexes. Women lose approximately 35% of their cortical bone and 50% of their trabecular bone, while men lose about two-thirds that amount. Bone loss occurs in two phases in women and involves both cortical and trabecular bone. The initial phase is slow and begins at about age 40 years. A rapid phase of bone loss with accelerated loss of trabecular bone takes place in some women immediately following menopause, especially if there is an abrupt withdrawal of estrogen, for example, following surgical oophorectomy [2].

It has been estimated that by age 60 years, bone mass will have fallen below the fracture threshold in 25% of all white females [3]. Type I postmenopausal osteoporosis becomes evident 10 to 15 years after menopause and is found mainly in females. The exact mechanism of production is not clear. Despite evidence of increased bone resorption, parathyroid hormone (PTH) production is decreased. Type II senile osteoporosis occurs in the elderly with a female-to-male ratio of 2 or 3 to 1. Type II osteoporosis is probably related to aging factors such as decreased calcium absorption and renal vitamin D activation, which in turn results in excessive PTH hormone activity.

Type I osteoporosis often results in fractures of trabecula-rich bones, including spinal vertebrae and distal radius. Type II osteoporosis tends to be associated with anterior wedging of vertebrae and/or hip fracture [2].

Vertebral compression fractures are by far the most common clinical problem in osteoporosis and, as was previously mentioned, can occur with minimal trauma, such as coughing, bending, sitting down in a low-set chair, or even lifting a light object. The lower thoracic and lumbar vertebral are most susceptible, and the pain of compression fracture is often severe. The patient can usually localize the pain to the fracture site, and this can be confirmed by even gentle percussion. The pain may radiate into the abdomen or flanks and can occasionally produce ileus, but nerve root compression is rare.

The patients lie on their back or side with knees and hips flexed. They often have to sit up or stand up from a lateral position. With bed rest and analgesics, acute pain usually subsides in six to eight weeks; however, patients frequently continue to have back pain. This usually results from paraspinal muscle spasm and spinal deformity. Patients lose height with each compression fracture, and in severe cases the ribs come to rest on the iliac crests. The abnormal skeletal mechanics can occasionally result in decreased respiratory compliance, early satiety and regurgitation of gastric contents, and a shuffling, unsteady gait due to altered pelvic tilt and hip muscle contractures [2].

Osteoporosis, like anemia, has many causes. The primary forms of osteoporosis should not be diagnosed before the secondary forms are ruled out. Following is a classification of the main causes of osteoporosis:

Primary, idiopathic causes

1. Early age onset
2. Elderly onset
   - Type I (postmenopausal osteoporosis)
   - Type II (senile osteoporosis)

Secondary causes

1. *Endocrinopathies:* hypogonadism (early oophorectomy, natural menopause, female athletes), hyperparathyroidism, hyperthyroidism, Cushing's syndrome
2. *Drugs:* glucocorticoids, anticonvulsants, heparin, alcohol
3. *B-cell neoplasia:* myeloma, Waldenstrom's macroglobulinemia, lymphoma (occasional T-cell lymphoma as well)
4. *Miscellaneous:* rheumatoid arthritis, intestinal malabsorption, postgastrectomy syndromes, chronic liver disease, systemic mastocytosis

2. TRUE

Although the patient appears to have primary osteoporosis by x-ray, it would be worthwhile to perform a technetium bone scan. The bone scan will help to determine whether the fracture is old and healed (will demonstrate normal isotope uptake) or recent and healing (increased isotope uptake). The scan may also help rule out metastatic carcinoma [4], which is a definite possibility because of the prior history of breast cancer. In metastatic malignancy, multiple sites of increased uptake in the spinal column or femora can be seen even though the routine x-ray shows no evidence of malignancy. The likelihood of a positive bone scan is greatly enhanced if clinical examination suggests prior history of malignancy, weight loss (frequently found in malignancy), or fever (frequently found in spinal infection) [5].

The characteristics of the pain are also important. Inflammatory back pain due to ankylosing spondylitis (mainly a disease of young adults) is characterized by pain and stiffness after prolonged inactivity. Mechanical back pain due to osteoporotic fractures or degenerative spinal disease is usually helped by rest but made worse by activity.

The pain of malignancy is often worse when the person lies still, especially when sleep is attempted. These patients often feel better pacing around [5].

3. FALSE

Most patients with myeloma have extensive bone destruction in the form of discrete osteolytic bone lesions, which may be confused with multiple metastasis as in breast and/or prostatic cancer. However, the bone lesions of myeloma occasionally produce generalized osteopenia that resembles idiopathic osteoporosis [6]. Despite the extensive bone destruction, hypercalcemia occurs in only 20% of cases of myeloma. The mechanism of bone destruction relates to the capacity of the plasma cells to synthesize a mediator that causes osteoclast activation [7].

Protein electrophoresis is a useful screening test for myeloma, since greater than 99% of cases have a monoclonal protein spike in serum and/or urine. Negative serum protein electrophoresis does not rule out myeloma, since 12% to 20% of cases will have Bence Jones protein (free light chain) in urine with no spike in serum [6].

The usual dip-stick analysis for protein in urine detects albumin, but not immunoglobulin or immunoglobulin light chains [6]. A high erythrocyte sediment rate and/or a low grade anemia suggests myeloma in patients with apparent osteoporosis but is not diagnostic. Myeloma can be truly diagnosed only by the detection of malignant plasma cell proliferation in either bone marrow or an extraskeletal site [6].

4. TRUE

It is not clear why only a percentage of postmenopausal women develop osteoporosis, since they are all estrogen deficient [2]. However, there is strong evidence that the provision of estrogens to estrogen-deficient women prevents the accelerated bone loss that occurs following loss of ovarian function [3]. Estrogen treatment will be more effective in preventing bone loss in persons with average bone mass, but it can also prevent further deterioration when the bone mass is below the fracture threshold.

Studies suggest that oral conjugated estrogens (*i.e.*, Premarin) at 0.625 mg per day prevent further bone loss in 90% of people. Recent data suggest that transdermal administration may be effective so long as significant blood levels of estrogen are obtained [3]. Some authorities recommend adjunct therapy such as 1000 to 1500 mg of calcium intake per day plus the equivalent in exercise of a five-mile walk per day [3]. Other investigators feel that high doses of calcium are of little value in the prevention of skeletal breakdown [8].

Progesterone added to estrogen is probably effective in reducing the total dose of estrogen required. This may result in decreased side effects, which include thrombosis, liver tumors, and cancer of the endometrium and, possibly, the breast [9].

Women who cannot or will not take estrogen may be given calcitonin. This peptide hormone will also reduce bone loss in osteoporosis. The subcutaneous route of calcitonin administration is somewhat impractical; the hormone can be effectively administered by the intranasal route [10].

5. TRUE

Cyclic etidronate therapy shows promise in the treatment of vertebral osteoporosis. Two recent studies have demonstrated that etidronate increases bone mass, and, more importantly, reduces vertebral fractures [11,12]. With etidronate there is an uncoupling of "coupling," that is, osteoclasts are inhibited by the etidronate, while osteoblasts continue to function producing more bone.

Etidronate is given cyclically in a dose of 400 mg per day for two weeks, followed by calcium for ten weeks. This regimen is then repeated. Preliminary follow-up of therapy that had continued for four years in this cyclical fashion has shown ongoing benefit. The only reported side effect noted with this therapy in osteoporosis is stomach upset. No ulcers have been reported with this therapy, however, and most patients are willing to put up with this minor discomfort.

6. TRUE

The use of sodium fluoride in the prevention and treatment of vertebral fractures remains controversial. While sodium fluoride is a bone-forming agent that increases trabecular bone mass in approximately 70% of cases, there is concern about the quality of new bone formed. In recent studies reported by the Mayo Clinic and Henry Ford Hospital, fluoride in relatively high doses (mean dose approximately 75 mg) was shown to increase bone mass, but did not reduce vertebral fracture rates[13,14]. Although patients complained of gastric upset, there was no actual increase in gastrointestinal bleeding. The investigators also found an increase in acute lower extremity pain syndrome, characterized by pain in the feet, ankles, and knees. This pain, in some instances, was felt to be due to incomplete fracture. In contrast, other studies using lower doses, intermittent therapy, or slower-release preparations have demonstrated both increases in bone mass and reductions in fracture rates [15,16].

Increased osteoid surfaces suggestive of osteomalacia may complicate sodium fluoride therapy. Adequate calcium intake and vitamin D supplementation in those who may be deficient may be useful in preventing excess osteoid accumulation.

At present, most experts in the field believe that further research in the use of fluoride therapy is required to establish the safest, most effective treatment regimen for osteoporosis.

Prevention is the only cost-effective approach to osteoporosis. Unless there is a history of hypercalciuria or kidney stones, the calcium content of the diet should be increased to 800 mg per day for adults and 1500 mg per day for adolescents. Weight-bearing exercise should be encouraged. Cigarette smoking should be stopped; alcohol and caffeine consumption should be curtailed. Hypogonadal young females should be evaluated and treated with estrogen if the problem persists. Estrogen replacement should be considered in high-risk persons at the time of menopause on an individualized basis [3].

REFERENCES

1. Lindsay R: Osteoporosis. *Clinics in Geriatric Medicine* (Saunders) 4:411, 1988.
2. Lyles KW: Osteoporosis. *In* WN Kelley (ed.) *Textbook of Internal Medicine.* Chap. 514, pp. 2601–2606. Philadelphia: Lippincott, 1989.
3. Lindsay R: Osteoporosis. Current strategy for management. *Geriatrics* 44:45, 1989.
4. Pelz DM, Haddad RG: Radiologic investigation of low back pain. *Journal of the Canadian Medical Association* 140:289, 1989.
5. Svarra CJ, Hadler N: Back pain. *Clinics in Geriatric Medicine* 4:395, 1988.
6. Cohen HJ: Monoclonal gammapathies and aging. *Hospital Practice* 23:75–100, 1988.
7. Garrett IR, Durie B, Nedwin G, *et al.*: Production of lymphotoxin, a bone-resorbing cytokine by cultured human myeloma cells. *New England Journal of Medicine* 316:173, 1987.
8. Riis B, Thomsen K, Christensen C: Does calcium supplementation prevent postmenopausal bone loss? *New England Journal of Medicine* 317:526, 1987.
9. Riggs BL, Melton III LJ: Involutional osteoporosis. *New England Journal of Medicine* 314:1676, 1986.
10. Reginster JY, Denis J, Albert A, *et al.*: A one-year randomized trial of prevention of early postmenopausal bone loss by intra-nasal calcitonin. *Lancet* 26:1481, 1987.

11. Storm T, Thamsborg G, Steiniche T, *et al.*: Effect of intermittent cyclical etidronate therapy on bone mass and fracture rate in women with postmenopausal osteoporosis. *New England Journal of Medicine* 322:1265–1271, 1990.
12. Watts NB, Harris ST, Genant HK, *et al.*: Intermittent cyclical etidronate treatment of postmenopausal osteoporosis. *New England Journal of Medicine* 323: 73–79, 1990.
13. Riggs BL, Hodgson SF, O'Fallon WM, *et al.*: Effect of fluoride treatment on fracture rate in postmenopausal women with osteoporosis. N*ew England Journal of Medicine* 322:802–809, 1990.
14. Kleerkoper M, Peterson E, Philips E, Nelson D, Tilley B, Parfitt AM. Continuous sodium fluoride therapy does not reduce vertebral fracture rate in postmenopausal osteoporosis. *Journal of Bone and Mineral Research* 4(suppl.1):S376, 1989.
15. Mamelle N, Meunier PJ, Dusan R, *et al.*: Risk-benefit ratio of sodium fluoride treatment in primary vertebral osteoporosis. *Lancet* 2:361–365, 1988.
16. Pak CYC, Sakhaee K, Kerwekh JE, Parcel C, *et al.*: Safe and effective treatment of osteoporosis with intermittent slow release sodium fluoride: Augmentation of vertebral bone mass and inhibition of fractures. *Journal of Clinical Endocrinology and Metabolism* 68:150–159, 1989.

Part VI

VASCULAR DISEASES

32 | HEART FAILURE

CASE PRESENTATION

Mr. J., a 79-year-old patient, presents to your office complaining of fatigue and insomnia. He has been unable to do his gardening this summer because of dyspnea on exertion. He complains of feeling "puffed out" when climbing the stairs from the basement to the second floor. At night, he has a nasty cough that wakes him two hours after going to bed and disappears after approximately 10 minutes of sitting up in bed.

He has been taking antihypertensive agents for eight years. Over the past four years, he has used hydrochlorothiazide (25 mg daily). Two years ago, he suffered a myocardial infarction (MI), which was uncomplicated except for a transient episode of congestive heart failure (CHF) that was treated with furosemide for one week. His other medications include levothyroxine and lorazepam (he forgot the doses). He denies any history of diabetes, or cardiac or pulmonary problems.

On examination, his pulse is regular at 100 bpm, and his BP is 165/80 mm Hg. He has an apical II/VI systolic ejection murmur. Carotid contour and volume are good. Chest auscultation reveals minimal bilateral basal crepitations.

You make the diagnosis of heart failure and send him for a chest x-ray, electrocardiogram, and blood tests. The radiologist reports that he had cardiomegaly and pulmonary vascular redistribution. The ECG shows

R. Jaeschke
M. Sauvé
D.W. Molloy

---

sinus tachycardia at a rate of 105 per minute, diffuse nonspecific ST-segment and T-wave abnormalities, small Q-waves in leads II and III (which were present two years ago), and a Q-wave in lead V_1 that was not present two years ago. Serum electrolytes are normal, and the results of the remaining blood work are pending.

Consider the following statements (true or false)

1. Appropriate management at this stage consists of initiating digoxin therapy in order to control symptoms.
2. The choice of therapy should be based only on the ability of a drug to control his symptoms.
3. With a new Q-wave in lead V_1, coronary artery disease (CAD) is the most likely cause of this abnormality (despite the fact that he has not had an episode of angina since his discharge from the hospital two years ago.)
4. This patient should not receive beta-blocker therapy because he suffered an episode of CHF at the time of his hospitalization for myocardial infarction.
5. Afterload reductions with angiotensin converting enzyme (ACE) inhibitors such as captopril are poorly tolerated in elderly patients.
6. It is not pressing to check the replacement dose of thyroid hormone that this patient is taking.

1. FALSE

The agent of choice for CHF is a subject of considerable debate. As of 1986, North American physicians chose diuretics (50%), diuretics with digoxin (33%), vasodilators (9%), and digoxin alone (7%) [1]. Nitrates were the most popular vasodilators (39%), followed by captopril (21%), and hydralazine alone (16%) or with nitrates (16%) [1].

Several recent well-designed studies have supplied new data that may change this pattern of practice. In a study comparing digoxin and captopril in patients with mild to moderate CHF, the ACE inhibitor was more effective than digoxin in increasing exercise tolerance, relieving symptoms, and improving functional class [2].

Studies comparing diuretics (combination of furosemide and amiloride) and captopril in CHF patients have shown that diuretics were more effective than captopril in relieving symptoms, improving exercise performance, and preventing decompensation [3,4].

The potency of different drugs in relieving CHF symptoms increases from digoxin through ACE inhibitors to diuretics. Therefore, diuretics are the agents of choice for initial symptom control. In this patient, increasing the dose of diuretic will result in the greatest degree of symptom relief. The dose of hydrochlorothiazide can be increased to 50 mg daily. If this proves ineffective in relieving symptoms, consider adding an ACE inhibitor.

2. FALSE

The prognosis associated with a new diagnosis of CHF remains very poor and is comparable with that of a variety of neoplasms. In the most recent report from the Framingham study, the four-year mortality rate for this condition was 55% for men and 24% for women [5]. This represents mortality figures six to seven times that of the general population of the same age.

Of the most widely used groups of drugs (digoxin, diuretics, and vasodilators), only vasodilators have been shown to favorably affect mortality rates. Although the combination of isosorbide dinitrate and hydralazine appears to improve survival [6], the most convincing reduction in CHF-related deaths was observed with the use of ACE inhibitors. This was confirmed for both enalapril [7] and captopril [8]. The six-month mortality rate was 44% on placebo *versus* 26% on enalapril. Corresponding figures for captopril and placebo were 21% *versus* 4%, respectively.

The effect of ACE inhibitors on the long-term survival of patients with mild CHF is now under study. However, a recent trial showed that captopril prevented progressive deterioration in left ventricular (LV) function, even in asymptomatic post-MI patients [9].

These data suggest that ACE inhibitors may become first-line therapy in newly diagnosed CHF patients, with diuretics added only if necessary for additional symptom control.

3. TRUE

Hypertension is a recognized cause of Q-waves in V_1 [10]. If the patient did not have a history of hypertension, silent MI would have been the most probable cause for these Q-waves. Silent MIs accounted for approximately 25% of infarctions in the Framingham study, and half of these were completely asymptomatic [11]. Hypertension and coronary artery disease (CAD) are the most common causes of heart failure in Western countries. As hypertension is a risk factor for CAD, it is often difficult to distinguish the primary mechanism leading to heart failure. The Framingham study showed that 50% of patients with cardiac failure had CAD and 70% had hypertension [5]. The fact that 90% of CAD patients who progressed to cardiac failure were hypertensive [5] supports the need for aggressive treatment of hypertension.

4. FALSE

Beta blockers are associated with reduced mortality rates in post-MI patients [12]; however, the use of beta blockers in patients with coexistent CHF is controversial. CHF is considered a contraindication for the use of beta blockers, although a study by Chadda *et al.* showed that beta blockers resulted in significant benefits in post-MI patients with CHF [13].

In this study, 710 patients were randomly assigned to standard therapy or to the same therapy plus propranolol (180 to 240 mg per day). The mortality rate in patients receiving propranolol was 13.3% compared to 18.4% in patients taking placebo. This 27% reduction was higher in CHF patients than in patients without CHF (25% reduction in three-year mortality).

The rate of withdrawal from the study due to decompensated CHF was similar in both groups (7.2% in the propranolol group and 6.6% in the placebo group). Therefore, beta blockers may be indicated in this patient.

5. TRUE

All drugs are more likely to produce higher incidences of side effects in the elderly than in younger patients. This is also true of drugs used in the treatment of CHF, such as digoxin, diuretics, and ACE inhibitors. Unfortunately, all large-scale trials of CHF therapy have excluded older patients or have included them only as a small proportion of the total population. The relative incidence of side effects must, therefore, be extrapolated from studies of younger patients.

In the study comparing the efficacy of captopril and digoxin, the rate of withdrawal due to side effects was 2.9% with captopril and 4.2% with digoxin [2]. However, the overall incidence of adverse reactions was higher with captopril (44%) than with digoxin (30%) or placebo (24%). Patients treated with captopril complained frequently of mild and transient dizziness or light-headedness. These symptoms were often alleviated by reducing the dose. As similar side effects may be associated with diuretic use, it is advisable in the elderly to institute diuretic therapy in low doses and monitor closely for possible side effects. Modify the dose or discontinue the drug if troublesome side effects appear.

6. FALSE

Factors such as anemia, fever, drugs, and iatrogenic fluid overload may precipitate CHF in the elderly. Inappropriate thyroid hormone replacement also should be considered in this patient. Both hyper- and hypothyroidism, even of relatively small magnitude, are associated with decreased LV performance and may contribute to CHF [14]. The patient's thyroid function tests should be checked to rule out the presence of hyper- or hypothyroidism. Patients with hyperthyroidism should have their thyroid hormone dosage reduced. In patients with hypothyroidism, determine whether they are complying with replacement therapy before attempting to increase the dose.

REFERENCES

1. Hlatky MA, Fleg JL, Hinton PC, *et al.*: Physician practice in the management of congestive heart failure. *J Am Coll Cardiol* 8:966, 1986.
2. The Captopril-Digoxin Multicenter Research Group: Comparative effects of therapy with captopril and digoxin in patients with mild to moderate heart failure. *JAMA* 259:539, 1988.
3. Cowley AJ, Stainer K, Wynne RD, *et al.*: Symptomatic assessment of patients with heart failure: Double-blind comparison of increasing doses of diuretics and captopril in moderate heart failure. *Lancet* II(8510):770, 1986.
4. Richardson A, Bayliss J, Scriven AJ, *et al.*: Double-blind comparison of captopril alone against furosemide plus amiloride in mild heart failure. *Lancet* II(8501): 709, 1987.
5. Kannel WB, Plehn JF, Cupples LA: Cardiac failure and sudden death in the Framingham study. *Am Heart J* 115:869, 1988.
6. Cohn JN, Archibald DG, Phil M, *et al.*: Effect of vasodilator therapy on mortality in chronic congestive heart failure: Results of a Veterans Administration cooperative study. *N Engl J Med* 314:1547, 1986.
7. The Consensus Trial Study Group: Effects of enalapril on mortality in severe congestive heart failure. *N Engl J Med* 316:1429, 1987.
8. Newman TJ, Maskin CS, Dennick LG, *et al.*: Effects of captopril on survival in patients with heart failure. *Am J Med* 84:140, 1988.
9. Sharpe N, Murphy J, Smith H, *et al.*: Treatment of patients with symptomless left ventricular dysfunction after myocardial infarction. *Lancet* I(8580):255, 1988.
10. Marriot HJL: *Practical Electrocardiography*. Baltimore: Williams and Wilkins, 1983.
11. Kannel WB, Abbott RD: Incidence and prognosis of unrecognized myocardial infarction. *N Engl J Med* 311:1144, 1984.
12. Frishman WH, Furberg CD, Friedewald WT: B-adrenergic blockade for survivors of acute myocardial infarction. *N Engl J Med* 310:830, 1984.
13. Chadda K, Goldstein S, Byington R, *et al.*: Effect of propranolol after acute myocardial infarction in patients with congestive heart failure. *Circulation* 3:503, 1986.
14. Forfar JC, Muir AL, Toft AD: Influence of thyroid hormones on left ventricular function—Evidence for impairment of myocardial contractility in both hyper- and hypothyroidism. *Ann Endocrinol* 43:42A, 1982.

33 | LOWER INTESTINAL BLEEDING

CASE PRESENTATION

A 75-year-old woman with iron deficiency anemia has been attending your office for three months. Her daughter confirms that she has been taking iron tablets every day. The patient has noted hematochezia (passage of bloody stools) twice in the past three months. She has not suffered abdominal pain but has a long history of constipation. She has undergone a barium meal and upper gastrointestinal tract endoscopy with normal results. A barium enema shows a few diverticula in the sigmoid colon. You feel that colonoscopy is required for diagnosis.

R. Clarnette
D.W. Molloy
R.H. Hunt

Consider the following statements (true or false)

1. Angiodysplasia and ischemic colitis are equally likely causes of this woman's blood loss.

2. The majority of patients' symptoms and/or radiologic changes from ischemic colitis occur only in the event of gangrene and/or perforation.

3. Angiodysplasia describes arteriovenous malformations in the gastrointestinal tract that occur predominantly in the right colon. Bleeding from these lesions may vary from massive to occult.

4. Angiodysplasia requires angiography for diagnosis since the lesions are too small to be seen on barium enema or colonoscopy.

5. Rectal blood loss due to diverticular disease is a diagnosis of exclusion.

1. FALSE

Ischemia of the bowel typically presents with mild to moderate crampy abdominal pain and is therefore less likely than angiodysplasia in this patient.

Ischemia of the bowel is a common cause of abdominal pain and rectal bleeding in the elderly [1]. The vascular supply to the intestine is derived from the celiac artery, superior mesenteric artery (SMA), and inferior mesenteric artery (IMA), which originate from the abdominal aorta. The mucosa receives most of the blood flow and is very susceptible to ischemia.

Ischemic colitis usually presents with a sudden onset of cramps in the left lower quadrant, but can occur anywhere in the abdomen. This is typically followed by bloody diarrhea and rectal bleeding. Cherry red blood is typical, but it may be altered [2]. "Transient ischemic colitis" is being recognized increasingly as a condition that is similar to ischemic colitis and resolves spontaneously. This condition may be under-diagnosed because, by the time these patients are investigated, symptoms and signs have resolved.

Radiologic studies are helpful and can confirm the diagnosis. On plain abdominal film the bowel may appear normal or may show a pattern suggestive of ileus. Barium enema may show thumbprinting of the colon or a series of smooth sacculations of the bowel wall, giving it a scalloped appearance. These are the pathognomonic signs of ischemia and are caused by mucosal edema or hemorrhage. Saw-tooth irregularity of the mucosa with ulceration and/or spasm of the involved segments may also be seen.

The watershed areas between the superior mesenteric artery (SMA) and the inferior mesenteric artery (IMA) and between the IMA and superior rectal artery are usually affected. The splenic flexure, descending colon, and sigmoid colon are most commonly involved, in decreasing order of frequency [3]. Colonoscopy is useful and is employed much earlier now in acute rectal bleeding. If barium enema is performed as the initial investigation, it interferes with subsequent colonoscopy and surgery, if they are indicated. Colonoscopy helps to rule out carcinoma.

Angiography is essential in the evaluation of small bowel ischemia but is generally unhelpful in patients with suspected colonic ischemia. Embolism is a rare cause of ischemic colitis due to the small caliber and oblique takeoff of the IMA. No specific occlusion can be identified in most cases at angiography, and the prognosis for ischemic colitis appears to be independent of the presence of arterial thrombi.

2. FALSE

In the majority of cases, ischemic colitis is a self-limiting disease, lasting only a few days and requiring only supportive therapy. One investigator reported 150 cases of colonic ischemia; 19% of the cases developed gangrene, 19% developed persistent colitis, and 42% had transient reversible colitis [1]. The outcome cannot be predicted on the basis of presenting symptoms or radiologic findings. Patients should receive supportive therapy and broad-spectrum antibiotics.

If fever, pain, leukocytosis, and abdominal tenderness persist after two or three days, serial abdominal films may help to diagnose perforation or megacolon. If there is little resolution of the x-ray findings, such as persistent edema "thumbprinting" with a dilated bowel, the prognosis for recovery is poor. Rectal bleeding is rarely profuse enough alone to require surgery.

As well as complete resolution and gangrene, stricture formation can

Table 33-1 Typical Findings in Acute Ischemic Bowel Disease.

	Small bowel	Large bowel
Age	More common with advancing age	
Precipitating cause	Hypotension	Usually none
Presentation	Central abdominal pain Diarrhea and/or hematochezia later	Lower abdominal pain Hematochezia and/or bloody diarrhea early
Diagnosis	Plain abdominal film Angiography (50% of patients have occlusion)	Plain abdominal film Barium enema Thumbprinting
Prognosis	Poor	Good
Complications	Perforation Gangrene (more common)	Stricture (usually asymptomatic) Gangrene, perforation (less common)

occur with ischemic colitis [4]. Strictures may develop acutely and can be followed with barium enema examinations. They rarely cause significant obstruction and rarely require surgery. The majority occur in the descending or sigmoid colon and tend to be longer and more symmetric than malignant strictures. Ischemic strictures are frequently found on the barium enema film of elderly patients who have no history of ischemic colitis. In these cases, colonoscopy is indicated to exclude carcinoma.

Ischemic ileitis also occurs more commonly in the elderly than in young adults. It may be preceded by an episode of hypotension due to cardiac failure, arrhythmia, or shock [5]. It presents with central abdominal pain, followed by diarrhea and/or hematochezia. Fifty percent have positive angiography, and the prognosis is worse than with ischemic colitis. Table 33-1 lists the features and characteristics of small and large bowel ischemia.

3. TRUE

The prevalence of colonic angiodysplasia increases with age and is frequently found in persons over age 60. Boley *et al.* examined the colons of patients in this age group who had undergone partial colectomy for colonic carcinoma [6]. None had a history of bleeding or colonic obstruction. A prevalence of mucosal ectasia (24%) and dilated mucosal veins (50%) was found. These disorders may precede the development of angiodysplasia.

The prevalence of angiodysplasia of the colon in asymptomatic elderly persons is unknown. In one series it was identified in 3% of over 3000 patients who underwent colonoscopy for rectal bleeding [7]. These lesions are vascular ectasias resulting from degenerative changes that accompany aging. They may be caused by chronic partial intermittent obstruction of the mucosal veins, where they pierce the submucosal layers of the colon. Repeated episodes may cause dilatation of veins and mucosal capillaries, with eventual loss of competency of the precapillary sphincters, resulting in an arteriovenous communication.

Lesions occur predominantly in the cecum and ascending colon. The prevalence of these lesions in the right colon can be attributed to the greater tension in the cecal wall than in other parts of the colon. According to Laplace's law $(P = T/D)$, for any given intraluminal pressure (P), the tension in the wall (T) is greatest in the portion of the bowel with the greatest diameter (D). Since raised wall tension produces the intermittent partial obstruction of the mucosal veins, the widest part of the cecum is the most common site for these vascular ectatic changes.

Angiodysplasia in the elderly differs from the usual congenital or neoplastic vascular abnormalities in the GI tract. It is not associated with angiomatous lesions of skin or of other viscera. It is associated with aortic valve stenosis. In one report the lesions stopped bleeding after aortic valve replacement [8].

Angiodysplastic lesions are usually less than 5 mm in diameter and range from 1 mm to 1 cm total size. There are often multiple lesions. They produce lower intestinal hemorrhage or anemia from chronic blood loss. Some patients have acute lower intestinal bleeding, which may be life-threatening. There is no characteristic bleeding pattern. It varies from massive life-threatening hemorrhage to slow occult bleeding. The same patient may exhibit different bleeding patterns on different occasions.

4. FALSE

If angiodysplasia is suspected, then colonoscopy is the investigation of choice [9]. Good bowel preparation and careful examination is required if lesions are to be seen. Coagulation of the lesions can be performed at the time of colonoscopy and may be curative. It is not possible to diagnose angiodysplasia with a barium enema.

Selective mesenteric angiography was the principal means of diagnosis before the advent of fiberoptic colonoscopy [10]. Since it is an invasive procedure and morbidity is increased in the elderly, angiography should be confined to those situations where the patient is still bleeding and colonoscopy has failed to provide a diagnosis.

If colonoscopic coagulation does not stop bleeding, then partial colectomy may be required. In a study of 26 patients who underwent colonoscopic coagulation, 11 had subsequent rebleeding [11]. Three patients underwent hemicolectomy as primary management because of extensive lesions. One patient required surgery for rebleeding and another because of coexistent carcinoma.

5. TRUE

The prevalence of diverticular disease of the colon correlates with advancing age in Western society [12]. It is clear that dietary habits have a pathogenetic role, especially the increased consumption of refined and

Table 33-2   Common Causes of Lower Gastrointestinal Bleeding in the Elderly.

Massive	*Occult*
Diverticular disease	Diverticular disease
Angiodysplasia	Angiodysplasia
Radiation proctitis	Colonic polyps
Colorectal carcinoma	Colorectal carcinoma
Colonic polyps	Hemorrhoids
Ischemic colitis	Fecal impaction
	Anal stricture
	Ischemic colitis

Source: Welch CE, Athanasoulis CA, Goldabini JJ: Hemorrhage from the large bowel with special reference to angiodysplasia and diverticular disease. *World J Surg* 2: 27–83, 1978.

processed food [13]. Most people with diverticular disease are asymptomatic throughout life. The patient may present with recurrent episodic left-sided abdominal pain, acute diverticulitis, or hemorrhage. The role that diverticula play in causing pain is not clear, and symptoms may be indistinguishable from irritable bowel syndrome.

Hemorrhage is a well-recognized complication of diverticular disease. Following the more widespread use of colonoscopy in the 1970s, it became clear that angiodysplasia was as common a cause of bleeding as diverticular disease, or even more common [14]. Therefore it is necessary to rule out angiodysplasia, carcinoma polyps, and colitis before bleeding is attributed to diverticular disease [15].

The investigative approach to a patient with colonic blood loss is determined by the most likely diagnosis after history and examination, the patient's condition, and the availability of facilities for testing. In general, colonoscopy is the procedure of choice after sigmoidoscopy has been performed. It has been shown to have greater sensitivity in detecting tumors greater than 5 mm in diameter in comparison to double contrast barium enema [16]. Management decisions should be based on consultation with the radiologist, endoscopist, surgeon, and nuclear medicine physician. The common causes of massive and occult lower intestinal bleeding are listed in Table 33-2.

REFERENCES

1. Boley SJ, Brandt LJ, Veith FJ: Ischemic disorders of the intestine. *Curr Prob Surg* 15:1, 1978.
2. Saegesser F, Sandblom P: Ischemic lesions of the distended colon. *Am J Surg* 129:309, 1975.
3. Marston A: Pattern of intestinal ischemia. *Lancet* 1:491, 1965.
4. Lea TM: Radiology—Plain films and barium studies of the ischemic bowel. *Clin Gastroenterol* 1:588–595, 1972.
5. Marston A: *Intestinal Ischemia.* London: Edward Arnold, 1977.
6. Boley SJ, Sammartano R, Adams A, *et al.*: On the nature and etiology of vascular ectasias of the colon. *Gastroenterol* 72:650–660, 1977.
7. Williams CB: Colonoscopy. *Br Med Bull* 42:265–269, 1986.
8. Cappell MS, Lebwohl O: Cessation of recurrent bleeding from gastrointestinal angiodysplasias after aortic valve replacement. *Ann Int Med* 105:54–57, 1986.
9. Hunt RH: Angiodysplasia of the colon. *In* Salmon P, ed.: *Growing Points in Endoscopy.* London: Chapman and Hall, 1982, p. 97.
10. Boley SJ, Sprayregan S, Sammartano RJ, Adams A, Kleinhause S: The pathophysiologic basis for the angiographic signs of vascular ectasias of the colon. *Diagn Radiol* 125:615–621, 1977.
11. Howard OM, Buchanan JD, Hunt RH: Angiodysplasia of the colon. Experience of 26 cases. *Lancet* 2:16–19, 1982.
12. Parks TG: Natural history of diverticular disease of the colon. *Clin Gastroenterol* 4:53–69, 1975.
13. Almy TP, Howell DA: Diverticular disease of the colon. *N Engl J Med* 302:324–331, 1980.
14. Welch CE, Athanasoulis CA, Galdabini JJ: Hemorrhage from the large bowel with special reference to angiodysplasia and diverticular disease. *World J Surg* 2:73–83, 1978.
15. Boley SJ, DiBiase A, Brandt LJ, Sammartano RJ: Lower intestinal bleeding in the elderly. *Am J Surg* 137:57–64, 1979.
16. Irvine EJ, O'Connor J, Frost RA, *et al.*: Prospective comparison of double contrast barium enema plus flexible sigmoidoscopy *vs.* colonoscopy in rectal bleeding. *Gut* 29:1188–1193, 1988.

34 | DEEP VENOUS THROMBOSIS

CASE PRESENTATION

A 73-year-old woman presents with a two-day history of right-calf swelling. She is fully ambulatory and has been well and asymptomatic up to two days ago. She suffers from arthritis in both knees and mild congestive heart failure (CHF), which has caused ankle edema in the past. She has no respiratory symptoms, and there is no history of trauma in the leg. On examination, you find that she has a reddened, swollen right calf and normal arterial pulses. Homans' sign is negative. You suspect that she may have deep venous thrombosis (DVT).

A. Panju
D.W. Molloy
R. Hull
J. Hirsh

Consider the following statements (true or false)

1. History and physical examination are reliable in diagnosing or excluding DVT.

2. Patients with suspected DVT should always have venography to confirm or rule out its presence.

3. A combination of impedance plethysmography (IPG) and fibrinogen leg scanning are as reliable as venography in diagnosing or excluding DVT.

4. Serial IPG detects clinically significant DVT and may be used instead of venography or the IPG and fibrinogen leg scanning combination.

5. About 50% of untreated patients with proximal DVT develop pulmonary embolism.

1. FALSE

For practical purposes, the clinician suspicious of DVT should always establish or exclude the diagnosis using objective tests. This is because patients with minimal leg symptoms may have extensive venous thrombosis and because classic signs and symptoms of pain, tenderness, and swelling of the leg are frequently caused by nonthrombotic disorders [1]. The factors that predispose to the formation of DVT are listed in Table 34-1.

In the vast majority of patients who present with clinically suspected DVT, the symptoms and signs are nonspecific, and in more than 50% of these patients, the clinical suspicion of venous thrombosis is not confirmed by objective testing [2,3]. This does not mean that a careful history

Table 34-1   Factors Increasing Risk and Predisposing to DVT Formation.

Immobility	Hematologic disorders (*e.g.,* thrombocytosis)
Congestive heart failure	
Neoplasia	Chronic obstructive pulmonary disease
Recent surgery	
Pregnancy	Obesity
Oral contraceptives (particularly in women over age 30)	Molecular abnormalities (A-T III, Protein C, Protein 5)
Intrinsic venous disease	

Table 34-2   Suspected DVT with Negative Venogram.

Cause	*Incidence*
Muscle strain from unaccustomed exercising	24%
Direct twisting injury to the leg	10%
Swelling in the paralyzed leg	9%
Venous reflex	7%
Lymphangitis, lymphatic obstruction	7%
Muscle tear	6%
Baker's cyst	5%
Cellulitis	3%
Internal knee derangement	2%
Unknown	26%

and physical examination should not be done, because they may uncover an alternative cause of the patient's symptoms, such as cellulitis, internal derangement of the knee, calf-muscle strain or tear, postphlebitic syndrome, ruptured Baker's cyst, calf-muscle hematoma, or lymphedema. The conditions that cause swelling, tenderness, or leg pain and are often mistaken for DVT are listed in Table 34-2. The possibility of venous thrombosis should always be excluded by objective testing.

2. FALSE

Three objective tests—venography, a combination of IPG and fibrinogen scanning, and serial IPG—have been subjected to rigorously designed clinical trials evaluating their ability to confirm or rule out a diagnosis of DVT. An approach to the use of these tests is described in Figure 34-1.

All three approaches are reliable if they are used appropriately [4]. The standard test for diagnosing venous thrombosis is venography. It has, however, a number of limitations, and for this reason alternative, less invasive objective tests are being used in Hamilton, Ontario.

Venography is invasive and relatively inconvenient to perform because it requires a fully equipped radiology suite. It may be painful, is relatively expensive, and cannot be performed conveniently on an outpatient basis. On rare occasions, it may be complicated by phlebitis. In addition, when done by an inexperienced radiologist, there is a higher incidence of inadequate venograms, which are impossible to interpret. Even when performed by expert radiologists, there is a 10% to 15% incidence of inadequate venograms. In spite of these limitations and potential problems, a negative venogram does rule out DVT in symptomatic patients [3].

3. TRUE

There is now good evidence that either a combination of IPG, fibrinogen leg scanning, or serial IPGs are as reliable as venography in confirming or excluding clinically important thrombosis in patients with suspected DVT [5,6]. IPG is sensitive and specific for thrombosis of the popliteal and more proximal veins (proximal venous thrombosis) in symptomatic patients. Fibrinogen leg scanning is sensitive to recent calf-vein thrombosis. Therefore, the diagnostic approach of IPG and leg scanning, used

Figure 34-1 Objective Testing in the Diagnosis of DVT.

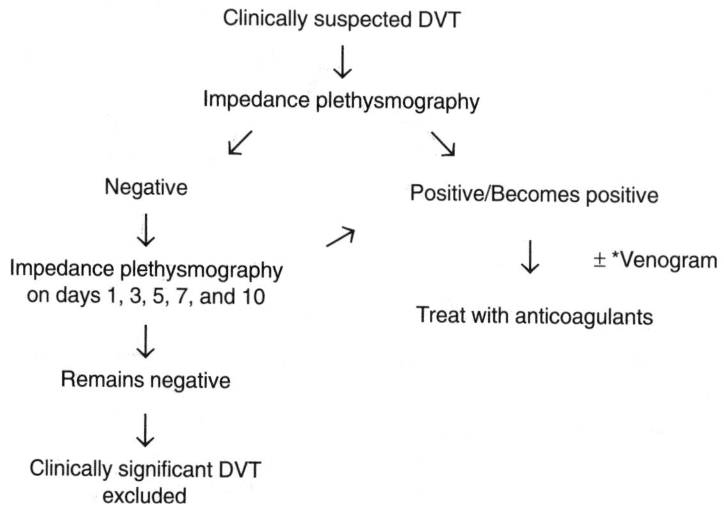

Clinically suspected DVT

↓

Impedance plethysmography

↙   ↘

Negative   Positive/Becomes positive

↓   ↗

Impedance plethysmography   ↓   ± *Venogram
on days 1, 3, 5, 7, and 10

↓   Treat with anticoagulants

Remains negative

↓

Clinically significant DVT
excluded

*If edema, poor test, or possibility of pelvic tumor, confirm with venogram.

Adapted from: Hull R, Raskob GE, LeClerc JR, *et al.*: The diagnosis of clinically suspected venous thrombosis. *Clin Chest Med* 5:439, 1984.

in combination, detects both proximal thrombosis and recent calf-vein
thrombosis. The combined approach of IPG and fibrinogen leg scanning
has been compared with venography and has been shown to be equivalent in sensitivity and specificity. It has also been demonstrated that it
is safe to leave patients untreated if the test results of this combined
approach are negative [3].

4. TRUE

Serial IPGs have been compared with a combination of IPG and leg
scanning (using clinical outcomes as the end points) and both methods
have been shown to be equivalent. If IPG is positive, there is a greater
than 95% chance that the patient has proximal vein thrombosis. If IPG

is negative and remains negative on serial testing, then it is safe to withhold therapy, as less than 2% of these patients will return with clinically important venous thrombosis or pulmonary embolism over the following 12 months.

IPGs will not detect calf-vein thrombosis. In less than 2% of patients with negative IPGs at presentation, calf-vein extension will occur during the period of testing. In theory, it is possible that a calf vein could extend rapidly and embolize before the IPG becomes positive. In practice, the use of serial IPGs in patients with clinically suspected DVT has now been used in many thousands of patients by five different research groups in three countries.

It is clear from these studies that patients with clinical symptoms compatible with DVT do not require treatment with anticoagulants, provided that the IPG is negative. The technique of serial IPGs is a safe way of following these patients, since there have been no cases of fatal pulmonary embolism and fewer than 0.2% of cases of symptomatic pulmonary embolism in the many thousands of patients followed this way [7]. IPGs are usually performed on day 0, day 1, day 3, day 5, day 7, and day 10. This repeated testing has the added advantage that repeated examination of the leg helps in the detection of alternative diagnoses (*e.g.*, cellulites or torn muscle). A false-positive test result with IPG may be obtained if the muscles of the legs are not relaxed or if there are any conditions that impair venous return or arterial flow. False-positive results may be obtained in patients with CHF, constrictive pericarditis, or pelvic masses. If the common femoral vein is compressed between the anterior thigh muscles and the inguinal ligament, or if the patient is positioned incorrectly or is not relaxed, the test may also yield false-positive results.

5. TRUE

The majority of calf-vein thrombi, which are detectable with fibrinogen leg scanning, are asymptomatic, but about 20% of untreated episodes lead to proximal extension. If untreated, about 50% of proximal vein thrombi embolize to the lung; and of these emboli, approximately 10% are fatal. It is estimated that about 10% of clinically detectable pulmonary emboli are fatal.

REFERENCES

1. Molloy DW, English J, O'Dwyer R, *et al.*: Clinical findings in the diagnosis of proximal deep vein thrombosis. *Ir Med J* 75:119, 1982.
2. Hull R, Carter C, Turpie, AGG, *et al.*: A randomized trial of diagnostic strategies for symptomatic deep vein thrombosis. *Thromb Haemost* 50:160, 1983.
3. Hull R, Hirsh J, Sackett DL, *et al.*: Clinical validity of a negative venogram in patients with clinically suspected venous thrombosis. *Circulation* 64:622, 1981.
4. Hull R, Raskob GE, LeClerc JR, *et al.*: The diagnosis of clinically suspected venous thrombosis. *Clin Chest Med* 5:439, 1984.

5. Hull R, Hirsh J, Sackett DL, *et al.*: Combined use of leg scanning and impedance plethysmography in suspected venous thrombosis: An alternative to venography. *N Engl J Med* 296:1497, 1977.
6. Hull R, Hirsh J, Sackett DL, *et al.* Replacement of venography in suspected venous thrombosis by impedance plethysmography and ^{125}I-fibrinogen leg scanning. *Ann Intern Med* 94:12, 1981.
7. Huisman MV, Buller HR, Tencate JW, *et al.*: Serial impedance plethysmography for suspected deep venous thrombosis in outpatients. *N Engl J Med* 314:823, 1986.

35 GIANT CELL ARTERITIS

CASE PRESENTATION

A 78-year-old woman presents with a two-month history of weight loss, anorexia, painful jaws when eating, generalized aches and pains, and fever. She also complains of intermittent blurring of vision. Routine investigations reveal a normochromic, normocytic anemia, hemoglobin of 101 g/l, normal white cell count (WBC), and erythrocyte sedimentation rate (ESR) of 96 mm/hr (Westergren). Chest x-ray, gastrointestinal series, plasma proteins, electrophoresis, and cultures are negative. She complains of aches and pains in her shoulders and hips. You suspect polymyalgia rheumatica or giant cell arteritis.

R. Clarnette
D.W. Molloy
E. Watson

Consider the following statements (true or false)

1. Men and women are equally affected by giant cell arteritis.

2. Headache is the initial manifestation of giant cell arteritis in more than 80% of patients.

3. Fever in giant cell arteritis is usually constant and low-grade.

4. Temporal artery biopsy is always necessary in the diagnostic work-up of the patient.

5. High-dose corticosteroids should be given for two weeks. The dose then must be reduced gradually. Prednisone may be stopped after 16 to 20 weeks in the majority of cases.

1. FALSE

The incidence of giant cell arteritis increases with age and peaks at 30 per 100,000 people in the eighth decade [1]. The disease is rare in blacks and Orientals but shows a striking predilection for caucasians. The disease is rare under age 50, and women are two to four times more likely to be affected than men [2].

Polymyalgia rheumatica (PMR) is a related condition that has many features in common with giant cell arteritis (GCA). PMR is four times more common than giant cell arteritis. The typical presentation of PMR is acute or gradual onset of pain that is felt more in the muscles than in the joints [3]. Morning stiffness is marked and is predominantly proximal in the shoulders and pelvic girdles. Physical examination may elicit mild tenderness in these muscles. There is no consistent muscle pathology associated with PMR. In patients who present with PMR, it is very important to rule out GCA, because GCA can present with symptoms suggestive of PMR.

2. FALSE

Many patients with GCA never complain of headache or tender temporal arteries. Almost 20% of patients present with polymyalgia rheumatica concurrently [3]. Giant cell arteritis may simply present with constitutional symptoms such as malaise, weight loss, and depression. These symptoms may last for many months before the diagnosis is made.

3. FALSE

Fever up to 38.5°C occurs in 30% of patients and may be associated with night sweats [4]. Permanent visual loss is the most common severe complication of the disease. Presenting visual symptoms range from sudden loss of vision, diplopia, and amaurosis fugax, to transient blurring. Once vision has been lost, the damage to the optic nerve is irreversible.

Other ischemic complications are much less common and include digital gangrene, stroke, and myocardial infarction [5]. Over one-third of patients with carotid territory disease have stroke, amaurosis fugax, or visual loss. Other neurologic presentations include dementia, mononeuritis, seizures, and myelopathy [6]. Table 35-1 lists the clinical and laboratory manifestations of GCA.

Table 35-1 Clinical and Laboratory Manifestations of Giant Cell Arteritis.

Clinical manifestations
    Polymyalgia rheumatica syndrome
    Headache
    Temporal artery tenderness
    Weight loss, flu-like illness, malaise
    Fever
    Visual manifestations
    Jaw claudication
    Aortic arch involvement

Laboratory manifestations
    Erythrocyte sedimentation rate >50 mm per hr (frequently >100 mm per hr)
    Normochromic/normocytic anemia
    Abnormal plasma proteins/electrophoresis (polyclonal increase in gamma
      globulins, or increase in alpha-2 globulins)
    Abnormal liver function tests
    Elevated haptoglobins
    Expect normal muscle enzymes (creatine phosphokinase, aldolase, serum
      glutamate oxaloacetate transaminase) electromyogram, muscle biopsy,
      rheumatoid factor

4. TRUE

A high degree of suspicion is required to diagnose giant cell arteritis. The presentation is often subtle, and the disease may be overlooked [6]. Consider GCA as soon as a patient's condition begins to deteriorate. Examine temporal, occipital, carotid, and more distal arteries for tenderness, bruits, or asymmetry. Temporal artery biopsy, where possible, will often confirm the diagnosis. Palpate the temporal artery and perform a biopsy of abnormal areas, since arteries are affected in a patchy distribution with normal portions intervening. The longer the portion of artery examined, the greater the chance of finding arteritis. Biopsy of the contralateral artery may be necessary if histologic examination of one artery is negative. It has been concluded that a positive biopsy correctly predicts the subsequent need for therapy in 94% of cases [7]. If the biopsy is negative but there is a very strong suspicion of the presence of disease, then treatment is indicated. Biopsy is performed to increase the certainty, as prolonged steroid therapy in this age group is not without risk and will certainly have significant effects on immune function, glucose metabolism, and bone density.

5. FALSE

Immediate administration of prednisone 40 to 60 mg orally is necessary if GCA is diagnosed clinically. A temporal artery biopsy can be obtained within the next two days. The initial dose should be maintained until symptoms and laboratory investigations improve (14 to 28 days). The response to steroids is usually rapid, and subjective improvement occurs within 24 hours. The dose of prednisone can be reduced gradually after the first month, for example, in 5-mg decrements to 20 mg and then 2.5-mg decrements to 5 mg. Maintenance doses are guided by improvement in clinical symptoms and results of serial ESR. Most patients require low-dose steroids for up to 24 months. Most patients recover fully, and the disease has no influence on overall survival [8].

The management of PMR is different in that nonsteroidal anti-inflammatory agents are useful as first-line therapy if the disease is mild. In refractory or severe cases, low-dose corticosteroid therapy is indicated, for example, 15 mg prednisone per day. Most patients recover from PMR, and the median duration of the disease is 11 months [9].

REFERENCES

1. Anderson R, Malmvall B-E, Bengtsson B-A: Long term survival in giant cell arteritis including temporal arteritis and polymyalgia rheumatica. *Acta Med Scand* 220:361–364, 1986.
2. Hauser WA, Ferguson RH, Holley KE, *et al.*: Temporal arteritis in Rochester, Minnesota, 1951 to 1974. *Mayo Clin Proc* 46:597, 1971.
3. Bengtsson B-A, Malmvall B-E: The epidemiology of giant cell arteritis including temporal arteritis and polymyalgia rheumatica. *Arthritis Rheum* 24:899–904, 1981.
4. Heasley LA, Wilske KR: *The Systemic Manifestations of Temporal Arteritis.* New York: Grune and Stratton, Inc., 1978.
5. Caselli RJ, Hunder GG, Whisnant JP: Neurologic disease in biopsy proven giant cell (temporal) arteritis. *Neurology* 38:352–359, 1988.
6. Molloy DW, Brooymans MA, Borrie MJ: Acute chest pain in an elderly woman. *Can J Cardiol* 4(3):144–145, 1988.
7. Hall S, Lie JT, Kurland LT, *et al.*: The therapeutic impact of temporal artery biopsy. *Lancet* 2:1217–1220, 1983.
8. Huston KA, Hunder GG, Lie JT, *et al.*: Temporal arteritis. A 25-year epidemiologic, clinical and pathologic study. *Ann Int Med* 88:162–167, 1978.
9. Chuang T-Y, Hunder GG, Ilstrup GM, *et al.*: Polymyalgia rheumatica: 10-year epidemiologic and clinical study. *Ann Int Med* 97:672–680, 1982.

36 | CEREBROVASCULAR DISEASE

CASE PRESENTATION

A previously independent 78-year-old woman was admitted to the hospital two weeks ago with mild right hemiparesis. Until the time of admission she had lived alone in a two-story house. She is presently on a general medical ward and has made good functional recovery. She cannot be discharged as she still has difficulty washing and dressing. She and her family ask you if she is going to continue to improve and if she would benefit from transfer to a stroke assessment unit. You had planned to discharge her with follow-up physiotherapy twice weekly in the outpatient department.

R. Clarnette
D.W. Molloy
R. Bloch

Consider the following statements (true or false)

1. In the elderly the risk of stroke rises in the presence of diastolic hypertension and hypercholesterolemia, but not systolic hypertension or diabetes.

2. In the elderly, over 80% of strokes are due to cerebral infarction, and the remainder are due to cerebral hemorrhage.

3. Immediately following a stroke, patients should be treated in a stroke intensive care unit, and rehabilitation should be delayed until consciousness and neurologic recovery occur.

4. Of stroke deaths, 50% occur within the first month. Of the survivors, 80% will have significant neurologic sequelae, but most will return home.

5. The degree of neurologic recovery two weeks after a stroke accurately predicts the patient's expected functional recovery. The latter may take two years to occur.

321

1. FALSE

Cerebrovascular disease is the third leading cause of death in Western communities; the annual incidence is 10 to 20 per 1000 persons in those over age 65 [1]. Hypertension is clearly associated with an increased risk of stroke, and longitudinal studies indicate that this is true for both diastolic and systolic hypertension [2,3]. The Framingham study, however, found that systolic hypertension was the best predictor of stroke [4]. In addition, pulse pressure and variability of blood pressure have predictive value [5].

There has been no demonstrated association between increased serum lipids and the incidence of strokes in the elderly [6]. Prospective epidemiologic studies examining the role of lipids in the pathogenesis of stroke have not shown consistent results in the elderly [7]. The Framingham data showed a positive relationship between serum lipid levels and stroke in those under 50 years of age. This did not occur in the over-50 age group [4].

Diabetes mellitus is associated with an increased incidence of atherosclerosis in the cerebral arteries which appears to be independent of the presence of hypertension [8]. The Framingham study noted a twofold increase in the incidence of stroke among diabetics [9]. There is evidence that hyperglycemia at the time of a stroke increases the amount of ischemic neuronal damage [10]. This makes tight control of blood glucose important in the acute phase of a stroke.

Patients with polycythemia have an increased incidence of stroke, and the incidence is directly related to the hematocrit level [11]. The mechanism may be an increase of blood viscosity, leading to decreased flow in small vessels. Men with hemoglobin exceeding 150 g/l and women with hemoglobin exceeding 140 g/l have double the incidence of cerebral infarction compared to normal controls [12].

2. TRUE

The incidence of cerebral infarction increases with age. Ostfeld *et al.* reported that 80% of all strokes in an elderly population were due to cerebral infarction. Intracerebral hemorrhage accounted for 12%. Of cerebral hemorrhages, 74% were due to subarachnoid hemorrhage and 26% were intracerebral [13]. Most of the latter are directly attributable to hypertension. In the elderly, however, amyloid angiopathy is a common cause of intracerebral hemorrhage and accounted for 19%, in patients over the age of 70, in one series [14]. Cortical vessels develop thickening due to infiltration with amyloid protein; the condition, though common in those with Alzheimer's disease, is benign until it causes intracerebral hemorrhage [15].

The majority of cerebral infarcts are caused by atheromatous disease of the internal carotid system and principally of the large vessels. Over 90% of such strokes are caused by thrombus formation with artery-to-artery embolism, rather than by large vessel occlusion alone [16].

Cerebral infarcts are also caused by lacunae and emboli of cardiac origin. The greatest risk factor for the former is hypertension [16]. In the elderly, cardiac emboli are usually related to the presence of atrial fibrillation (AF). In those over the age of 80, the prevalence of AF is greater than 10% [17]. The risk of stroke diminishes with length of duration of AF; annual stroke risk for chronic AF is 5% [16].

Artery-to-artery embolism may also give rise to transient cerebral ischemic attacks (TIA). Population surveys show that 9% of cerebral infarcts are preceded by a TIA. This figure is as high as 35% in some hospital series [18]. Patients who present following carotid distribution TIAs are often considered for endarterectomy. Although this is a common procedure, particularly in North America, its efficacy has yet to be established in a well-designed trial [19]. Studies that address this issue are currently under way.

Trials of the use of anticoagulants in treating TIAs have failed to show an effect on future stroke occurrence [20]. Anticoagulants should be used only when it is clear that a cardiac source for the embolism is present.

Antiplatelet therapy is now the preferred treatment for TIAs. The weight of evidence is certainly in favor of using aspirin [21]. Unfortunately, there are methodologic problems with the majority of the trials that have examined this issue [22]. The beneficial effects of aspirin therapy appear to be confined to males [21]. Possible reasons for the lack of effect in females include low TIA incidence, methodologic discrepancies in the trials, and a true biologic difference between the sexes. It is accepted that females should not be denied treatment with aspirin following a TIA. The current recommended dose of aspirin is 325 mg daily [23]. Studies do not support the use of dipyridamole in the prevention of stroke [24].

3. FALSE

Treating patients in stroke intensive care units, compared to general medical wards, has not been shown to affect the high early mortality rate [25]. It has, however, been shown to improve morbidity by reducing the number of complications in survivors [26].

Rehabilitation should be started as soon as possible, since delay is associated with increased disability. Even while the patient is unconscious and the involved limbs are flaccid, an organized rehabilitation program can do much to prevent stroke complications such as contractures, pressure sores, aspiration, pneumonia, deep vein thrombosis, urinary retention and infection, fecal impaction, dehydration, malnutrition, and depression [27].

4. TRUE

Up to 50% of patients who die from a stroke do so within the first three weeks. Advanced age is associated with higher acute mortality [28]. If the patient survives the acute event, the prognosis is good, and there is a fairly constant subsequent mortality rate of about 8% per year. The cause of death in up to two-thirds of stroke victims is myocardial infarction, not a second stroke. Stroke victims, unlike survivors of myocardial infarction, are more likely to have a high level of dependency as a result of their disability.

Of those who survive one month, 10% recover almost completely and spontaneously, 10% are so severely disabled that no improvement can be expected, and the remaining 80% have significant impairment but are not totally disabled. The latter group benefits most from rehabilitation [29]. Of patients completing a rehabilitation program, 75% have achieved enough independence and mobility to be discharged home. This figure is maintained at one-year follow-up [30,31].

It is useful to distinguish between impairment, disability, and handicap. "Impairment" describes the deficits in neurologic and physiologic function. "Disability" refers to reduced ability in pursuing normal activities of daily living, such as self-care, walking, communicating, and executive functions such as money management. "Handicap" indicates an alteration in social role, be it personal, within the family, economic, or vocational.

Recovery of impairment is largely spontaneous and is determined by the natural history of the disease. Rehabilitation is mainly directed at minimizing disability resulting from a given impairment. Carefully planned social interventions and support can minimize handicap following disability.

The World Health Organization has defined rehabilitation as "the combined and coordinated use of medical, social, educational, and vocational measures for training or retraining individuals to the highest possible level of functional ability." Given the cost of chronic institutionalization and the fact that stroke victims at present take up more acute hospital beds than any other disease group, rehabilitation after a stroke is cost-effective.

5. FALSE

The outcome of a rehabilitation program for a stroke patient is determined by length of hospital stay, independence in activities of daily living, and the presence of an appropriate place for discharge. There are a number of well-recognized predictors that correlate negatively with satisfactory outcome. These are:

1. *Persistent incontinence*: Not all incontinence following stroke is organic. Before a patient is labeled as incontinent, he or she should have a good trial of scheduled voiding. Indwelling catheters and diapers should be avoided as much as possible.
2. *Poor motivation/depression*: Depression is often overlooked after stroke [32,33]. There are both situational and organic factors predisposing stroke patients to depression. In lethargic, poorly motivated patients, a trial of an antidepressant such as nortriptyline is indicated.
3. *Prolonged unconsciousness*
4. *Cognitive impairment*
5. *Perceptual or sensory loss*
6. *Homonymous hemianopia*
7. *Severe weakness*
8. *Previous stroke*
9. *Large or deep lesions on CT scan*

In 1977 Feigenson and colleagues investigated the value of prescreening patients for admission to a stroke rehabilitation unit [34]. Criteria for inclusion into the program included patients under the age of 80 who were motivated, with no deficits in orientation or perception, had no homonymous hemianopia, and had severe weakness for more than 30 days, and a caregiver involved in discharge planning.

The study found that preadmission screening did not improve overall outcome or length of stay. The best indicator of a patient's ability to benefit from a rehabilitation program was his/her response to a two- or three-week trial of intensive therapy.

Intrinsic recovery following a stroke is usually noted in the first 3 to 6 months. By 6 months the majority of motor recovery has occurred. Aphasia may take longer to recover. Only 5% of patients show continuing recovery one year after the stroke. If full recovery is to occur, then some improvement of the affected limb is usually seen within the first month. Therefore, a patient with significant weakness and/or sensory deficit at 18 months is not going to improve significantly two years after the stroke. Unfortunately, this is the unrealistic expectation many patients and their families have when given the two-year recovery frame. This expectation can interfere significantly with the ability to "get on with life" and to acquire adaptive techniques for performing day-to-day activities.

REFERENCES

1. Kurtzke JF, Kurland LT: The epidemiology of neurologic disease. *In* Baker AB, Baker LH (eds.): *Clinical Neurology*, Vol. 4. Philadelphia: Harper and Row, 1984, pp. 1–143.
2. Shekelle RB, Ostfeld AM, Klawans HK: Hypertension and risk of stroke in an elderly population. *Stroke* 5:71–75, 1974.
3. Baker AB, Resch JA, Loewenson RB: Hypertension and cerebral atherosclerosis. *Circulation* 39:701–710, 1969.
4. Kannel S, Dawber T, Sorlie P, *et al.*: Components of blood pressure and risk of atherothrombotic brain infarction: The Framingham study. *Stroke* 7:327–331, 1976.
5. Kannel S, Dawber T, Sorlie P, *et al.*: Components of blood pressure and risk of atherothrombotic brain infarction: The Framingham study. *Stroke* 5:71–75, 1974.
6. Wolf PA: Risk factors for stroke. *Stroke* 16:359, 1985.
7. Ostfeld AM, Shekelle RB, Klawans H, *et al.*: Epidemiology of stroke in an elderly welfare population. *Am J Public Health* 64:450–458, 1974.
8. Aronson SM: Intracranial vascular disease in diabetes mellitus. *J Neuropath Exp Neurol* 32:183–196, 1973.
9. Garcia MJ, McNara PM, Gordon T, *et al.*: Morbidity and mortality in diabetics in the Framingham population. *Diabetes* 23:104–111, 1974.
10. Pulsinelli WA, Waldman S, Rawlinson D, Plum F: Moderate hyperglycemia augments ischemic brain damage: A neuropathologic study in the rat. *Neurology* 32:1239–1246, 1982.

11. Thomas DJ, Du Boulay AH, Marshall J, *et al.*: Effect of hematocrit on cerebral blood flow in man. *Lancet* 2:941–943, 1977.
12. Elwood PC, Waters WE, Benjamin IT, Sweetnam PM: Mortality and anemia in women. *Lancet* 1:891–894, 1974.
13. Sacco RL, Wolf PA, Barucha NE, *et al.*: Subarachnoid hemorrhage and intracerebral hemorrhage: Natural history, prognosis and precursive factors in the Framingham study. *Neurology* 34:847–854, 1984.
14. Lee SS, Stemmerman GN: Congophilic angiopathy and intracerebral hemorrhage. *Arch Pathol Lab Med* 102:317–321, 1978.
15. Nadeau SE, Bebin J, Smith E: Nonspecific dementia, cortical blindness, and congophilic angiopathy. A clinicopathologic report. *J Neurol* 234:14–18, 1987.
16. Nadeau SE: Stroke. *Med Clin North Am* 73:1351–1369, 1989.
17. Wolf PA, Abbott RD, Kannel WB: Atrial fibrillation: A major contributor to stroke in the elderly. The Framingham study. *Arch Int Med* 147:1561–1564, 1987.
18. Whisnant JP: The decline of stroke. *Stroke* 15:160–168, 1984.
19. Dyken ML, Pokras R: The performance of endarterectomy for disease of the extracranial arteries of the head. *Stroke* 15:948–950, 1984.
20. Brust JCM: Transient ischemic attacks: Natural history and anticoagulation. *Neurology* 27:701–707, 1977.
21. Mirsen TR, Hachinski VC: Transient ischemic attacks and stroke. *Can Med Assoc J* 138:1099–1105, 1988.
22. Sackett DL: Rational therapy in the neurosciences: The role of the randomized trial. *Stroke* 17:1323–1329, 1986.
23. UK TIA Study Group. The United Kingdom transient ischemic attack aspirin trial: Interim results. *Br Med J* 296:316–320, 1988.
24. Grotta JC: Current medical and surgical therapy for cerebrovascular disease. *N Engl J Med* 317:1505–1511, 1987.
25. Kennedy FB, Pozen TJ, Gabelman EH, *et al.*: Stroke intensive care: An appraisal. *Am Heart J* 80:188, 1970.
26. Drake WE, Hamilton MJ, Carlsson M, *et al.*: Acute stroke management and patient outcome: The value of neurovascular care units. *Stroke* 4:933, 1973.
27. Hayes SH, Carroll SR: Early intervention care in the acute stroke patient. *Arch Phys Med Rehab* 67:319, 1986.
28. Wade DT, Hewer RC: Stroke: Association with age, sex and side of weakness. *Arch Phys Med Rehab* 67:540, 1986.
29. Steinberg FU: Rehabilitating the older stroke patient: What is possible? *Geriatrics* 5:85, 1986.
30. Lehmann JF, DeLateur BJ, Fowler RS: Stroke: Does rehabilitation affect outcome? *Arch Med Phys Rehab* 56:375, 1975.
31. Steinburg FU: The stroke registry: A prospective method of studying stroke. *Arch Med Phys Rehab* 54:31, 1973.
32. Feibel JH, Springer CJ: Depression and failure to resume social activities after stroke. *Arch Phys Med Rehab* 63:276–278, 1982.
33. Robinson RG, Stow LB, Vubos KL, Price TR: A two year longitudinal study of post stroke mood disorders: Findings during the initial evaluation. *Stroke* 14:736–741, 1983.
34. Feigenson JS, McDowell FH, *et al.*: Factors influencing outcome and length of stay in a stroke rehabilitation unit. *Stroke* 8:651, 1977.

Part VII

GENERAL

37 | MAGNESIUM METABOLISM

CASE PRESENTATION

A 72-year-old retired sea captain was admitted to the emergency department three days ago with a myocardial infarction. He had been taking digoxin (0.125 mg/day) and furosemide (40 mg/day) for many years for congestive heart failure. Upon admission, a serum magnesium test was performed, as the skipper was known to like his rum. Test results showed 0.24 mEq/l. The normal range is 0.6–1.2 mEq/l. Since admission he has had frequent multifocal ventricular ectopic beats, in spite of infusions and boluses of lidocaine. A nurse has just informed you that he is experiencing ventricular tachycardia.

D.W. Molloy
L. Rees
E. Alemeyehu
A. Cranney

Consider the following statements (true or false)

1. Normal, healthy elderly patients experience a gradual decline in serum magnesium levels with advancing age.

2. Chronic alcoholics have normal or raised serum magnesium levels because alcohol causes increased magnesium re-uptake in the distal tubule.

3. Long-term diuretic use is associated with hypomagnesemia.

4. Serum magnesium is a sensitive index of intra- and extracellular magnesium in the body.

5. Severe hypomagnesemia causes a slowing in atrioventricular conduction that results in heart block and asystole.

1. FALSE

Magnesium is the fourth most abundant cation in the body and the second most abundant intracellular cation in the body [1]. Dietary deficiency of magnesium is rare, as magnesium is found in a wide range of foods. Serum magnesium levels are unaffected by age [2,3], but up to 25% of elderly patients admitted to a hospital have mild hypomagnesemia [4]. There is no direct correlation between serum albumin levels and serum magnesium levels [4,5]. When dietary intake is low, the kidney almost completely reabsorbs magnesium. Aging results in a fall in urinary magnesium excretion, which probably reflects a decreased intake [6]. In adults, small variations in dietary magnesium do not produce hypomagnesemia. Hypercalcemia, malignancy, and primary hyperparathyroidism cause increased excretion of magnesium.

2. FALSE

Although hypomagnesemia from dietary deficiency is rare, it may occur in association with malnutrition, chronic alcoholism, or prolonged parenteral feeding with magnesium-deficient foods. A daily intake of 140 mg is sufficient to maintain magnesium balance in normal adults. Magnesium is absorbed primarily from the small intestine, but may be absorbed from the duodenum or colon. Approximately 3% to 5% of the 2 grams of magnesium filtered daily is excreted by the kidneys.

Hypomagnesemia is a common disorder, occurring in 2% of hospital patients. Approximately 30% to 37% of chronic alcoholics and up to 80% of alcoholics with delirium tremens may have magnesium deficiency [7]. McLeod *et al.* found that 20% of elderly men and 40% of elderly women living at home were taking less than 0.3 mEq/kg of magnesium per day [8]. The intake below which adults experience negative balance is 0.5 mEq/kg/day. Lim and Jacob reported diminished skeletal muscle magnesium levels in 9 out of 10 alcoholics tested for magnesium deficiency. None of these patients had abnormal bone values, and only 2 patients had low serum magnesium levels [9]. Common causes of hypomagnesemia are listed in Table 37-1.

3. TRUE

Martin *et al.* first reported hypomagnesemia as a complication of ammonium chloride and meralluride therapy [10]. Since then, ethacrynic acid,

Table 37-1 Causes of Magnesium Deficiency.

Dietary	*Renal loss*
Reduced intake	Osmotic diuresis
Malnutrition	Renal insufficiency
Prolonged parenteral feeding	*Endocrine*
Gastrointestinal	Primary hyperaldosteronism
Malabsorption	Hyperthyroidism
Chronic diarrhea	Hypothyroidism
Bowel resection of fistula	Hyperparathyroidism
Acute pancreatitis	Hypoparathyroidism
Drugs	Hypophosphatemia
Alcohol	
Diuretics	
Cardiac glycosides	
Gentamicin	
Cisplatin	

furosemide, and thiazide diuretics also have been associated with an increased incidence of hypomagnesemia. Long-term diuretic therapy may cause hypomagnesemia in both young and elderly patients [5,11]. Digitalis therapy and secondary hyperaldosteronism also may contribute to magnesium deficiency. Digitalis toxicity may be precipitated by hypomagnesemia, as digitalis reduces renal reabsorption of magnesium, and hypomagnesemia increases the myocardial uptake of digoxin.

Diuretics are one of the most commonly prescribed drugs in the elderly. Approximately one-third of institutionalized and noninstitutionalized patients aged 65 years or older take some form of maintenance diuretic therapy [12,13]. Therefore, elderly patients with heart failure are at increased risk for developing hypomagnesemia because of secondary hyperaldosteronism and diuretic and cardiac glycoside use—all of which increase magnesium excretion.

4. FALSE

It is not clear whether serum levels or muscle magnesium levels provide the most accurate assessment of magnesium deficiency states. Serum magnesium measures extracellular magnesium, while muscle magnesium measures intracellular magnesium. Half of the body's magnesium is stored in bone, and half is stored in both muscular and nonmuscular soft tissue. Of the magnesium in bone, 70% is nonexchangeable and 30% is freely exchangeable.

The body's ability to mobilize magnesium decreases with age. Less than 1% of the body's magnesium is found in the blood, 0.2% is found in plasma, and 0.4% is found in red blood cells. In serum, more than half of the magnesium is ionized, and posture and prolonged stasis during venipuncture may affect measured serum magnesium levels.

Many studies have reported an inconsistent relationship between serum and muscle magnesium levels. Serum magnesium levels may be an insensitive index of total body magnesium. Lim and Jacob reported low skeletal muscle magnesium levels in 5 of 10 patients on long-term diuretic therapy [11]. Only 2 of these patients had low serum magnesium levels. Much of the confusion surrounding magnesium levels in serum, muscle, bone, and other body stores results from our ignorance of the relationship of these stores to each other and from the lack of standardization between different biopsy techniques and laboratory measurements.

5. FALSE

Symptoms and signs of hypomagnesemia relate poorly to clinical signs until profound hypomagnesemia occurs, and even then there is no characteristic pattern [14]. Clinical manifestations of hypomagnesemia

Table 37-2   Clinical Manifestations of Hypomagnesemia.

Neuromuscular	*Central nervous system*
Chvostek's sign, tremors	Generalized weakness
Muscle fasciculation	Nystagmus
Muscle spasticity	Vertigo
Muscle weakness	Ataxia
Muscle wasting	Increased irritability
	Confusion
Gastrointestinal tract	Behavioral abnormalities
Anorexia	
Dysphagia	*Cardiac*
Vomiting	Ventricular ectopic beats
Nausea	Ventricular tachycardia
	Venticular fibrillation

are listed in Table 37-2. Hyponatremia and hypokalemia frequently accompany hypomagnesemia and may complicate the clinical picture. Hypomagnesemia has been linked with ischemic heart disease, coronary artery spasm, and arrhythmias [15]. Hypomagnesemia also is associated with muscle weakness and may cause a characteristic myopathy [16]. Alcoholic cardiomyopathy may be multifactorial in origin, but experimental magnesium deficiency produces similar histologic and electrocardiographic abnormalities. We measured respiratory muscle strength in patients with hypomagnesemia and randomly treated them with magnesium or placebo. We found a significant improvement in respiratory muscle strength in patients who received magnesium compared to patients who received placebo therapy [17].

Magnesium therapy is indicated for life-threatening arrhythmias, in particular ventricular fibrillation and tachycardia that have not responded to anti-arrhythmics or cardioversion and especially for arrhythmias associated with prolonged QT intervals (torsades de pointes) [18].

Magnesium should be considered in patients with digoxin-induced tachyarrythmias, multifocal atrial tachycardia, and supraventricular tachycardia associated with magnesium deficiency [19]. There is recent evidence to suggest that magnesium administration during acute myocardial infarction may decrease tachyarrythmias and intrahospital mortality [20]. The recommended dose in patients wihout renal impairment is 2 gm of magnesium sulfate (4 ml of 50% $MGSO_4$) over 1 minute, followed by 10 gm over 5–8 hours (500 cc of 2% $MGSO_4$ solution). Patients should be monitored with ECG recordings, deep tendon reflexes, blood pressure, and serum potassium and magnesium levels [19].

REFERENCES

1. Wacker WEC, Parisi AF: Magnesium metabolism. *N Engl J Med* 278:656, 1968.
2. Lim P, Jacob E, Dong S, *et al.*: Value for tissue magnesium as a guide in detecting magnesium deficiency. *J Clin Pathol* 22:417, 1969.
3. Landhal S, Graffner C, Jagenberg R, *et al.*: Prevalence and treatment of hypomagnesemia in the elderly. *Aktuele Gerontologie* 9:397, 1980.
4. McConway NG, Martin BJ, Nugent N, *et al.*: Magnesium status in the elderly on hospital admission. *Journal of Clinical and Experimental Gerontology* 3:367, 1981.
5. Thomas AJ, Hodkinson HM: Which diuretics cause hypomagnesemia? A study of elderly inpatients. *Journal of Clinical and Experimental Gerontology* 3:269, 1981.
6. Nordin BEC: *Calcium, Phosphate and Magnesium Metabolism: Clinical Physiology and Diagnostic Procedures.* Edinburgh: Churchill Livingstone, 1976.

7. Sullivan JF, Wolpert PW, Williams R, *et al.*: Serum magnesium in chronic alcoholism. *Ann NY Acad Sci* 162:947, 1969.
8. McLeod CC, Judge TG, Caird Fl: Nutrition of the elderly at home III: Intake of minerals. *Age and Ageing* 4:49, 1975.
9. Lim P, Jacob E: Magnesium status of alcoholic patients. *Metabolism* 11:1045, 1972.
10. Martin HE, Mehl J, Wertman AB: Clinical studies of magnesium metabolism. *Med Clin North Am* 36:1157, 1952.
11. Lim P, Jacob E: Magnesium deficiency in patients on long term diuretic therapy for heart failure. *Br Med J* 3:620, 1972.
12. Myers MG, Kearns PA, Kennedy DS, *et al.*: Postural hypotension and drug therapy in the elderly. *Can Med Assoc J* 119:581, 1978.
13. Skoll SL, August RJ, Johnson GE: Drug prescribing for the elderly in Saskatchewan during 1976. *CMAG* 121:1074, 1979.

14. Shils ME: Experimental human magnesium depletion. *Medicine* 1:61, 1969.
15. Iseri LT, Freed J, Bures AR: Magnesium deficiency and cardiac disorders. *Am J Med* 58:837, 1975.
16. Molloy DW: Hypomagnesemia and respiratory muscle weakness in the elderly. *Geriatric Medicine Today* 6:53, 1987.
17. Molloy DW, Dhingra S, Solven F, *et al*.: Hypomagnesemia and respiratory muscle power. *Am Rev Respir Dis* 129:497, 1984.
18. Roden DM: Magnesium treatment of ventricular arrhythmias. *Am J Cardiol* 63:43G, 1989.
19. Iseri LT: Role of magnesium in cardiac tachyarrhythmias. *Am J Cardiol* 65:47K, 1990.
20. Schekter M, Hanoch H, Marks N, *et al*.: Beneficial effects of magnesium sulfate in acute myocardial infarction. *Am J Cardiol* 66: 271, 1990.

38 | HIP FRACTURES

CASE PRESENTATION

You receive an urgent call from the daughter of a 75-year-old patient who is concerned that her mother has not answered the phone for 24 hours. When you gain entry to the house, you find her lying on the floor unable to move because of pain in her right hip. Although somewhat confused, she tells you that she fell the previous night. She is dehydrated and has an irregular pulse with a carotid bruit. Examination of the hip reveals a shortened external rotator and a slightly flexed right hip.

X-rays at a local hospital show a displaced subcapital fracture of her right hip. The orthopedic surgeon recommends an operative procedure. The patient's daughter asks you about the risks involved in surgery and whether it is necessary.

D.W. Molloy
M. Gross
E. Alemeyehu

Consider the following statements (true or false)

1. Osteoporosis is associated with more than 90% of hip fractures in the elderly.

2. Osteoporosis prevents successful healing of hip fractures.

3. Subcapital fractures result in higher incidences of complications such as avascular necrosis than do intertrochanteric fractures.

4. The best predictor of outcome in patients with hip fractures is the patient's mental status prior to the event.

5. The mortality rate in elderly hip fracture patients is determined by the type of hip fracture.

1. FALSE

Studies show that osteopenia, defined as radiographically visible bone demineralization, occurs in 80% of white women by the age of 69. The principal cause of morbidity in osteoporosis is vertebral compression fractures, a condition that affects up to 25% of white women over the age of 65 [1].

The ribs also demonstrate a propensity for spontaneous fracture. Osteoporosis patients also are more prone to fractures of the distal radius and hip fractures after falls than are healthy patients. In white women, aged 75 and over, the incidence of hip fracture is 16 per 1000 per year [2]. The causes of falls in the elderly are numerous and include postural hypotension, arrhythmias, and unsteady gait. Environmental hazards (stairs, poor lighting, loose objects on the floor) may account for 40% of falls in the elderly with femoral neck fractures [3–5]. Patients presenting with hip fractures should be investigated for the cause or causes of falls.

2. FALSE

Osteoporosis *per se* does not prevent successful healing of hip fractures, although it may complicate their operative management. Healing of fractured bone is determined by the blood supply and the degree of reduction and immobilization occurring between the fracture fragments. Osteoporotic bone is often weaker than normal bone due to the loss of the trabeculae within the cancellous bone. This process generally is irreversible once the trabeculae have disappeared. At least 30% of bone loss has to occur before it becomes evident on x-rays. The degree of osteoporosis can be classified by the Singh index [6], although this is an insensitive measurement with poor observer agreement [7].

3. TRUE

Blood supply to the femoral head is maintained by blood vessels that supply the posterior aspect of the femoral neck. Blood also reaches the femoral head through trabecular bone in the intertrochanteric area and from the ligamentum teres, which supplies a very small part of the head.

The posterior blood supply is interrupted by subcapital fractures or fractures through the neck of the femur. The greater the displacement of the femoral head in relation to the femoral neck, the more likely there is to be a complete disruption of the blood supply. Even with adequate reduction and firm fixation of the femoral head on the femoral neck, there is still a high incidence of avascular complications such as avascular necrosis.

Intertrochanteric fractures do not cause problems with blood supply, as blood can reach both sides of the fracture. With this fracture there often is a large amount of exposed bone, which increases the potential for bone healing.

The rationale for surgical procedures on subcapital fractures is to achieve an anatomic reduction of the femoral head on the femoral neck, to hold it with secure fixation and to monitor the patient for avascular necrosis. If avascular necrosis develops, the patient may require hip replacement (when the hip becomes painful enough to cause disability). Very old patients often have their femoral head replaced with an artificial joint such as the Moore or Thomson arthroplasty. In very old patients with reduced life expectancies, joint replacement may be the intervention of choice so they will only undergo one operation and are unlikely to suffer long-term complications.

To treat intertrochanteric fractures, bones are usually held in position with a screw and plate device. The bones are pruned to prevent varus angulation at the fracture site, leg shortening, and malrotation.

This implant serves as an internal splint while fracture healing occurs. Complications associated with this procedure are the result of osteoporosis. The screw device may fall out, or the surgeon may be unable to obtain an adequate purchase in the femoral head.

4. TRUE

In elderly patients, the best predictor of outcome following a fractured femur is the patient's mental state prior to the event [8,9]. Elderly patients undergoing hip replacement are at risk of developing infection, confusion, or adverse drug reactions in the postoperative period [10]. Surgery adversely affects cognitive functioning in the early postoperative period following emergency procedures [11]. The effects of elective surgery on cognitive function appear to be minimal [12]. Medical problems such as cardiac failure, stroke, and hypertension may affect surgical risk, but do not affect long-term outcome. There are variable changes in mental function in the elderly after acute or elective hip surgery [13–16].

5. FALSE

Although mental status is the best predictor of outcome in patients with hip fractures [8], antecedent medical complications such as arrhythmias, myocardial infarction in the last three months, and recovery from pneumonia, will influence the course of the procedure and postoperative recovery. Surgery is performed as early as possible after the patient has been stabilized to maximize mobilization following surgery and to prevent recumbency complications such as skin ulcers, pneumonia, constipation, and deep venous thrombosis.

REFERENCES

1. Smith RW, Eyelr WR, Mellinger RL: The incidence of osteoporosis. *Ann Intern Med* 52:773, 1960.
2. Bollett A, Engh G, Parson W: Epidemiology of osteoporosis; sex and race incidence of hip fractures. *Arch Intern Med* 116:191, 1965.
3. Sheldon JH: On the natural history of falls in old age. *Br Med J* 2:1685, 1960.
4. Brocklehurst JC, Exton-Smith AN, *et al.*: Fracture of the femur in old age: A two centre study of associated clinical factors and the course of the fall. *Age and Ageing* 7:7, 1978.
5. Dias JJ: An analysis of the nature of injury in fractures of the neck at the femur. *Age and Ageing* 16:373, 1987.

6. Singh M, Magrath AR, Maini PS: Changes in trabecular pattern in the upper end of the femur as an index of osteoporosis. *JBJS* 52A:457, 1970.

7. Hyman O, *et al.*: Determination of osteoporosis in patients with fractured femoral neck using the singh index. A Jerusalem study. *Clin Orthop* 156:189, 1981.

8. Grimley Evans J: Fractured proximal femur in Newcastle-Upon-Tyne. *Age and Ageing* 8:16, 1979.

9. Mesulem MM, Geschwind N: Disordered mental states in the post-operative period. *Urol Clin North Am* 3:199, 1976.

10. Sheppeard H, Cleak DK, Ward DJ, O'Connor BJ: A review of early mortality and morbidity in elderly patients following Charnley total hip replacement. *Arch Orthop Trauma Surg* 97:243, 1980.

11. Bedford PD: Adverse cerebral effects of anesthesia on old people. *Lancet* 2:259, 1955.

12. Simpson BR, William M, Scott JF, *et al.*: The effects of anesthesia and elective surgery on old people. *Lancet* 2:887, 1961.

13. Hughes D, Bowes JB, Brown MN: Changes in memory following general or spinal anesthesia for hip arthroplasty. *Anesthesia* 43:114, 1988.

14. Bigle D, Adelhoj B, Petring OU, *et al.*: Mental function and morbidity after acute hip surgery during spinal and general anesthesia. *Anesthesia* 40:672, 1985.

15. Riis J, Lomholt B, Haxholdt O, *et al.*: Immediate and long-term mental recovery from general varus epidural anesthesia in elderly patients. *Acta Anaesthesiol Scand* 27:44, 1983.

16. Hole A, Tevjesen T, Breivik H: Epidural versus general anaesthesia for total hip arthroplasty in elderly patients. *Acta Anaesthesiol Scand* 24:279, 1980.

39 | SURGICAL RISK

CASE PRESENTATION

Dr. A. M. Putee, a surgeon, asks you to assess Mrs. Smith, a 72-year-old retired nurse who is scheduled for elective left knee replacement tomorrow. She has severe, painful osteoarthritis which limits her mobility.

She had a myocardial infarction 10 years ago and has experienced dyspnea on walking half a block until limited by claudication in the last 6 months, and two pillow orthopnea in the last year. She reduced cigarette smoking to half a pack a day. She has no diabetes or hypertension. Her only medication is digoxin, 0.125 mg daily.

On examination, she has an S4, no edema, absent right pedal pulses, a grade 1/6 systolic ejection murmur, JVP 6 cm above the sternal angle, and a few bibasilar crackles. FEV1 = 1.41 per second, FVC = 2.21, CXR shows very mild interstitial edema. EKG shows left bundle branch block and atrial fibrillation with a ventricular rate of 90 per min. CBC, BUN, electrolytes, and sugar are normal.

M.D. Sauvé
R. Jaeschke
D.W. Molloy

Consider the following statements (true or false)

1. The independent risk factors for perioperative cardiac complications in Mrs. Smith are: (1) age over 70 years, (2) past history of myocardial infarction, (3) presence of peripheral vascular disease, (4) atrial fibrillation, (5) smoking, and (6) congestive heart failure.

2. The general complication rate for this operation is the best estimate we can make of the risk of complication for any given patient (*i.e.*, there is no way to quantify and individualize risk assessment for each patient).

3. Aortic stenosis should be considered; however, clinical assessment excludes this within reason.

4. The surgeon requests some further evaluations given the physical findings that you have documented. A gated blood pool cardiac scan will best assess her cardiac function.

5. Mrs. Smith's risk of perioperative cardiac complications (MI, death, CHF, coronary insufficiency) is about 45% if she is operated on now.

345

1. FALSE

Age

Age greater than 70 years was found to be a predictor of perioperative cardiac complications in both univariate [38,39] and multivariate analysis (where we can conclude that the risk factor independently predicts outcome) [2,20,35]. The relative risk for those aged greater than 70 years, calculated from Goldman's series [2], is 12.8 for dying perioperatively and 4.8 for suffering a perioperative myocardial infarction [14]. See Table 39-1.

CHF

The two strongest predictors of perioperative cardiac complications are MI within the last three (or even six) months and uncompensated congestive heart failure (CHF) [1,2,9,36–39]. Mrs. Smith has the latter. From Goldman's series of 1001 patients, we can review the risk of uncompensated failure. See Table 39-2.

Mrs. Smith has congestive heart failure (elevated JVP, basal crepitations, cardiomegaly). She should have surgery postponed until she is treated and her failure has resolved. Compensated CHF carries only a marginally increased risk. Surgery should be postponed until she is stabilized.

Arrhythmia

Atrial fibrillation, rhythm other than sinus, more than five ventricular premature beats on any ECG preoperatively, or sinus rhythm with atrial premature beats on the last preoperative electrocardiogram, increase the risk of perioperative complications [2].

History of MI

Remote MI (more than five years ago) was not an independent predictor of perioperative cardiac complications [2]. None of Goldman's 13 patients with MI more than five years before this operation had postoperative infarction or death. The largest studies have come from the Mayo Clinic, where MI more than six months before surgery was associated with a 4% to 5% risk of reinfarction [1,9]. The data were not broken down for remote surgery (over five years before surgery), and the risk could have been attributable to other coexistent factors.

Therefore, in summary, age greater than 70 years, congestive failure, MI in the previous six months, and arrhythmia independently increase Mrs. Smith's preoperative risk (see Tables 39-3 and 39-4). History of smoking and peripheral vascular disease are not independent risk factors

Table 39-1 Effect of Age on Risk of Perioperative MI or Death.

Complication	Age <70	Age >70	Relative Risk
MI	6/777	12/324	4.8
Death	3/777	16/324	12.8

Table 39-2 Effect of Cardiac Failure (Elevated JVP Gallop Rhythm) on Perioperative Risk, Death, or MI.

Risk factor	Complication	Incidence	Relative risk
S3 or JVP*	MI or death	Not available	Reported ≈20
S3	death 3/17	18%	10.8
JVP	death 5/23	22%	15.2
S3	MI 1/17	6%	3.4
JVP	MI 1/23	4%	2.5

* JVP = elevated JVP.
Source: Calculated from [2] using [3].

Table 39-3 Independent Risk Factors for Perioperative Cardiac Complications, in Order of Decreasing Significance.

1. Uncompensated congestive heart failure (S3 or jugular vein distention preoperatively)
2. Coronary artery disease (MI within the last six months, unstable angina [40], or Canadian Cardiovascular Society (CCS) angina class 3 or 4)
3. Arrhythmia (defined as rhythm other than sinus, or PACs on preoperative ECG, or >5 PVCs on routine preoperative ECG)
4. Intra-abdominal or intrathoracic surgery
5. Age over 70 years (see text for risk assessment)
6. Severe aortic stenosis
7. Emergency surgery
8. Poor general medical status (serious lung, liver, or renal disease, K+ <3.0 mEq/l, or bedridden patient)
9. Unplanned prolonged intra-operative hypotension (>33% drop for >10 min.)

Adapted from [2, 10, 11, 20].

Table 39-4   Independent Risk Factors for Perioperative Infarction.

1. Age >70
2. Shortness of breath, orthopnea or pulmonary edema
3. Grade 2/6 or louder murmur of mitral regurgitation*
4. Over 5 PVCs per min. any time preoperatively
5. Tortuous or calcific aorta on CXR

*Only factors with >4% incidence of MI.
Source: from [2].

Table 39-5   Risk Factors Not Associated with Cardiac Complications.

1. S4
2. Stable angina (CCS class 1 or 2)
3. Diabetes, hyperlipidemia, smoking
4. Hypertension or LVH
5. Grade 2/6 or greater systolic ejection murmur (without aortic stenosis)
6. Body build

Source: from [2,20].

Table 39-6   Estimate of Any Patient's Pre-Examination Risks of Cardiac Complication.

Based on the type of operation to be performed at the Toronto General Hospital.

Type of Surgery	Pre-Exam Risk of Cardiac Complications	
	AWFUL: Death, MI, pulmonary edema	ALL: Awful group plus CHF and coronary insuf- ficiency (unstable angina)
Major Surgery		
Vascular	13%	21%
Aortic	16%	25%
Carotid	15%	19%
Peripheral	6%	18%
Orthopedic	14%	18%
Intrathoracic or intraperitoneal	8%	13%
Head and neck	3%	8%
Minor Surgery		
TURPs, Cataracts, etc.	2%	8%

(see Table 39-5).

One might think that hyperlipidemia, diabetes, hypertension, or smoking predispose patients to cardiac events perioperatively, yet several studies show that patients with these risk factors have no increased perioperative cardiac risk [2,6,9].

2. FALSE

In patients with cardiac disease who undergo noncardiac (major) surgery, the risk of cardiac complications is in the range of 5% to 15% [2,10,15,16,21–23,29,30,33,36,41] (see Table 39-6). Yet on multivariate analysis, it did not come out as an independent predictor of complications [2]. The factors that are known to increase the preoperative risk, with a numeric value in each case, are listed in Table 39-7.

Detsky published a nomogram that allows the risk assessment to be tailored for each individual patient [10] (see Figure 39-1).

In our clinical setting, the average perioperative cardiac complication rate (pretest probability) for orthopedic surgery is about 15% [2,10,41].

3. FALSE

An S4 and a systolic murmur with a history of pulmonary edema should caution against surgery until aortic stenosis is excluded. The reliability and validity of clinical features such as pulsus parvus or tardus for predicting critical aortic stenosis is questionable [7]. An excellent noninvasive technique for assessing critical aortic stenosis is Doppler echocardiography [8]. Mrs. Smith should certainly have a Doppler echocardiogram before surgery to exclude significant aortic stenosis.

4. FALSE

Gated blood pool cardiac scan (RNA, MUGA, or LV gated scan) is an excellent tool to assess resting ventricular function and gives a precise measurement of ejection fraction. Yet for the purpose of assessing the ability of a patient to sustain a surgical stress, its value is limited [33,42,43]. An excellent, more specific, and sensitive tool is dipyridamole thallium scanning [12,19,24–27,29,33]. The dipyridamole thallium scan will allow detection of myocardial ischemia and areas at risk. Cost is an issue, and Eagle advised and validated an algorithm where thallium

Table 39-7   Numeric Values Assigned to the Factors Known to Increase Preoperative Risk.

	Points
Evidence of coronary heart disease	
Myocardial infarction within last 6 months	10
Myocardial infarction more than 6 months ago	5
Stable angina	
Walking less than 2 blocks or climbing less than 1 flight of stairs (Class 3)	10
On any physical activity (Class 4)	20
Unstable angina within last 6 months	
Less than 1 month and with minimal exertion, or at rest, or crescendo, or with coronary insufficiency	10
Alveolar pulmonary edema	
Within past week	
Physical signs (S3, respiratory distress, crackles or jugulars more than 3 cm vertical distance above the sternal angle with the patient at 45°) *and* a positive chest film for alveolar pulmonary edema	10
Ever	
History of respiratory distress, explained (by an M.D. at the time) as consistent with pulmonary edema, and relieved by diuretics	5
Valvular heart disease	
Critical aortic stenosis	
Syncope on exertion, slow and low carotid upstroke despite vigorous left ventricle, and LVH on ECG	20
Arrhythmias	
Any rhythm other than sinus (with or without APBs) on pre-op ECG	5
More than 5 PVCs per minute on any ECG or exam	5
Poor general medical status	
pO_2 less than 60 mm Hg; pCO_2 more than 50 mm Hg; K less than mmol/l; HCO_3 less than 20 mmol/l; urea more than 18 mmol/l; creat. more than 260 mmol/l; abnormal SGOT, chronic liver disease; bedridden from noncardiac cause	5
Age over 70	5
Emergency operation	10
Total	120

Figure 39-1 The Likelihood Ratio Nomogram.

Anchor straight edge at value on pretest side of nomogram determined by surgical procedure. Run line through point in center column reflecting patient's score from Table 39-7 (patient's index score and likelihood ratio). Now, the point where this line intersects the right-hand column is the patient's position probability, that is, the patient's risk of perioperative cardiac complication. A. General risk pretest probability (scored from Table 39-6, depends on the procedure). B. Index score of likelihood ratio (scored from Table 39-7). C. Post-test probability of perioperative cardiac complication.

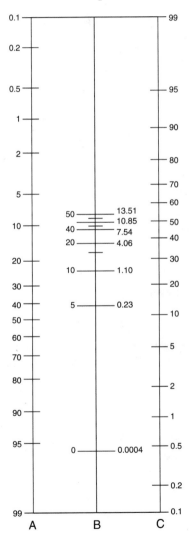

scan was done only in patients with a history of angina, myocardial infarction, congestive heart failure, diabetes, or Q waves on ECG [12] (see Figure 39-2). Exercise stress testing is useful in only about 30% of patients [17,32,41], mostly because of inability to complete the test. Holter is promising [34] but not yet validated.

Figure 39-2　Data Supporting Screening Selected Patients With Dipyridamole Thallium Imaging, from Eagle [12].

Algorithm applied to validation set of 50 patients undergoing vascular surgery. ECG indicates electrocardiogram.

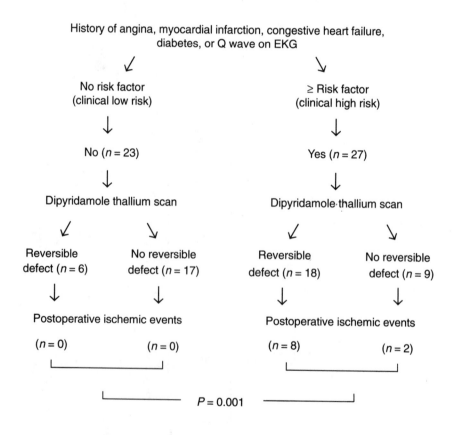

History of angina, myocardial infarction, congestive heart failure, diabetes, or Q wave on EKG

No risk factor (clinical low risk)	≥ Risk factor (clinical high risk)
No ($n = 23$)	Yes ($n = 27$)
Dipyridamole thallium scan	Dipyridamole thallium scan

Reversible defect ($n = 6$)	No reversible defect ($n = 17$)	Reversible defect ($n = 18$)	No reversible defect ($n = 9$)
Postoperative ischemic events		Postoperative ischemic events	
($n = 0$)	($n = 0$)	($n = 8$)	($n = 2$)

$P = 0.001$

Table 39-8   Mrs. Smith's Score From the Information We Have Been Given.

	Points	Mrs. Smith's Score
Evidence of coronary heart disease		
Myocardial infarction within last 6 months	10	0
Myocardial infarction more that 6 months ago	5	5
Stable angina		
Walking less than 2 blocks or climbing less than 1 flight of stairs (Class 3)	10	0
On any physical activity (Class 4)	20	0
Unstable angina within last 6 months		
Less than 1 month and with minimal exertion, or at rest, or crescendo, or with coronary insufficiency	10	0
Alveolar pulmonary edema		
Within past week		
Physical signs (S3, respiratory distress, crackles or jugulars more than 3 cm vertical distance above the sternal angle with the patient at 45°) *and* a positive chest film for alveolary pulmonary edema	10	10
Ever		
History of respiratory distress, explained (by an M.D. at the time) as consistent with pulmonary edema, and relieved by diuretics	5	0
Valvular heart disease		
Critical aortic stenosis		
Syncope on exertion, slow and low carotid upstroke despite vigorous left ventricle, and LVH on ECG	20	0
Arrhythmias		
Any rhythm other than sinus (with or without APBs) on pre-op ECG	5	5
More than 5 PVCs per minute on any ECG or exam	5	0
Poor general medical status		
pO_2 less than 60 mm Hg; pCO_2 more than 50 mm Hg; K less than mmol/l; HCO_3 less than 20 mmol/l; urea more than 18 mmol/l; creat. more than 260 mmol/l; abnormal SGOT, chronic liver disease; bed-ridden from noncardiac cause	5	0
Age over 70	5	5
Emergency operation	10	0
Total	120	25

Figure 39-3   Mrs. Smith's Post-Exam Risk of Cardiac Complications, Found Using the Nomogram of Figure 39-1.

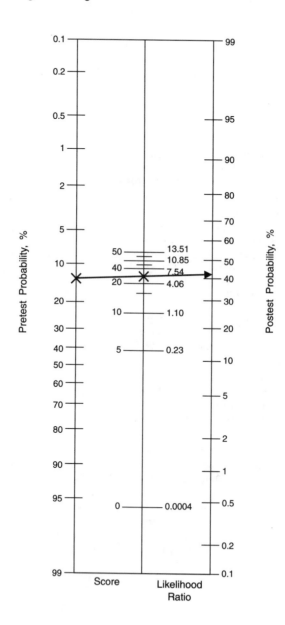

5. TRUE

Mrs. Smith's risk of perioperative cardiac complications can now be assessed using some of the information already given. Look back at the nomogram in Figure 39-1. You will need two pieces of information to assess her probability of complications perioperatively.

First obtain the pretest probability from the type of surgery she is about to have (see Table 39-6). She will have orthopedic surgery (risk 14%). This puts us at 14 on the left column of Figure 39-1. Now we must individualize her risk. Assess what score she had from Table 39-7. Her score is shown on Table 39-8 (total 25) (please note that we are assuming that she does not have critical aortic stenosis). Now before you turn to Figure 39-3, what is her risk? The correct answer is about 45%.

REFERENCES

1. Steen PA, Tinker JH, Tarhan S: Myocardial reinfarction after anesthesia and surgery. *JAMA* 239:2566–2570, 1978.
2. Goldman L, Caldera DL, Southwick FS, *et al.*: Cardiac risk factors and complications in noncardiac surgery. *Medicine* 57:357–370, 1978.
3. Clinical epidemiology rounds: The interpretation of diagnostic data: V. How to do it with simple math. *CAMJ* 129:947–954, 1983.
4. Rao TK, Jacobs KH, El-Etr AA: Reinfarction following anesthesia in patients with myocardial infarction. *Anesthesiology* 59:499–505, 1983.
5. Robin ED: The cult of the Swan-Ganz catheter. Overuse and abuse of pulmonary flow catheters. *Ann Intern Med* 103(3):445–449, 1985.
6. Cooperman M, Pflug B, Martin E, *et al.*: Myocardial infarction after general anesthesia. *JAMA* 220:1451–1454, 1972.
7. Lombard JT, Selzer A: Valvular aortic stenosis. *Ann Intern Med* 106:292–298, 1987.
8. Currie PJ, Saward JB, Reeder GS, *et al.*: Continuous wave Doppler echocardiography assessment of severity of calcific aortic stenosis: A simultaneous Doppler-catheter correlative study in 100 adult patients. *Circulation* 71:1162–1169, 1985.
9. Tarhan S, Moffit EA, Taylor WF, *et al.*: Myocardial infarction after general anesthesia. *JAMA* 220:1451–1454, 1972.
10. Detsky AS, Abrams HB, Forbath N, Scott JG, *et al.*: Cardiac assessment for patients undergoing noncardiac surgery: A multifactorial clinical risk index. *Arch Intern Med* 146:2131–2134, 1986.
11. Detsky A: Predicting cardiac complications in patients undergoing non-cardiac surgery. *J Gen Intern Med* 1:211–219, 1986.
12. Eagle KA, Singer DE, Brewster DC, Darling RC, Mulley AG, Boucher CA: Dipyridamole-thallium scanning in patients undergoing vascular surgery. Optimizing preoperative evaluation of cardiac risk. *JAMA* 257(16):2185–2189, 1987.
13. Coriat P: Prevention of perioperative myocardial ischemia with continuous nitroglycerine infusion. *Ann Fr Anesth Rean* I:47–52, 1982.
14. Sackett DL, Haynes RB, Tugwell P: *Clinical Epidemiology—A Basic Science for Clinical Medicine*, 1st ed. Chapter 7. Boston: Little, Brown and Co., 1985.

15. Thompson JE, Garrett WV: Peripheral-arterial surgery. *N Engl J Med* 302:491–503, 1980.
16. Hertzer NR: Fatal myocardial infarction following lower extremity revascularization. Two hundred seventy-three patients followed six to eleven postoperative years. *Ann Surg* 193:492–498, 1981.
17. McPhail N, Calvin JE, Shariatmadar A, Barber GG, Scobie TK: The use of preoperative exercise testing to predict cardiac complications after arterial reconstruction. *J Vasc Surg* 7:60–68, 1988.
18. Cutler BS, Wheeler HB, Paraskos JA, Cardullo PA: Applicability and interpretation of electrocardiographic stress testing in patients with peripheral vascular disease. *Am J Surg* 141:501–506, 1981.
19. Boucher CA, Brewster DC, Darling RC, Okada RD, Strauss HW, Pohost GM: Determination of cardiac risk by dipyridamole thallium imaging before peripheral vascular surgery. *N Engl J Med* 312:389–394, 1985.
20. Goldman L, Caldera D, Nussbaum SR, *et al.*: Multifactorial index of cardiac risk in non-cardiac surgical procedures. *N Engl J Med* 297:845–850, 1977.
21. Johnston KW, Scobie TK: Multicenter prospective study of nonruptured abdominal aortic aneurysms. I. Population and operative management. *J Vasc Surg* 7(1): 69–81, 1988.
22. Rutherford RB: *Vascular Surgery*, 2nd ed. Philadelphia: Saunders, 1984.
23. Calvin JE, Kieser TM, Walley VM, McPhail NV, Barber GG, Scobie TK: Cardiac mortality and morbidity after vascular surgery. *Can J Surg* 29:93–97, 1986.
24. Okada RD, Boucher CA, Kirschenbaum HK, *et al.*: Improved diagnostic accuracy of thallium-201 stress test using multiple observers and criteria derived from interobserver analysis of variance. *Am J Cardiol* 46:619–624, 1980.
25. Ruddy TD, Dighero HR, Newell JB, Pohost GM, Strauss HW, Okada RD, Boucher CA: Quantitative analysis of dipyridamole thallium images for the detection of coronary artery disease. *J Am Coll Cardiol* 9:25A, 1987.
26. Callahan RJ, Froelich JW, McKusick KA, *et al.*: A modified method for the *in vivo* labeling of red blood cells with TC-99m. *J Nucl Med* 23:315–318, 1982.
27. Ruddy TD, Yasuda T, Gold HK, Leinbach RC, Newell JR, McKusick KA, Boucher CA, Strauss HW: Anterior ST segment depression in acute inferior myocardial infarction as a marker of greater inferior, apical and posterolateral damage. *Am Heart J* 112:1210–1216, 1986.
28. Yousif H: Perioperative myocardial ischemia: Its relation to perioperative infarction. *Br Heart J* 58:9–14, 1987.
29. Leppo J, Plaga G, Gionet M, Tumolo J, Paraskos JA, Cutler BS: Noninvasive evaluation of cardiac risk before elective vascular surgery. *J Am Coll Cardiol* 9(2): 269–276, 1987.

30. Hertzer NR: Fatal myocardial infarction following peripheral vascular operations: A study of 951 patients followed 6 to 11 years post operatively. *Clev Clin Quart* 19:1–11, 1982.
31. Thomson IR: Failure of intravenous nitroglycerine to prevent intraoperative myocardial ischemia during fentanyl-pancuronium anesthesia. *Anesthesiology* 61:385–393, 1984.
32. Arous IL, Baum PL, Cutler BS: The ischemic exercise test in patients with peripheral vascular disease. *Arch Surg* 119:280–288, 1981.
33. Ruddy TD, McPhail NV, Calvin JE, Davies RA, Vigus LL, Barber GG, Cole CW, Scobie TK: Noninvasive prediction of cardiac complications in patients undergoing vascular surgery. *Clin Invest Med* 11(5):171, 1988.
34. Raby KE, Creager MA, Goldman L, Cook EF, Udvarhelyi IS, Barry J, Selwin AP: Detection of preoperative ischemia to assess cardiac risk in peripheral vascular surgery. *N Engl J Med* 321:1296–1302, 1989.
35. Goldman L: Cardiac risk and complication of noncardiac surgery. *Ann Int Med* 98:504–513, 1983.
36. Jamieson WRE, Janusz MT, Miyagishima RT, *et al.*: Influence of ischemic heart disease on early and late mortality after surgery for peripheral vascular occlusive disease. *Circ* 66:192–197, 1982.
37. Baker HW, Grismer JT, Wise RA: Risk of surgery in patients with myocardial infarction. *Arch Surg* 70:739, 1955.
38. Atkins R, Smessaert AA, Hicks RG: Mortality and morbidity in surgical patients with coronary artery disease. *JAMA* 190:485, 1964.
39. Skinner JF, Pearce ML: Surgical risk in the cardiac patient. *J Chronic Dis* 17:57, 1964.
40. National Cooperative Study Group: Unstable angina pectoris: National Cooperative Study to compare surgical and medical therapy. II. In hospital experience and follow up results in patients with one, two and three vessel disease. *Am J Cardiol* 42:839, 1978.
41. McPhail N, Menkis A, Shariatmadar A, Calvin J, Barber G, Scobie K, White P: Statistical prediction of cardiac risk in patients who undergo vascular surgery. *Can J Surg* 28:404–406, 1985.
42. Kazmers A, Cerqueira MD, Zierler RE: The role of preoperative radionuclide left ventricular ejection fraction for risk assessment in carotid surgery. *Arch Surg* 123(4):416–419, 1988.
43. Morise AP, McDowell DE, Savrin RA, Goodwin CA, Gabrielle OF, Oliver FN, Nullet FR, Bekheit S, Jain AC: The prediction of cardiac risk in patients undergoing vascular surgery. *Am J Med Sci* 293(3):150–158, 1987.

40 | ANEMIA

CASE PRESENTATION

An 85-year-old man presents at your office for an annual health examination. He feels healthy and takes no medications. His weight is stable, and he has no gastrointestinal (GI) symptoms. The physical examination is normal. His hemoglobin level is 116 g/l.

C.J. Patterson
D.W. Molloy
A.M. Benger

Consider the following statements (true or false)

1. His hemoglobin level is normal for a man of his age.

2. The prevalence of anemia among elderly patients admitted to the hospital is 25%.

3. Iron deficiency in the elderly is unlikely if serum ferritin is normal (18 to 300 pg/l).

4. Vitamin B_{12} deficiency, folic acid deficiency, hypothyroidism, hemolysis, β-thalassemia trait, or dysmyeloplastic syndrome (preleukemic syndrome) may cause a macrocytic anemia in the elderly.

5. Refractory sideroblastic anemias are common in extremely old people.

1. FALSE

Anemia does not occur in the elderly in the absence of a deficiency or disease. Although the hemoglobin level tends to fall with advancing age, anemia cannot be attributed to age alone (Table 40-1) [1]. The prevalence of diseases likely to cause anemia (bleeding GI lesions, chronic inflammatory conditions, chronic renal failure) increases with age, making anemia more common in the elderly, although never a normal finding. Anemia in an older person should arouse the same degree of suspicion as in a younger patient.

Reviewing red cell indices to see whether the patient has a macrocytic, normocytic, or microcytic disease will help determine the specific cause of anemia. In elderly patients the most likely causes are iron deficiency secondary to chronic GI blood loss, a chronic disease, or secondary anemia from renal impairment or chronic inflammatory disease, and vitamin deficiency (B_{12} or folate).

His hemoglobin level cannot be attributed to age alone.

2. TRUE

Anemia is common in the hospitalized elderly [2]. The World Health Organization defines anemia as a hemoglobin level of less than 130 g/l in men and 120 g/l in women. Many geriatricians consider these levels too rigorous, and use levels of 120 g/l in men and 110 g/l in women.

Table 40-1 Common Causes of Anemia.

Structure	Cause
Hypochromic microcytic	Iron deficiency Secondary (chronic disease) Thalassemia
Normochromic normocytic	Acute blood losses Early stage of iron deficiency secondary to chronic disease Hypothyroidism

Macrocytic	Megaloblastic (i.e., vitamin B_{12} deficiency,
	  folate deficiency)
	Nonmegaloblastic (i.e., hemolysis,
	  dysmyeloplastic syndrome, liver disease,
	  hypothyroidism)

Using these criteria, surveys show that between 20% and 30% of patients in geriatric units are anemic.

3. FALSE

The diagnosis of iron deficiency anemia usually is made on the basis of a microcytic hypochromic picture, low serum iron, elevated total iron binding capacity, and subnormal ferritin levels. Serum ferritin is frequently elevated, however, in inflammatory conditions and liver disease. Patients with inflammatory conditions who are iron deficient may have normal serum ferritin levels. These normal levels do not exclude iron deficiency anemia. Subnormal serum ferritin is a specific but relatively insensitive diagnostic feature of iron deficiency in the elderly [3]. Iron deficiency is likely if serum ferritin is below 45 pg/l and very unlikely if it is greater than 100 [5].

4. FALSE

Vitamin B_{12} and folic acid deficiency produce a megaloblastic picture characterized by macrocytosis and changes in blood cells and bone marrow consistent with abnormal maturation of both myeloid and erythrocyte series. Dysmyeloplastic syndrome is characterized by anemia and neutropenia that may be present several years before the development of acute myeloid leukemia. Erythrocytes usually are macrocytic. Hypothyroidism may cause either normochromic, normocytic anemia, or less commonly, a macrocytic but nonmegaloblastic picture.

Hemolysis produces a brisk reticulocyte response. As reticulocytes are slightly larger than mature red cells, automated hematology analysis machines may indicate macrocytosis.

β-thalassemia trait, however, is usually associated with microcytosis [4].

5. FALSE

Sideroblastic anemias are often refractory (not responsive to pyridoxine). Ringed sideroblasts, the hallmark of this anemia, are found as part of dysmyelopoetic syndrome, but occasionally may be found in other conditions (rheumatoid arthritis, carcinomas, multiple myeloma, alcoholism and lead poisoning). Although many of these conditions occur more frequently in the very elderly, sideroblastic anemias are uncommon in this age group.

REFERENCES

1. Hale WE, Stewart RB, Marks RG: Hematological and biochemical laboratory values in an ambulatory elderly population. An analysis of the effects of age, sex and drugs. *Age and Ageing* 12:275, 1983.
2. Sneath P, Chanarin I, Hodkinson HM, *et al.*: Folate status in a geriatric population and its relation to dementia. *Age and Ageing* 2:177, 1973.
3. Patterson C, Turpie ID, Benger AM: Assessment of iron stores in anemic geriatric patients. *J Am Geriatr Soc* 33:764, 1985.
4. Williams HW, Beutler E, Erslev AJ, *et al.* (eds.): *Hematology*. New York: McGraw-Hill, 1983, p. 434.
5. Guyatt G, Patterson C, Ali M, *et al.*: Diagnosis of iron deficiency anemia in the elderly. *Am J Med* 88:205–209, 1990.

Appendixes

Appendix A

STANDARDIZED MINI–MENTAL STATE EXAMINATION

DIRECTIVES FOR ADMINISTATION

1. Before the questionnaire is administered try to get the subject to sit down facing you. Assess the subject's ability to hear and understand very simple conversation, for example, "What is your name?" If the subject uses hearing or visual aids, try to provide these before starting.

2. Introduce yourself and try to get the subject's confidence. Before you commence, get the subject's permission to ask questions; for example, "Would it be all right to ask you some questions about your memory?" This helps to avoid catastrophic reactions.

3. Ask each question a maximum of three times. If the subject does not respond, score 0.

4. If the subject answers incorrectly, score 0. Do not hint, prompt, or ask the question again. For example, if you ask, "What year is this?" and the answer is 1952, accept that answer; do not ask the question again, hint, or provide any physical clues, such as head shaking, *etc.*

5. The following equipment is required to administer the instrument: a watch, a pencil, a piece of paper with "close your eyes" written in large letters, two five-sided figures intersecting to make a four-sided figure, and some blank paper.

6. If the subject answers "What did you say?" do not explain or engage in conversation, merely repeat the same directions (*e.g.*, "What year is this?") to a maximum of three times.

7. If the subject interrupts, saying, for example, "What's this for?" just reply, "I will explain in a few minutes when we are finished. Now if we could just proceed please . . . we are almost finished."

364

STANDARDIZED MINI-MENTAL STATE EXAM (SMMSE)

I am going to ask you some questions and give you some problems to solve. Please try to answer as best you can.

		Score	*Max Score*
1.	*(Allow 10 seconds for each reply)*		
a)	WHAT YEAR IS THIS? (Accept exact answer only)	_____	_1_
b)	WHAT SEASON IS THIS? (During last week of the old season or first week of a new season, accept either season)	_____	_1_
c)	WHAT MONTH OF THE YEAR IS THIS? (On the first day of the new month, or last day of the previous month, accept either)	_____	_1_
f)	WHAT IS TODAY'S DATE? (Accept previous or next date, e.g., on the 7th accept 6th or 8th)	_____	_1_
a)	WHAT DAY OF THE WEEK IS THIS? (Accept exact answer only)	_____	_1_
2.	*(Allow 10 seconds for each reply)*		
a)	WHAT COUNTRY ARE WE IN? (Accept exact answer only)	_____	_1_
b)	WHAT PROVINCE (STATE) ARE WE IN? (Accept exact answer only)	_____	_1_
c)	WHAT CITY ARE WE IN? (Accept exact answer only)	_____	_1_
d)	WHAT IS THE NAME OF THIS HOSPITAL/ BUILDING? (Accept exact name of hospital or institution only)	_____	_1_
e)	WHAT FLOOR OF THE BUILDING ARE WE ON? (Accept exact answer only)	_____	_1_

TOTAL FOR THIS PAGE   _____   _10_

	Score	Max Score

3. I AM GOING TO NAME THREE OBJECTS. AFTER I HAVE SAID ALL THREE OBJECTS, I WANT YOU TO REPEAT THEM. REMEMBER WHAT THEY ARE BECAUSE I AM GOING TO ASK YOU TO NAME THEM AGAIN IN A FEW MINUTES. (Say them slowly at approximately one-second intervals)

   APPLE   TABLE   PENNY

   PLEASE REPEAT THE THREE ITEMS FOR ME. (Score 1 point for each correct reply on the first attempt. Allow 20 seconds for reply. If subject did not repeat all three, repeat until they are learned or up to a maximum of five times) _____ _3_

4. SPELL THE WORD "WORLD." (You may help subject to spell "world" correctly) Say NOW SPELL IT BACKWARDS PLEASE. (Allow 30 seconds to spell backwards. If the subject cannot spell "world" even with assistance, score 0) _____ _5_

5. NOW WHAT WERE THE THREE OBJECTS THAT I ASKED YOU TO REMEMBER?

   APPLE   TABLE   PENNY

   (Score 1 point for each correct response regardless of order. Allow 10 seconds) _____ _3_

6. Show wristwatch. Ask, WHAT IS THIS CALLED? (Accept "wristwatch" or "watch." Do not accept "clock," "time," *etc.*) _____ _1_

7. Show pencil. Ask WHAT IS THIS CALLED? (Accept "pencil" only; score 0 for "pen") _____ _1_

8 I'D LIKE YOU TO REPEAT A PHRASE AFTER ME: "NO IF'S, AND'S, OR BUT'S."

   (Allow 10 seconds for response. Score 1 point for a correct repetition. Must be exact, *e.g.*, for "No if's or but's," score 0.) _____ _1_

TOTAL FOR THIS PAGE _____ _14_

	Score	Max Score

9. READ THE WORDS ON THIS PAGE AND THEN DO WHAT IT SAYS. (Hand the subject a sheet with "Close your eyes" on it)

   CLOSE YOUR EYES

   (If subject just reads and does not close eyes, you may repeat "Read the words on this page and then do what it says" to a maximum of three times. Allow 10 seconds, score 1 point only if subject closes eyes. Subject does not have to read aloud) _____ __1__

10. Ask if the subject is right- or left-handed. Alternate right/left hand in statement; for example, if the subject is *right-handed*, say, "Take this paper in your *left* hand . . ." Take a piece of paper, hold it up in front of subject and say the following: TAKE THIS PAPER IN YOUR RIGHT/LEFT HAND, FOLD THE PAPER IN HALF WITH BOTH HANDS, AND PUT THE PAPER DOWN ON THE FLOOR.

	Score	
Takes paper in correct hand	_____	__1__
Folds it in half	_____	__1__
Puts it on the floor	_____	__1__

   (Allow 30 seconds. Score 1 point for each instruction correctly executed) _____ __3__

11. (Hand subject a pencil and paper)

   WRITE ANY COMPLETE SENTENCE ON THAT PIECE OF PAPER. (Allow 30 seconds. The sentence should make sense. Ignore spelling errors) _____ __1__

12. COPY THIS DESIGN PLEASE. (Place design, pencil, eraser, and paper in front of subject. Allow multiple tries until patient is finished and hands it back. Maximum time, 1 minute)

   (Score 1 point for correctly copied diagram. The subject must have drawn a four-sided figure between the two five-sided figures) _____ __1__

   TOTAL FOR THIS PAGE _____ __6__

   TOTAL TEST SCORE _____ _30__

Scoring " WORLD" Backwards

- Correct response: DLROW.   Score 5 points.

- Omission of one letter, for example,
  DLRW; DLOW; DROW; DLRO.   Score 4 points

- Omission of two letters, for example,
  DLR; LRO; DLW.   Score 3 points

- Reversal of two letters, for example,
  DLORW; DRLOW; DLRWO; DLWOR   Score 3 points

- Omission/reversal of three letters, for example,
  DORLW; DL; OW.   Score 2 points

- Reversal of four letters, for example,
  DRLWO, LDRWO.   Score 1 point.

Scoring the Figure

The subject must draw two five-sided figures intersected by a four-sided figure.

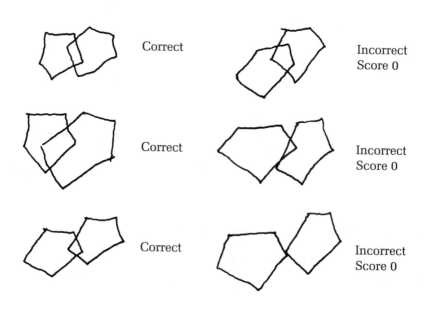

Correct

Incorrect
Score 0

Correct

Incorrect
Score 0

Correct

Incorrect
Score 0

Serial Sevens

The calculation task (serial sevens) may be used in place of Question 4. Decide at the start to use serial sevens or "world." Do not use serial sevens if the subject is unable to spell "world" and vice versa.

	Score	*Max Score*
4. SUBTRACT 7 FROM 100 AND KEEP SUBTRACTING 7 FROM WHAT'S LEFT UNTIL I TELL YOU TO STOP. (You may repeat three times if subject pauses. Just repeat the same instruction. Allow 1 minute)	_____	_5_

Scoring of Serial Sevens

Once the subject starts, do not interrupt. Allow the subject to proceed until five subtractions have been made. If the subject stops before five subtractions have been made, repeat the original instruction, "Keep subtracting seven from what's left" (maximum three times).

Score as follows:

- 93, 86, 79, 72, 65   5 points (all correct)
- 93, 88, 81, 74, 67   4 points (4 correct, 1 wrong)
- 92, 85, 78, 71, 64   4 points (4 correct, 1 wrong)
- 93, 87, 80, 73, 64   3 points (3 correct, 2 wrong)
- 92, 85, 78, 71, 63   3 points (3 correct, 2 wrong)
- 93, 87, 80, 75, 67   2 points (2 correct, 3 wrong)
- 93, 87, 81, 75, 69   1 point (1 correct, 4 wrong)

Total SMMSE Scores

- 24 – 30   Normal
- 20 – 24   Mild cognitive impairment
- 10 – 20   Moderate cognitive impairment
- 0 – 10   Severe cognitive impairment

Appendix B

DYSFUNCTIONAL BEHAVIOR RATING INSTRUMENT (DBRI)*

INSTRUCTIONS FOR CAREGIVER SCORING THE DBRI

Thank you for taking the time to complete the DBRI. The DBRI is used to measure the frequency of _____'s behavior problems and your reaction to each of these problems. Please read each item carefully and CIRCLE just ONE number in each column.

First look in the FREQUENCY column. If the behavior NEVER occurs, CIRCLE 0. If the behavior DOES occur, CIRCLE ONLY ONE NUMBER between 1 and 5.

Now look in the REACTION column. If the behavior is NOT a problem, CIRCLE 0. If the behavior IS a problem, CIRCLE ONLY ONE NUMBER between 1 and 5.

Thank you for taking the time to complete this questionnaire. I will help us to treat you and _____ better. It is important that you fill this out as honestly as possible. If you have any questions or are unsure about any of the items, please do not hesitate to ask.

---

* Molloy DW, McIlroy WE, Guyatt G, Rees L, Lever JA. Validity and reliability of the Dysfunctional Behavior Rating Instrument. *Acta Psych Scand* (in press).

How often has [PATIENT'S NAME] had any of the following behaviors in the last few weeks?
Circle the number that best applies:

FREQUENCY

How often does this occur?

0 Never
1 About every two weeks
2 About once a week
3 More than once a week
4 At least once daily
5 More than five times a day

REACTION

How much of a problem is this?

0 No problem
1 Very little problem
2 Little problem
3 Somewhat of a problem
4 Moderate problem
5 Great deal of a problem

		FREQUENCY							REACTION					
1.	Asked same questions over and over	0	1	2	3	4	5		0	1	2	3	4	5
2.	Repeated stories over and over	0	1	2	3	4	5		0	1	2	3	4	5
3.	Became angry	0	1	2	3	4	5		0	1	2	3	4	5
4.	Was withdrawn (did not speak or do anything unless asked)	0	1	2	3	4	5		0	1	2	3	4	5
5.	Was demanding	0	1	2	3	4	5		0	1	2	3	4	5
6.	Was afraid to be left alone	0	1	2	3	4	5		0	1	2	3	4	5
7.	Was aggressive	0	1	2	3	4	5		0	1	2	3	4	5
8.	Was hiding things	0	1	2	3	4	5		0	1	2	3	4	5

FREQUENCY

How often does this occur?

0 Never
1 About every two weeks
2 About once a week
3 More than once a week
4 At least once daily
5 More than five times a day

REACTION

How much of a problem is this?

0 No problem
1 Very little problem
2 Little problem
3 Somewhat of a problem
4 Moderate problem
5 Great deal of a problem

	FREQUENCY	REACTION
9. Was suspicious	0 1 2 3 4 5	0 1 2 3 4 5
10. Had temper outbursts	0 1 2 3 4 5	0 1 2 3 4 5
11. Had delusions, that is, thought that:		
• Spouse was "not my wife/husband"	0 1 2 3 4 5	0 1 2 3 4 5
• Home was "not my home"	0 1 2 3 4 5	0 1 2 3 4 5
• There were "people in the house"	0 1 2 3 4 5	0 1 2 3 4 5
• "People were stealing things"	0 1 2 3 4 5	0 1 2 3 4 5
• Other: _____	0 1 2 3 4 5	0 1 2 3 4 5
12. Had hallucinations:		
• Saw things that were not there	0 1 2 3 4 5	0 1 2 3 4 5

Item													
• Heard things or people that were not there	0	1	2	3	4	5		0	1	2	3	4	5
• Other: _____	0	1	2	3	4	5		0	1	2	3	4	5
13. Was agitated, for example, pacing	0	1	2	3	4	5		0	1	2	3	4	5
14. Was crying	0	1	2	3	4	5		0	1	2	3	4	5
15. Was frustrated	0	1	2	3	4	5		0	1	2	3	4	5
16. Wandered, got lost in house, on property, or elsewhere	0	1	2	3	4	5		0	1	2	3	4	5
17. Was up at night	0	1	2	3	4	5		0	1	2	3	4	5
18. Wanted to leave	0	1	2	3	4	5		0	1	2	3	4	5
19. Kept changing mind	0	1	2	3	4	5		0	1	2	3	4	5
20. Refused to cooperate	0	1	2	3	4	5		0	1	2	3	4	5
21. Embarrassing behavior in public	0	1	2	3	4	5		0	1	2	3	4	5
22. Are there any other behaviors not mentioned above that [PATIENT'S NAME] had?													
• _____	0	1	2	3	4	5		0	1	2	3	4	5
• _____	0	1	2	3	4	5		0	1	2	3	4	5
• _____	0	1	2	3	4	5		0	1	2	3	4	5

Appendix C

BOWEL/BLADDER RECORD

INSTRUCTIONS FOR USE

The purpose of this record is to describe the pattern and severity of urine and fecal incontinence. It is understood that, even though the times are written for every hour, it is not always possible to check patients at that time. So please fill in only the times when the patient was acually checked. Do not backdate or guess. Do not write in numbers to fill in the record if the patient was not checked at that time. It is better to have an accurate, half-filled record than an inaccurate, filled one.

Please write in all numbers that apply. For instance,

- a patient who was incontinent of a small volume of urine and a small amount of feces: 2,4

- a patient who was incontinent of a large volume of urine and a large amount of feces: 3,5

- a patient who voided urine (350 cc) and was incontinent of a small amount of urine (350 cc) shortly after: 6,2.

Patient's name: _____

Date: _____

Person completing form: _____

374

BOWEL/BLADDER RECORD

Write in one or more numbers each time the patient is checked.

1. Continent (dry)
2. Incontinent urine (small)
3. Incontinent urine (large)

4. Incontinent bowel (small)
5. Incontinent bowel (large)
6. Voided urine (volume)
7. Voided bowel

	Mon.	Tues.	Wed.	Thurs.	Fri.	Sat.	Sun.
6:00 a.m.							
7:00 a.m.							
8:00 a.m.							
9:00 a.m.							
10:00 a.m.							
11:00 a.m.							
12:00 p.m.							
1:00 p.m.							
2:00 p.m.							
3:00 p.m.							
4:00 p.m.							
5:00 p.m.							
6:00 p.m.							
7:00 p.m.							
8:00 p.m.							
9:00 p.m.							
10:00 p.m.							
11:00 p.m.							
12:00 p.m.							
1:00 a.m.							
2:00 a.m.							
3:00 a.m.							
4:00 a.m.							
5:00 a.m.							

INDEX

PROPERTY OF WASHINGTON
SCHOOL OF PSYCHIATRY
LIBRARY